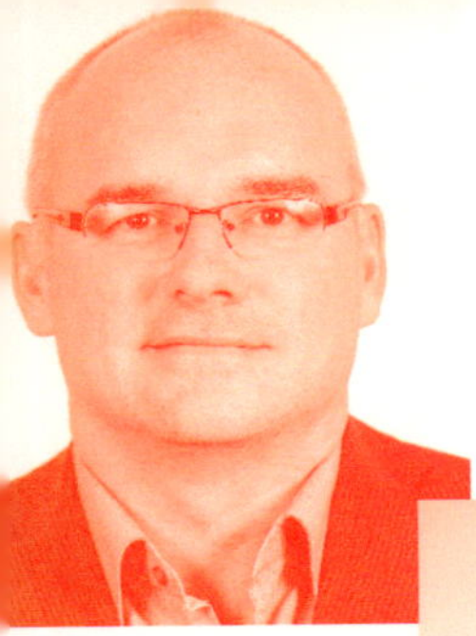
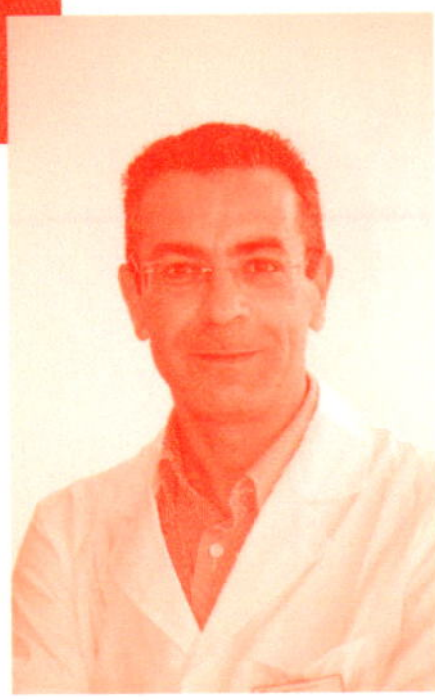
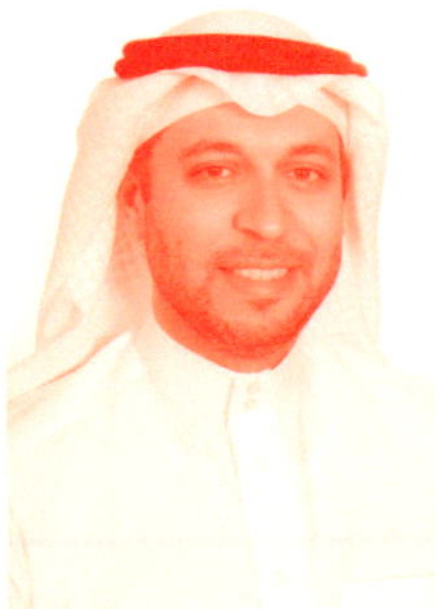
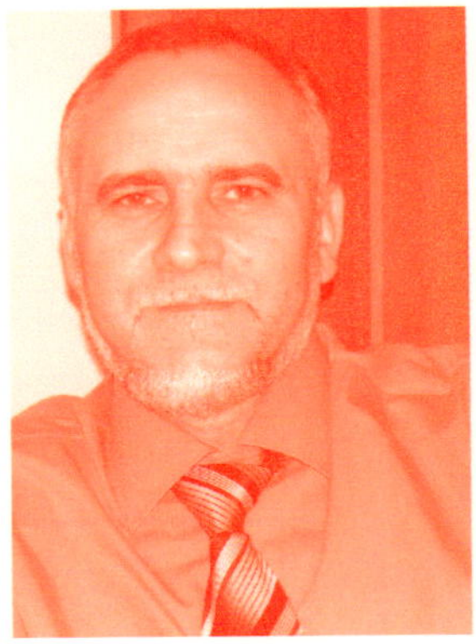
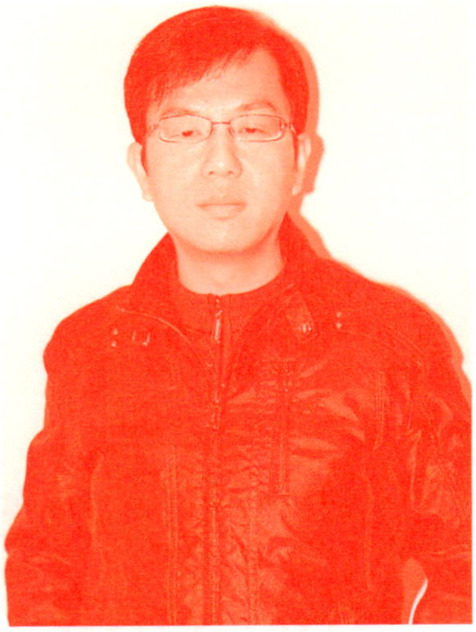
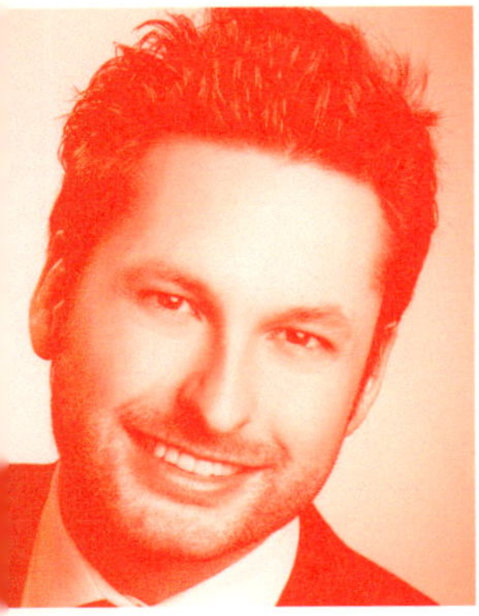
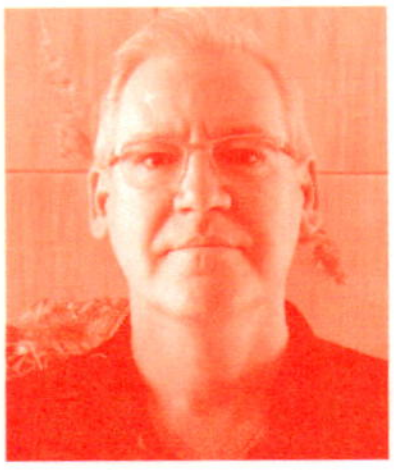

IntechOpen

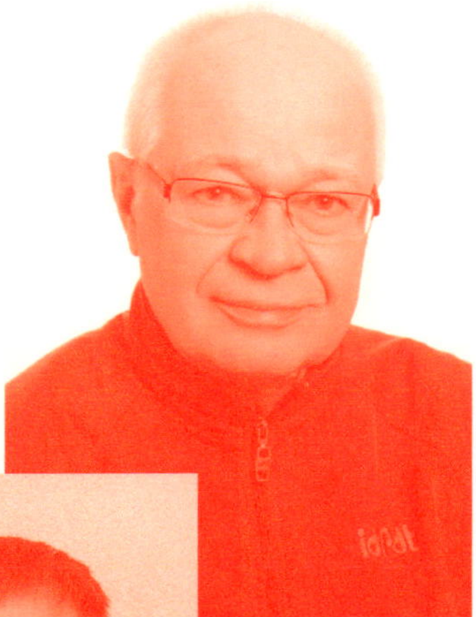
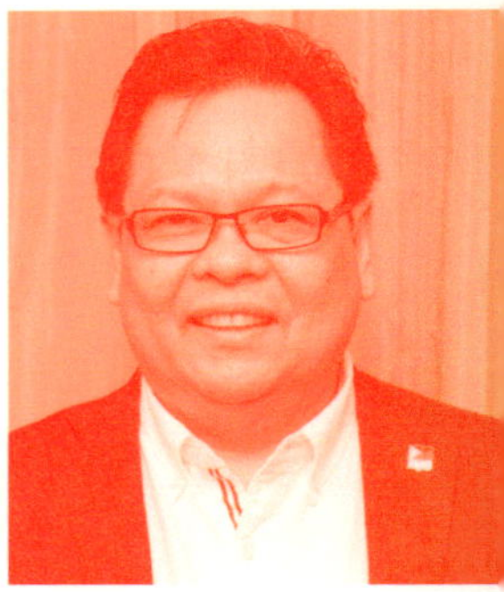
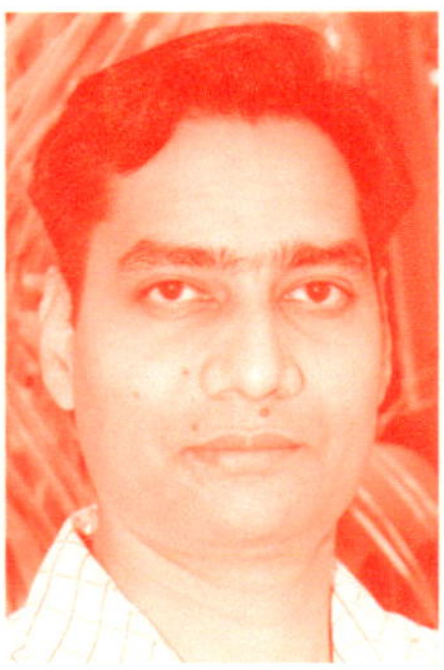
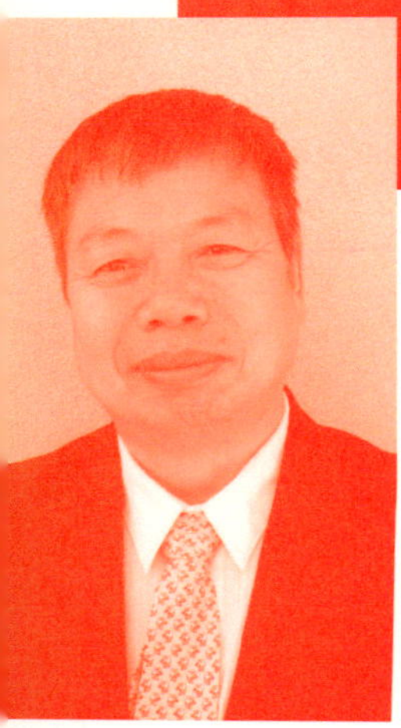
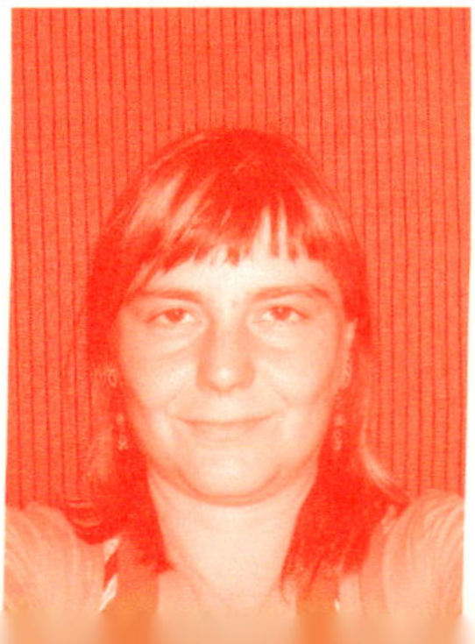
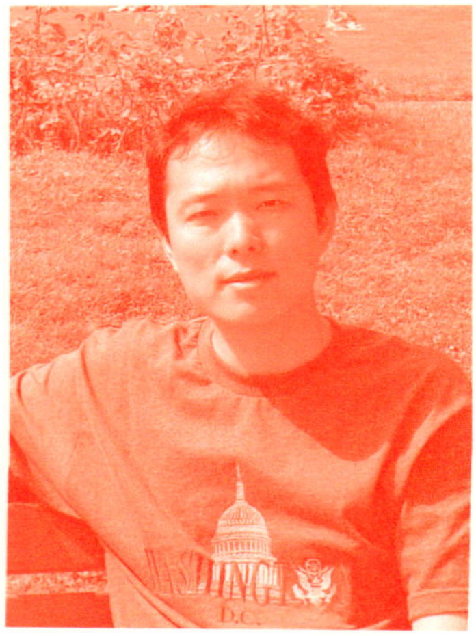

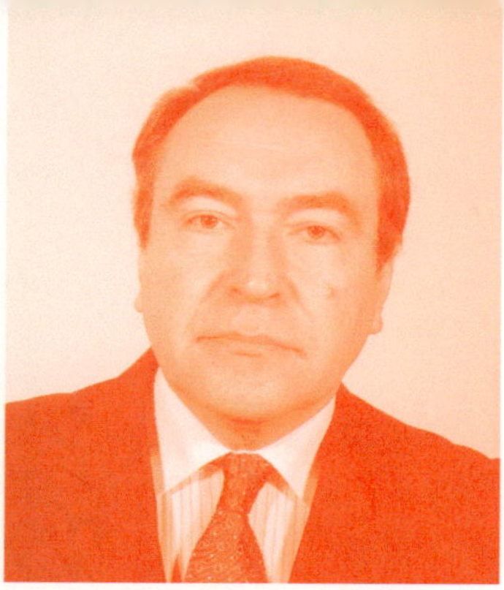

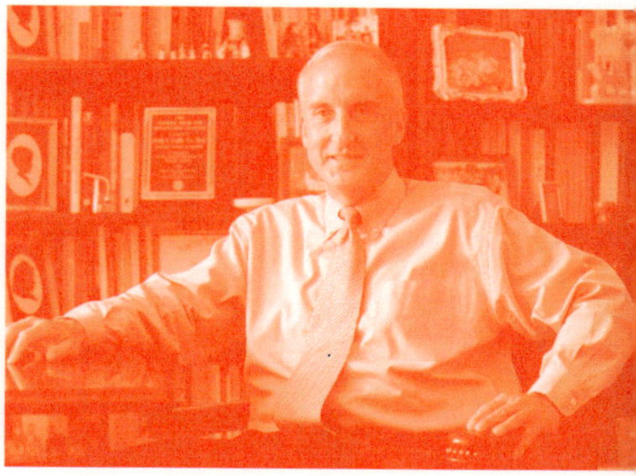

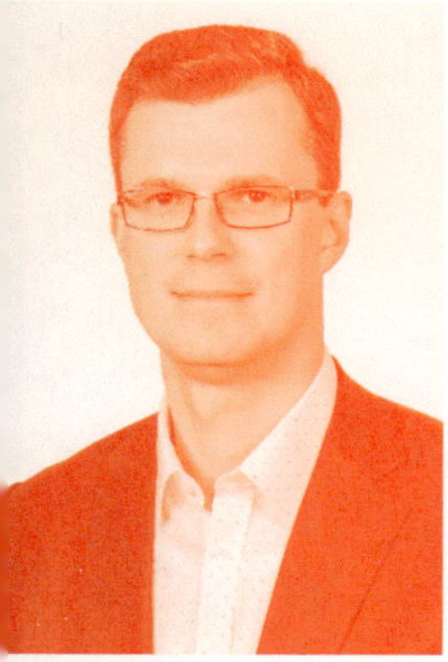

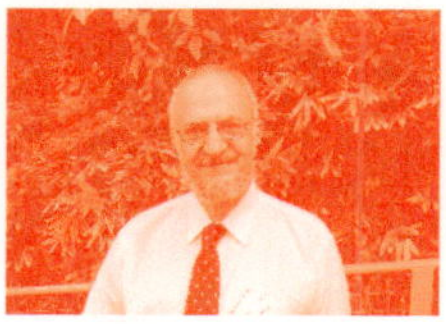

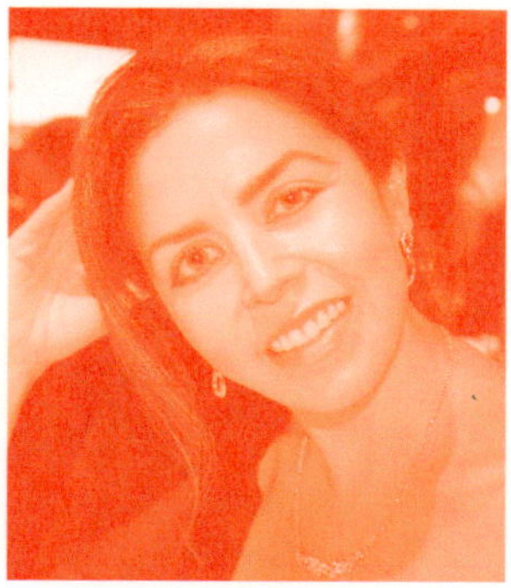

Supporting open minds since 2005

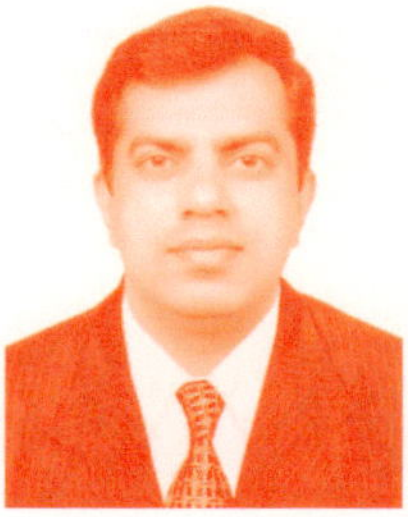

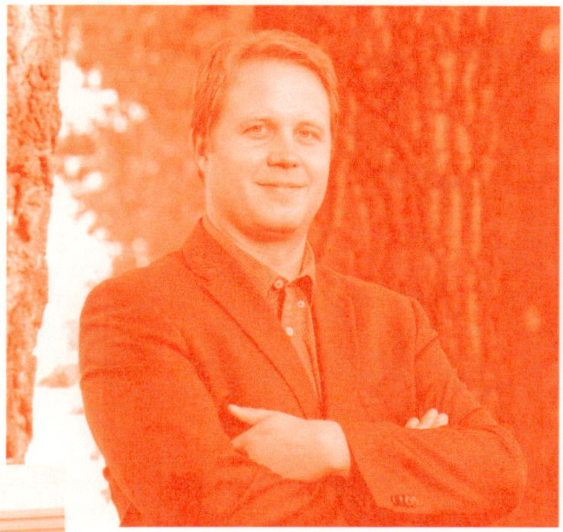

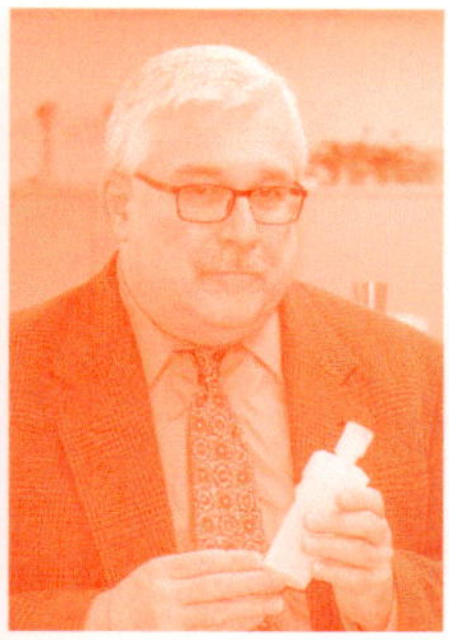

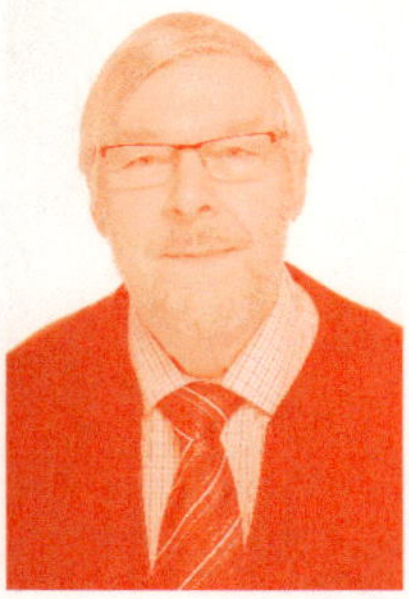

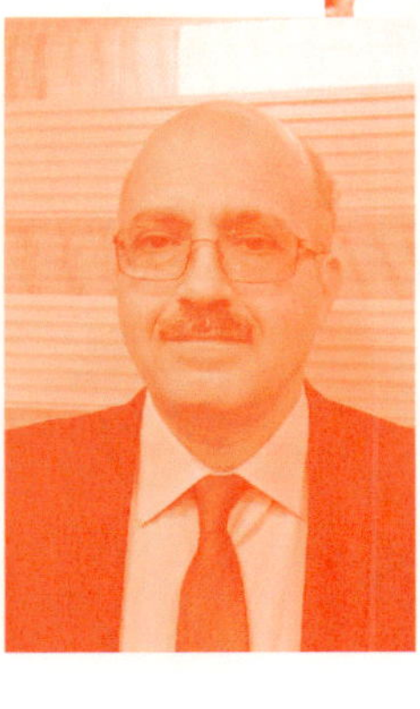

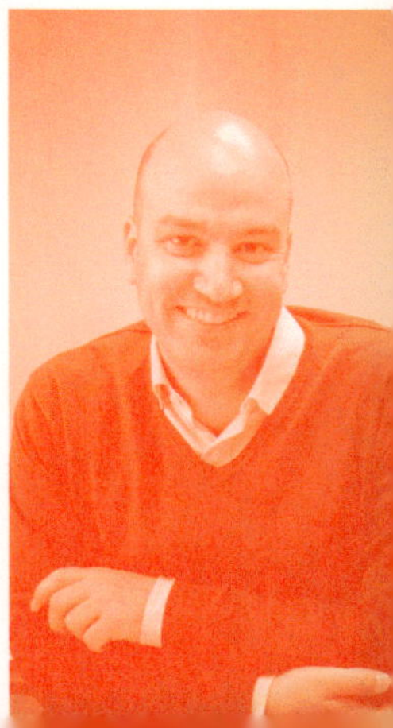

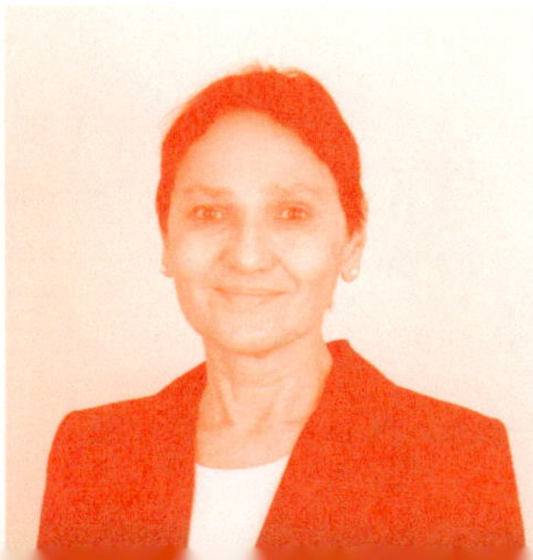

Current Topics and Emerging Issues in Malaria Elimination
http://dx.doi.org/10.5772/intechopen.87323
Edited by Alfonso J. Rodriguez-Morales

Part of IntechOpen Book Series: Infectious Diseases, Volume 8
Book Series Editor: Shailendra K. Saxena

Contributors
Kingsley Badu, Kwadwo Boampong, Amma Aboagyewa Larbi, Arantxa Roca-Feltrer, Ann-Sophie Stratil, James K. Tibenderana, Ilunga-Ilunga Félicien, Leveque Alain, Dramaix Michèle, Mbuyi Kanyinda Veve, Mbikayi Muya Jean Paul, Yahaya Mohammed Mohammed Katagum, Faisal Bin Ibrahim, Hayati Binti Kadir Shahar, Anisah Baharom, Rafee Baharudin, Chukwudi Michael Michael Egbuche, Alexandre Costa, Anna Caroline Campos Aguiar, Dhelio Batista Pereira, Angelina Moraes Silva, Isaac K. Quaye, Larysa Aleksenko, Liwang Cui, Awtum Brashear, Lynette Menezes, John Adams, Anupam Nath Jha, Upasana Pathak, Sanchaita Rajkhowa, Abhichandan Das, Francis S.O Ugwu, Cheikh Cambel Dieng, Eugenia Lo, Jennifer Huynh, Yaw A. Afrane, Linda E. Amoah, Colby T. T. Ford, Daniel A Janies, Susanta Ghosh, Chaitali Ghosh, Mary Oboh, Mamadou Ndiath, Olumide Ajibola, Kolapo Oyebola, Alfred Amambua-Ngwa, Sarat K. Dalai, Nikunj U Tandel, Alfonso J. Rodriguez-Morales, Jaime A. Cardona-Ospina, D. Katterine-Bonilla-Aldana, Luis Andrés Salas-Matta, Wilmer E. Villamil-Gómez, Juan Pablo Escalera-Antezana, Lucia E. Alvarado-Arnez, Carlos Franco-Paredes, Juan-Carlos Navarro, Tomas Orduna, José A. Suárez

First published in London, United Kingdom, 2021 by IntechOpen
IntechOpen is the global imprint of INTECHOPEN LIMITED, registered in England and Wales, registration number: 11086078, 5 Princes Gate Court, London, SW7 2QJ, United Kingdom
Printed in Croatia

British Library Cataloguing-in-Publication Data
A catalogue record for this book is available from the British Library

Additional hard and PDF copies can be obtained from orders@intechopen.com

Current Topics and Emerging Issues in Malaria Elimination
Edited by Alfonso J. Rodriguez-Morales
p. cm.
Print ISBN 978-1-83968-483-8
Online ISBN 978-1-83968-484-5
eBook (PDF) ISBN 978-1-83968-485-2
ISSN 2631-6188

For EU product safety concerns:
IN TECH d.o.o., Prolaz Marije Krucifikse Kozulić 3, 51000 Rijeka, Croatia, info@intechopen.com or visit our website at intechopen.com.

IntechOpen Book Series
Infectious Diseases
Volume 8

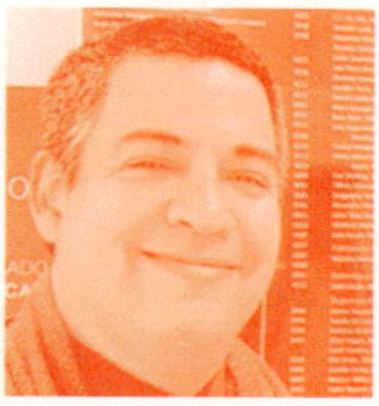

Dr. Alfonso J. Rodriguez-Morales received his MD from Universidad Central de Venezuela, Caracas, and his MSc in Protozoology/Parasitology from Universidad de Los Andes, Trujillo, Venezuela. He received his Diploma in Tropical Medicine & Hygiene (DTM&H) from Universidad Peruana Cayetano Heredia, Lima, Peru, and the University of Alabama at Birmingham, Alabama, USA. He also holds a DipEd. Dr. Rodriguez-Morales is a fellow of the Royal Society for Tropical Medicine & Hygiene (FRSTMH), London, United Kingdom; of the Faculty of Travel Medicine (FFTM) of the Royal College of Physicians and Surgeons of Glasgow (RCPSG), Glasgow, Scotland, United Kingdom; of the American College of Epidemiology (FACE), USA; and of the International Society for Antimicrobial Chemotherapy (FISAC). He has a HonDSc from Universidad Privada Franz Tamayo (UniFranz), Cochabamba, Bolivia. He is also the president of the Travel Medicine Committee and Pan American Infectious Diseases Association, and the vice president of the Colombian Infectious Diseases Association (2019–2021). He is a Member of the Council (2020-2026), International Society for Infectious Diseases (ISID). He is a senior researcher of Colciencias (2015–2021), and a professor at the Fundación Universitaria Autónoma de las Américas, Pereira, Risaralda, Colombia, and the Universidad Cientifica del Sur, Lima, Peru. He is an external professor for the Master in Research of Tropical Medicine and International Health, University of Barcelona, Spain, and a visiting professor at multiple national and international universities.

Editor of Volume 8:
Alfonso J. Rodriguez-Morales
Grupo de Investigación Biomedicina, Faculty of Medicine,
Fundación Universitaria Autónoma de las Américas, Pereira, Risaralda, Colombia

Book Series Editor:
Shailendra K. Saxena
King George's Medical University

Scope of the Series

The series will give a most comprehensive overview of recent trends in various infectious diseases (as per the most recent Baltimore classification), as well as general concepts of infections, immunopathology, diagnosis, treatment, epidemiology and etiology to current clinical recommendations in management of infectious diseases, highlighting the ongoing issues, recent advances, with future directions in diagnostic approaches and therapeutic strategies. This book series will focus on various aspects and properties of infectious diseases whose deep understanding is very important for safeguarding human race from more loss of resources and economies due to pathogens.

Contents

Preface

Malaria is one of the most important tropical diseases in the history of the world. This vector-borne disease has been a significant cause of morbidity and mortality in tropical countries of Africa, Asia, and Latin America. Like most tropical diseases, this parasitic disease is strongly associated with environmental and social conditions along with other factors whose improvement leads to a reduction in the disease. This effect has been observed in multiple countries where the development and control of the disease have resulted in the reduction and outright elimination of malaria, as evidenced in El Salvador and Argentina [1–16]. Conversely, adverse or poor environmental and social conditions may trigger reemergence, persistence, and an increase in diseases like malaria, as is the unfortunate situation in Venezuela. This once rich country is now the worst economy of South America and is witnessing the reemergence of multiple vector-borne diseases, especially malaria, as well as vaccine-preventable diseases such as measles, diphtheria, pertussis, and yellow fever, among others [17–20].

Keeping these issues in mind, this book presents research and clinical topics related to malaria elimination in the world. The book's fifteen chapters are organized in four major sections: "Advances in Diagnosis"; "Epidemiology and Surveillance"; "Policy and Prevention"; and "Prevention, Vector Control and Vaccines."

Commissioning of this book by IntechOpen is related in part to my long commitment to vector-borne, zoonotic, and neglected tropical diseases. I am co-chair of the Working Group on Zoonoses of the International Society for Chemotherapy (WGZ-ISC), as well as of the Committee on Tropical Medicine, Zoonoses and Travel Medicine of the Colombian Association of Infectious Diseases (Asociación Colombiana de Infectología; ACIN). Since January 2016, I have also been the chair of the Colombian Collaborative Network of Research on Zika (Red Colombiana de Colaboración en Zika; RECOLZIKA). RECOLZIKA has contributed in many ways to the research on Zika in Colombia and other countries in Latin America, including research on congenital Zika syndrome and Guillain-Barré syndrome, among other clinical consequences of this arboviral disease.

I have been involved in tropical diseases for the last two decades, including not only malaria but also leishmaniasis, Chagas disease, and dengue, and since 2014, chikungunya and emerging arboviruses, such as Zika and Mayaro. Since moving from Venezuela to Colombia in 2011, I have been involved in research of tropical diseases in Risaralda. Part of all this is a clear reflection of the work impulse at the Public Health and Infection Research Group, Faculty of Health Sciences, Universidad Tecnológica de Pereira, directed by Dr. Guillermo Javier Lagos-Grisales. Dr. Lagos-Grisales is not just a partner, a colleague, and a friend, but also an extreme believer in our work in vector-borne and zoonotic diseases. I must also recognize the beginning of significant collaboration with Dr. Wilmer Ernesto Villamil-Gómez, whom I met in Cartagena in 2013 during the Colombian Congress of Infectious Diseases. He is also part of the former Committee of Zoonoses and Hemorrhagic Fevers of the Colombian Association of Infectious Diseases (Asociación Colombiana de Infectología, ACIN), now called Committee of Zoonoses and Tropical Medicine. Dr. Villamil-Gómez is my most important collaborator on arboviruses, including Zika and malaria. In addition, since 2002 I have been involved in tropical medicine and travel medicine, participating in multiple studies on malaria, Chagas disease, leishmaniasis, and other tropical diseases. Currently in Colombia, we continue studying most of them, including their assessment in internally displaced populations.

Following the same philosophy we used for my ten previous books with IntechOpen [21–29], this book is not intended to be an exhaustive compilation. Many related topics are covered in a previous book, Current Topics in Malaria [24]; however, this updated book presents complementary topics in chapters written by new contributors with new perspectives.

I would like to give a very special thanks to IntechOpen, particularly Author Service Managers Mateo Pulko and Maja Bozicevic and Commissioning Editor Andrea Koric for the opportunity to edit this interesting and important book, as well for their constant support.

I want to take the appropriate time and space to dedicate this book to my beloved family distributed geographically among Venezuela, Chile, and Colombia (Aurora, Alfonso José, Alejandro, and Andrea, the neurologist). Katterine, my fiancé, makes every day special. I love her more than anything and I am happy to have her lovely existence in my life. I love you more and more every day.

I would also like to extend thanks to my friends and my undergraduate and postgraduate students in Colombia, Venezuela, and Latin America. Thanks also go to my colleagues at the Working Group on Zoonoses, International Society for Chemotherapy, and the Committee on Zoonoses, Tropical Medicine and Travel Medicine and a large list of members of RECOLZIKA (www.RECOLZIKA.org). Special thanks again to my friend and colleague Dr. Lagos-Grisales. Members of our research group and incubator consist of young and enthusiastic medical students, some veterinary medical students, and young medical doctors, all of whom are pursuing significant improvements in the understanding of the epidemiology of zoonotic, vector-borne, parasitic, and infectious diseases. The idea for this book came in 2019, but in 2020, we faced the COVID-19 pandemic, which affected multiple life processes including the development of this book. In light of this new pathogen, we created the LANCOVID network for research and collaboration (www.LANCOVID.org). In 2019, I also began to work at the Fundacion Universitaria Autonoma de las Americas, Pereira, Risaralda, Colombia, a new "home" that brings me support and trust in my new endeavors in research and teaching. I have to give special thanks in that order to Drs. Maria Monica Murillo, our dean at the Faculty of Medicine, as well as to our School of Medicine Director Dr. Jaime Cardona-Ospina, a long-time friend and fellow.

Finally, I hope our readers enjoy this publication as much as I enjoyed putting it together with my talented and knowledgeable collaborators.

Prof. Alfonso J. Rodriguez-Morales
MD, MSc, DTM&H, DipEd, FRSTMH(Lon), FFTM RCPS(Glasg), FACE, FISAC, HonDSc
Senior Researcher, Grupo de Investigación Biomedicina, Faculty of Medicine, Fundación Universitaria Autónoma de las Américas, Pereira, Risaralda, Colombia

Lecturer, Universidad Científica del Sur, Lima, Peru

Chair, Grupo de Colaboración en Enfermedades Transmitidas por Vectores y Zoonóticas de Risaralda (GETZ), Pereira, Risaralda, Colombia

Co-Chair, Working Group on Zoonoses, International Society for Chemotherapy (ISC)

Vicepresident, Colombian Association of Infectious Diseases (ACIN)

Member of the Committee on Tropical Medicine, Zoonoses and Travel Medicine, ACIN

President, Committee on Travel Medicine, Pan-American Association of Infectious Diseases.

References

[1] Mihreteab S, Lubinda J, Zhao B, Rodriguez-Morales AJ, Karamehic-Muratovic A, Goitom A, Shad MY, Haque U. Retrospective data analyses of social and environmental determinants of malaria control for elimination prospects in Eritrea. Parasit Vectors. 2020 Mar 12;13(1):126. doi: 10.1186/s13071-020-3974-x.

[2] Rodríguez-Morales AJ, Suárez JA, Risquez A, Cimerman S, Valero-Cedeño N, Cabrera M, Grobusch MP, Paniz-Mondolfi A. In the eye of the storm: Infectious disease challenges for border countries receiving Venezuelan migrants. Travel Med Infect Dis. 2019 Jul-Aug;30:4-6. doi: 10.1016/j.tmaid.2019.05.014.

[3] Rodríguez-Morales AJ, Suárez JA, Risquez A, Villamil-Gómez WE, Paniz-Mondolfi A. Consequences of Venezuela's massive migration crisis on imported malaria in Colombia, 2016-2018. Travel Med Infect Dis. 2019 Mar-Apr;28:98-99.

[4] Grobusch MP, Rodríguez-Morales AJ, Schlagenhauf P. The Primaquine Problem-and the Solution? Point-of-care Diagnostics for Glucose 6-Phosphate Dehydrogenase Deficiency. Clin Infect Dis. 2019 Sep 27;69(8):1443-1445.

[5] Rodríguez-Morales AJ, Suárez JA, Risquez A, Delgado-Noguera L, Paniz-Mondolfi A. The current syndemic in Venezuela: Measles, malaria and more co-infections coupled with a breakdown of social and healthcare infrastructure. Quo vadis? Travel Med Infect Dis. 2019 Jan-Feb;27:5-8. doi: 10.1016/j.tmaid.2018.10.010.

[6] Franco-Herrera D, González-Ocampo D, Restrepo-Montoya V, Gómez-Guevara JE, Alvear-Villacorte N, Rodríguez-Morales AJ. Relationship between malaria epidemiology and the human development index in Colombia and Latin America. Infez Med. 2018 Sep 1;26(3):255-262. PMID: 30246769.

[7] Chowdhury FR, Ibrahim QSU, Bari MS, Alam MMJ, Dunachie SJ, Rodriguez-Morales AJ, Patwary MI. The association between temperature, rainfall and humidity with common climate-sensitive infectious diseases in Bangladesh. PLoS One. 2018 Jun 21;13(6):e0199579. doi: 10.1371/journal.pone.0199579. Erratum in: PLoS One. 2020 Apr 21;15(4):e0232285.

[8] Faccini-Martínez ÁA, Pérez-Díaz CE, Botero-García CA, Benítez-Baracaldo FC, Rodríguez-López AE, Rodríguez-Morales AJ. Role of the blood smear in febrile returning travelers: Beyond malaria. Travel Med Infect Dis. 2016 Sep-Oct;14(5):515-516.

[9] Medina-Morales DA, Montoya-Franco E, Sanchez-Aristizabal VD, Machado-Alba JE, Rodríguez-Morales AJ. Severe and benign Plasmodium vivax malaria in Emberá (Amerindian) children and adolescents from an endemic municipality in Western Colombia. J Infect Public Health. 2016 Mar-Apr;9(2):172-80. doi: 10.1016/j.jiph.2015.09.001.

[10] Rodríguez-Morales AJ, Orrego-Acevedo CA, Zambrano-Muñoz Y, García-Folleco FJ, Herrera-Giraldo AC, Lozada-Riascos CO. Mapping malaria in municipalities of the Coffee Triangle region of Colombia using Geographic Information Systems (GIS). J Infect Public Health. 2015 Nov-Dec;8(6):603-11. doi: 10.1016/j.jiph.2015.05.011. Epub 2015 Jun 20. PMID: 26106039.

[11] Munoz-Urbano M, Lopez-Isaza AF, Hurtado-Hurtado N, Gomez-Suta D, Murillo-Abadia J, Delgado-Osorio N, Lagos-Grisales GJ, Villegas S,

Medina-Morales DA, Rodriguez-Morales AJ. Scientific research in malaria: bibliometric assessment of the Latin-American contributions. Recent Pat Antiinfect Drug Discov. 2014;9(3):209-15. doi: 10.2174/1574891x10666150410165038.

[12] Rodríguez-Morales AJ, Paniz-Mondolfi AE. Venezuela's failure in malaria control. Lancet. 2014 Aug 23;384(9944):663-4. doi: 10.1016/S0140-6736(14)61389-1. PMID: 25152269.

[13] Rodriguez-Morales AJ, Giselle-Badillo A, Manrique-Castaño S, Yepes MC. Anemia and thrombocytopenia in Plasmodium vivax malaria is not unusual in patients from endemic and non-endemic settings. Travel Med Infect Dis. 2014 Sep-Oct;12(5):549-50.

[14] Oróstegui-Pinilla D, Rodríguez-Morales AJ. Neonatal Plasmodium vivax malaria. Trop Biomed. 2011 Aug;28(2):339-42.

[15] Rodriguez-Morales AJ, Ferrer MV, Barrera MA, Pacheco M, Daza V, Franco-Paredes C. Imported cases of malaria admitted to two hospitals of Margarita Island, Venezuela, 1998-2005. Travel Med Infect Dis. 2009 Jan;7(1):44-8. doi: 10.1016/j.tmaid.2008.09.006.

[16] Rifakis PM, Hernandez O, Fernández CT, Rodriguez-Morales AJ, Von A, Franco-Paredes C. Atypical Plasmodium vivax malaria in a traveler: bilateral hydronephrosis, severe thrombocytopenia, and hypotension. J Travel Med. 2008 Mar-Apr;15(2):119-21.

[17] Rodríguez-Morales AJ, Sánchez E, Arria M, Vargas M, Piccolo C, Colina R, Franco-Paredes C. Haemoglobin and haematocrit: the threefold conversion is also non valid for assessing anaemia in Plasmodium vivax malaria-endemic settings. Malar J. 2007 Dec 17;6:166. doi: 10.1186/1475-2875-6-166.

[18] Rodriguez-Morales AJ, Benítez JA, Arria M. Malaria mortality in Venezuela: focus on deaths due to Plasmodium vivax in children. J Trop Pediatr. 2008 Apr;54(2):94-101. doi: 10.1093/tropej/fmm074.

[19] Rodríguez-Morales AJ, Sánchez E, Vargas M, Piccolo C, Colina R, Arria M. Anemia and thrombocytopenia in children with Plasmodium vivax malaria. J Trop Pediatr. 2006 Feb;52(1):49-51. doi: 10.1093/tropej/fmi069.

[20] Rodriguez-Morales AJ. (Editor). Current Topics in Tropical Medicine. ISBN 978-953-51-0274-8. InTech, Croatia, March 2012. Available at: http://www.intechopen.com/books/current-topics-in-tropical-medicine

[21] Rodriguez-Morales AJ. (Editor). Current Topics in Public Health. ISBN 978-953-51-1121-4. InTech, Croatia, May 2013. Available at: http://www.intechopen.com/books/current-topics-in-public-health

[22] Rodriguez-Morales AJ. (Editor). Current Topics in Echinococcosis. ISBN 978-953-51-2159-6. InTech, Croatia, September 2015. http://www.intechopen.com/books/current-topics-in-echinococcosis

[23] Rodriguez-Morales AJ. (Editor). Current Topics in Chikungunya. ISBN 978-953-51-2595-2. InTech, Croatia, August 2016. http://www.intechopen.com/books/current-topics-in-chikungunya

[24] Rodriguez-Morales AJ. (Editor). Current Topics in Malaria. ISBN 978-953-51-2790-1. InTech, Croatia, November 2016. http://www.intechopen.com/books/current-topics-in-malaria

[25] Rodriguez-Morales AJ. (Editor). Current Topics in Giardiasis. ISBN

978-953-51-5260-6. InTech, Croatia, December 2017. http://www.intechopen.com/books/current-topics-in-giardiasis

[26] Rodriguez-Morales AJ. (Editor). Current Topics in Zika. ISBN 978-1-78923-271-4. InTech, United Kingdom, June 2018. https://www.intechopen.com/books/current-topics-in-zika

[27] Rodriguez-Morales AJ. (Editor). Current Topics in Tropical Emerging Diseases and Travel Medicine. ISBN 978-1-78984-824-3. InTech, United Kingdom, December 2018. https://www.intechopen.com/books/current-topics-in-tropical-emerging-diseases-and-travel-medicine

[28] Rodriguez-Morales AJ. (Editor). Current Topics in Neglected Tropical Diseases. ISBN 978-1-78923-890-7. InTech, United Kingdom, December 2019. Available at: https://www.intechopen.com/books/current-topics-in-neglected-tropical-diseases

[29] Rodriguez-Morales AJ. (Editor). Current Concepts in Zika Research. ISBN 978-1-83880-876-1. InTech, United Kingdom, February 2021. Available at: https://www.intechopen.com/books/current-concepts-in-zika-research

Section 1

Advances in Diagnosis

Chapter 1

Introductory Chapter: Malaria Elimination - A Challenge with Multiple Emerging Ecosocial Challenges

Alfonso J. Rodriguez-Morales, Jaime A. Cardona-Ospina, D. Katterine Bonilla-Aldana, Luis Andrés Salas-Matta, Wilmer E. Villamil-Gómez, Juan Pablo Escalera-Antezana, Lucia E. Alvarado-Arnez, Carlos Franco-Paredes, Juan-Carlos Navarro, Tomas Orduna and José A. Suárez

1. Introduction

Malaria has been a major parasitic disease affecting humankind over centuries, with a disproportionate impact among populations, regions of the world and living conditions [1–5]. Caused by five well-accepted species, *Plasmodium falciparum, P. vivax, P. malariae, P. ovale,* and *P. knowlesi* [6] malaria remains a global public health threat due to multiple reasons [7, 8] including biological, social and climatic factors [3, 9–13] influencing the distribution of *Anopheles* vectors, especially *A. darlingi* in the Americas [14, 15]. There is an ongoing debate regarding the potential role of *Plasmodium cynomolgi* as the sixth etiological species of human malaria [16, 17]. The etiological diagnosis and the epidemiological and clinical management of malaria remains a major challenge in many settings, populations, and during specific clinical scenarios including cases of severe malaria in travelers [18–20].

2. Major challenges in malaria elimination: social and economic downturn in Latin America and the role of climate change

Over decades, especially in the 20th century, malaria has been a major cause of morbidity and mortality at national and regional level in Latin America and the Caribbean (LAC) [21, 22]. The epidemiological transition and improvement of social conditions (i.e. social determinants of disease) have concomitantly reduced malaria-associated morbidity and mortality in many countries [1, 5, 23–25]. Since 2000, drastic reductions in the incidence of malaria occurred in countries with the highest burden of disease (i.e., Brazil) [26–28]. Between 1962 and 1973 other countries in the region such as Grenada, Dominica, Barbados, Chile (a country where never was confirmed the occurrence of autochthonous transmission) [29], Saint Lucia, and Trinidad and Tobago received official certification as malaria-free, after the implementation of specific control measures. More recently, Argentina,

Bahamas, Antigua and Barbuda, Paraguay, Saint Kitts and Nevis, Saint Vincent and the Grenadines, Uruguay (another country that never has autochthonous malaria) [30], and lately El Salvador, were added to the list [31]. Experiences in malaria elimination, such as those of El Salvador, have been of significant impact. In other countries of the region, such as Ecuador, malaria had fallen to very low levels between 2000-2009, with transmission increasing again between 2014 and 2020, due to carelessness in the control campaigns in traditional outbreaks, as well as due to the mobilization and immigration from both the northern and southern borders [32, 33]. The starting point was the elimination of foci in each municipality, where active detection was included (searching of malaria cases), considering the DTIR strategy (Detection, Diagnosis, Treatment, Intervention and Response), so that more cases are diagnosed instead of stopping after the index case detection. Specific activities at the local level were monitored and evaluated for an overall impact that led the country to elimination [34].

Unfortunately, factors such as climate change represents a major negative factor that could potentially favor the spread of malaria-to-malaria-free areas [9, 35–40]. Mass deforestation, landscape change, wildfires, and other anthropogenic threats [41] influence the distribution of vector-borne diseases such as malaria [42]. Furthermore, the etiological agents of human malaria have been already detected in non-human primates, especially in Asia [17, 43–50], but also in LAC, particularly in Brazil [51–53] illustrating the risk of humans amplifying the spread of malaria to animal species.

Malaria transmission depends on several weather conditions including rainfall patterns, humidity and temperature (i.e., the ideal environmental characteristics of the malaria transmission are present in the Amazon Basin) and also depends of occurrence of water bodies and associated floating or emerging vegetation, as well as the surrounding forest cover that provides shade on the edges of lagoons. Malaria is associated with climate change [54] because the environmental consequences are linked to specific conditions that would benefit *Anopheles* population, and not only the life and distribution of the vector but the possibility of transmission of malaria too. The influence of climate change is highly relevant as the mosquitoes are ectotherm hosts [55]. To increase the knowledge of what could happen in the future, Intergovernmental Panel on Climate Change (IPCC) Fifth Assessment Report (AR5) provides an interesting review and evaluation of the science of the climate change and their multiple future scenarios (https://www.ipcc.ch/report/ar5/syr/). In general, all depends on the real trajectory of the greenhouse gases (GHG) but the development of the global warming is always related with increasing average temperatures and changes in precipitation patterns that has an effect on malaria causal factors [56, 57]. In spite of what acknowledgment we probably want to reach, there are several possible effects as potential scenarios, therefore estimation models are required to approach the most potential situation [58]. To directly associate the increasing of the average temperature with malaria, is known that the distribution of species as *P. falciparum* would expand depending on the increase of the temperatures even in greater latitudes and altitudes [59]. In the case of the changes in precipitation patterns, it is related with the zones where the mosquito breeding proliferates due to water levels decreasing and forming pools after the extreme increase of rivers because of the rain or other reasons like ice melting of the mountains. Nonetheless, species like *Anopheles darlingi* which appears to be directly associated with high levels of precipitation [60], would decrease their population on several scenarios in the future, so the study of climate change and malaria should be specifics owing to the effects of temperature and precipitations could be different if we evaluate combined possibilities [61]. Even in Europe, some studies have pointed out that climate change is a significant factor associated with reemergence of malaria in southern areas of the continent [62–64].

Two recent initiatives, the World Health Organization (WHO) Strategic Advisory Group on Malaria Eradication and the Lancet Commission on Malaria Eradication, have assessed the feasibility of achieving global malaria eradication and proposed strategies to succeed at it. Both reports (WHO and Lancet Commission) rely on a climate-driven model of malaria transmission to conclude that long-term trends in climate will assist eradication efforts overall and, consequently, neither prioritize strategies to manage the effects of climate variability and change on malaria programming [65]. Climate change associated factors and consequences is key for the consideration of ecosocial and integrative vector control strategies, as has been proposed for decades by the WHO. In the case of Latin America, there is still a long road to improve the associated situation, mitigation, and adaption on climate change according to the Intergovernmental Panel on Climate Change (IPCC) [66–73]. Then, climate change, is definitively a "stone in the shoe" in the control and elimination of malaria in LAC.

In addition, multiple social factors are still present in the region with a complex interplay, such as uncontrolled mining, poverty, the recent impact of Coronavirus Disease 2019 (COVID-19), political, economic, and social crisis, in countries from different ideological political positions, such as Brazil, Argentina, Peru, Bolivia, but especially Venezuela. The situation in the latter, once considered as the richest in the region, started to fall into a spiral of social devastation since 1998, impacting especially all the health aspects. Malaria control, in the past highlighted as the best program (1930s–1960s), today raises many concerns. Venezuela is the main focus of malaria in LAC, amid a humanitarian crisis, that also impacted Colombia and Brazil, as neighboring countries, but also to distant nations in South and Central America, even generating imported cases to Argentina or Mexico [3, 8, 11–13, 21, 22, 74]. The humanitarian crisis has led to a reemergence of multiple infectious diseases, but also the persistence and increase of multiple endemic diseases including malaria. In this context the forced migration occurring to multiple countries also constitute a challenge in the control of malaria in endemic and even not-endemic countries in LAC. Imported cases may be associated with local transmission by multiples routes, vector and not-vector-borne (e.g., blood transfusion, transplantation, congenital). Unfortunately, such crisis will not be solved in the near future, therefore it lies to the other countries in the region to prioritize the best strategy in managing imported cases, assuring early diagnosis and treatment to avoid potentially associated consequences, and to enhance surveillance and consider the importance of specific programs targeting migrant populations.

Regarding the COVID-19 pandemic, this has posed multiples challenges, including coinfections (SARS-CoV-2/*Plasmodium*), in the efforts of malaria elimination. During 2019–2020, malaria cases increased by 26%, in the countries where malaria is targeted for elimination in the Americas. In particular, there was increased malaria transmission in three countries of Mesoamerica: Nicaragua, Honduras, Panama. With a reduced number of laboratory samples and diagnostic tests, reduced mobility of people and disruption of health services, limited field operations due to social restriction gaps in ensuring personal protective equipment, malaria elimination is facing multiple difficulties. These existing gaps in malaria case detection and treatment may translate into increased chaos by 2021, added to the regional situation above mentioned of Venezuela [75].

3. Conclusions

We face multiple and perennial challenges when controlling tropical infectious diseases, such as malaria [42]. Despite many achievements in malaria control efforts during the last few decades, there are many countries in LAC where malaria transmission remains or revert to being a major public health concern for the region. In other regions of the world, such as Africa and Asia, the recent emergence of zoonotic species of *Plasmodium*, coupled with the impacts of climate change, economic downturn post-COVID-19, and globalization are also causing significant concern. There is an urgent need for local, national, and international health authorities to strengthen surveillance and multisectorial control approaches to advance the noble effort of malaria control and elimination in LAC and other regions.

Author details

Alfonso J. Rodriguez-Morales[1,2,3,4,5,6*], Jaime A. Cardona-Ospina[1,4], D. Katterine Bonilla-Aldana[3], Luis Andrés Salas-Matta[2], Wilmer E. Villamil-Gómez[5,7], Juan Pablo Escalera-Antezana[8], Lucia E. Alvarado-Arnez[6], Carlos Franco-Paredes[9], Juan-Carlos Navarro[10], Tomas Orduna[11] and José A. Suárez[12]

1 Grupo de Investigación Biomedicina, Faculty of Medicine, Fundación Universitaria Autónoma de las Américas, Pereira, Risaralda, Colombia

2 Universidad Cientifica del Sur, Lima, Peru

3 Semillero de Investigación en Zoonosis, Grupo BIOECOS, Fundación Universitaria Autónoma de las Américas, Pereira, Colombia

4 Emerging Infectious Diseases and Tropical Medicine Research Group, Instituto para la Investigación en Ciencias Biomédicas-Sci-Help, Pereira, Colombia

5 Infectious Diseases and Infection Control Research Group, Hospital Universitario de Sincelejo, Sincelejo, Sucre, Colombia

6 Coordinación Nacional de Investigación, Universidad Privada Franz Tamayo (UNIFRANZ), La Paz, Bolivia

7 Programa del Doctorado de Medicina Tropical, SUE Caribe, Universidad del Atlántico, Barranquilla, Colombia

8 Direction of Second Level Hospitals, Secretaría Municipal de Salud, Gobierno Autónomo Municipal de Cochabamba, Cochabamba, Bolivia

9 Department of Medicine, Division of Infectious Diseases, School of Medicine, University of Colorado Denver, Aurora, CO, United States of America

10 Research Group of Emerging Diseases, Ecoepidemiology and Biodiversity, Health Sciences Faculty, Universidad Internacional SEK, Quito, Ecuador

11 Hospital de Infecciosas FJ Muñiz, Buenos Aires, Argentina

12 Investigador SNI Senacyt Panamá, Instituto Conmemorativo Gorgas de Estudios de la Salud (ICGES), Panama

*Address all correspondence to: ajrodriguezmmd@gmail.com

References

[1] Rodriguez-Morales AJ, Benitez JA, Arria M. Malaria mortality in Venezuela: focus on deaths due to Plasmodium vivax in children. J Trop Pediatr. 2008;54(2):94-101.

[2] Rodriguez-Morales AJ, Sanchez E, Vargas M, Piccolo C, Colina R, Arria M. Anemia and thrombocytopenia in children with Plasmodium vivax malaria. J Trop Pediatr. 2006;52(1): 49-51.

[3] Rodriguez-Morales AJ, Paniz-Mondolfi AE. Venezuela's failure in malaria control. Lancet. 2014;384 (9944):663-664.

[4] Rodriguez-Morales AJ, Sanchez E, Arria M, Vargas M, Piccolo C, Colina R, et al. Haemoglobin and haematocrit: the threefold conversion is also non valid for assessing anaemia in Plasmodium vivax malaria-endemic settings. Malar J. 2007;6:166.

[5] Mihreteab S, Lubinda J, Zhao B, Rodriguez-Morales AJ, Karamehic-Muratovic A, Goitom A, et al. Retrospective data analyses of social and environmental determinants of malaria control for elimination prospects in Eritrea. Parasit Vectors. 2020;13(1):126.

[6] Rodriguez-Morales AJ. Malaria: an eradicable threat? J Infect Dev Ctries. 2008;2(1):1-2.

[7] Hotez PJ, Bottazzi ME, Franco-Paredes C, Ault SK, Periago MR. The neglected tropical diseases of Latin America and the Caribbean: a review of disease burden and distribution and a roadmap for control and elimination. PLoS Negl Trop Dis. 2008;2(9):e300.

[8] Grillet ME, Hernandez-Villena JV, Llewellyn MS, Paniz-Mondolfi AE, Tami A, Vincenti-Gonzalez MF, et al. Venezuela's humanitarian crisis, resurgence of vector-borne diseases, and implications for spillover in the region. Lancet Infect Dis. 2019;19(5):e149-ee61.

[9] Chowdhury FR, Ibrahim QSU, Bari MS, Alam MMJ, Dunachie SJ, Rodriguez-Morales AJ, et al. The association between temperature, rainfall and humidity with common climate-sensitive infectious diseases in Bangladesh. PLoS One. 2018;13(6):e0199579.

[10] Gutierrez-Ocampo E, Villamizar-Pena R, Holguin-Rivera Y, Molina-Ortiz K, Puerta-Laverde V, Rodriguez-Morales AJ. Malaria in Bogota, Colombia (2007-2017) - An analysis of notified domestic and international cases. Travel Med Infect Dis. 2020;33:101560.

[11] Rodriguez-Morales AJ, Suarez JA, Risquez A, Cimerman S, Valero-Cedeno N, Cabrera M, et al. In the eye of the storm: Infectious disease challenges for border countries receiving Venezuelan migrants. Travel Med Infect Dis. 2019;30:4-6.

[12] Rodriguez-Morales AJ, Suarez JA, Risquez A, Delgado-Noguera L, Paniz-Mondolfi A. The current syndemic in Venezuela: Measles, malaria and more co-infections coupled with a breakdown of social and healthcare infrastructure. Quo vadis? Travel Med Infect Dis. 2019;27:5-8.

[13] Rodriguez-Morales AJ, Suarez JA, Risquez A, Villamil-Gomez WE, Paniz-Mondolfi A. Consequences of Venezuela's massive migration crisis on imported malaria in Colombia, 2016-2018. Travel Med Infect Dis. 2019;28: 98-99.

[14] Maldonado V, Finol HJ, Navarro JC. Anopheles aquasalis eggs from two Venezuelan localities compared by scanning electron microscopy. Mem Inst Oswaldo Cruz. 1997;92(4):487-491.

[15] Dantur Juri MJ, Moreno M, Prado Izaguirre MJ, Navarro JC, Zaidenberg MO, Almiron WR, et al. Demographic history and population structure of Anopheles pseudopunctipennis in Argentina based on the mitochondrial COI gene. Parasit Vectors. 2014;7:423.

[16] Hartmeyer GN, Stensvold CR, Fabricius T, Marmolin ES, Hoegh SV, Nielsen HV, et al. Plasmodium cynomolgi as Cause of Malaria in Tourist to Southeast Asia, 2018. Emerg Infect Dis. 2019;25(10):1936-1939.

[17] Bykersma A. The New Zoonotic Malaria: Plasmodium cynomolgi. Trop Med Infect Dis. 2021;6(2).

[18] Garcia J, Seijo A, Benchetrit A, Couto E, Echazarreta S, Lloveras S, et al. [Failure to radical cure in Plasmodium vivax malaria]. Rev Chilena Infectol. 2016;33(4):468-471.

[19] Gallego V, Berberian G, Lloveras S, Verbanaz S, Chaves TS, Orduna T, et al. The 2014 FIFA World Cup: communicable disease risks and advice for visitors to Brazil--a review from the Latin American Society for Travel Medicine (SLAMVI). Travel Med Infect Dis. 2014;12(3):208-218.

[20] Gallego V, Berberian G, Siu H, Verbanaz S, Rodriguez-Morales AJ, Gautret P, et al. The 2019 Pan American games: Communicable disease risks and travel medicine advice for visitors to Peru - Recommendations from the Latin American Society for Travel Medicine (SLAMVI). Travel Med Infect Dis. 2019;30:19-24.

[21] Griffing SM, Villegas L, Udhayakumar V. Malaria control and elimination, Venezuela, 1800s -1970s. Emerg Infect Dis. 2014;20(10): 1697-1704.

[22] Gabaldon-Figueira JC, Villegas L, Grillet ME, Lezaun J, Pocaterra L, Bevilacqua M, et al. Malaria in Venezuela: Gabaldon's legacy scattered to the winds. Lancet Glob Health. 2021;9(5):e584-e5e5.

[23] Franco-Herrera D, Gonzalez-Ocampo D, Restrepo-Montoya V, Gomez-Guevara JE, Alvear-Villacorte N, Rodriguez-Morales AJ. Relationship between malaria epidemiology and the human development index in Colombia and Latin America. Infez Med. 2018;26(3):255-262.

[24] Munoz-Urbano M, Lopez-Isaza AF, Hurtado-Hurtado N, Gomez-Suta D, Murillo-Abadia J, Delgado-Osorio N, et al. Scientific research in malaria: bibliometric assessment of the Latin-American contributions. Recent Pat Antiinfect Drug Discov. 2014;9(3):209-215.

[25] Risquez A, Echezuria L, Rodriguez-Morales AJ. Epidemiological transition in Venezuela: relationships between infectious diarrheas, ischemic heart diseases and motor vehicles accidents mortalities and the Human Development Index (HDI) in Venezuela, 2005-2007. J Infect Public Health. 2010;3(3):95-97.

[26] Nekkab N, Lana R, Lacerda M, Obadia T, Siqueira A, Monteiro W, et al. Estimated impact of tafenoquine for Plasmodium vivax control and elimination in Brazil: A modelling study. PLoS Med. 2021;18(4):e1003535.

[27] Bezerra JMT, Barbosa DS, Martins-Melo FR, Werneck GL, Braga EM, Tauil PL, et al. Changes in malaria patterns in Brazil over 28 years (1990-2017): results from the Global Burden of Disease Study 2017. Popul Health Metr. 2020;18(Suppl 1):5.

[28] Melo JO, Padilha MAO, Barbosa RTA, Alonso WJ, Vittor AY, Laporta GZ. Evaluation of the malaria elimination policy in Brazil: a systematic review and epidemiological analysis study. Trop Biomed. 2020;37(2):513-535.

[29] United Nations. Argentina está libre de malaria y su caso es ejemplo para el continente. https://news.un.org/es/story/2019/05/1456411

[30] Ceruzzi O, Paparamborda M, Coppola J. Malaria en el Uruguay: vigilancia de los casos posteriores al regreso de misiones a zonas endémicas. Parasitol Día. 1996;20(1/2):4-9.

[31] WHO. Countries and territories certified malaria-free by WHO. https://www.who.int/malaria/areas/elimination/malaria-free-countries/en/ 2019

[32] Martin JA, Hendershot AL, Saá Portilla IA, English DJ, Woodruff M, Vera-Arias CA, Salazar-Costa BE, Bustillos JJ, Saénz FE, Ocaña-Mayorga S, Koepfli C, Lobo NF. Anopheline and human drivers of malaria risk in northern coastal, Ecuador: a pilot study. Malar J. 2020 Oct 2;19(1):354. doi: 10.1186/s12936-020-03426-y

[33] Gunderson AK, Kumar RE, Recalde-Coronel C, Vasco LE, Valle-Campos A, Mena CF, Zaitchik BF, Lescano AG, Pan WK, Janko MM. Malaria Transmission and Spillover across the Peru-Ecuador Border: A Spatiotemporal Analysis. Int J Environ Res Public Health. 2020 Oct 13;17(20):7434. doi: 10.3390/ijerph17207434.

[34] BID. El Salvador, primer país de Mesoamérica libre de malaria. https://blogs.iadb.org/salud/es/el-salvador-libre-de-malaria/ 2021

[35] Poveda G. Concomitant malaria, dengue and COVID-19: an extraordinary challenge for Colombia's public health system. Curr Opin Environ Sustain. 2020;46:23-26.

[36] Lubinda J, Haque U, Bi Y, Shad MY, Keellings D, Hamainza B, et al. Climate change and the dynamics of age-related malaria incidence in Southern Africa. Environ Res. 2021;197:111017.

[37] de Azevedo TS, Lorenz C, Chiaravalloti-Neto F, Sallum MAM. Kerteszia cruzii and extra-Amazonian malaria in Brazil: Challenges due to climate change in the Atlantic Forest. Infect Genet Evol. 2020;85:104456.

[38] Alimi TO, Fuller DO, Qualls WA, Herrera SV, Arevalo-Herrera M, Quinones ML, et al. Predicting potential ranges of primary malaria vectors and malaria in northern South America based on projected changes in climate, land cover and human population. Parasit Vectors. 2015;8:431.

[39] Lubinda J, Haque U, Bi Y, Hamainza B, Moore AJ. Near-term climate change impacts on sub-national malaria transmission. Sci Rep. 2021;11(1):751.

[40] Siraj AS, Santos-Vega M, Bouma MJ, Yadeta D, Ruiz Carrascal D, Pascual M. Altitudinal changes in malaria incidence in highlands of Ethiopia and Colombia. Science. 2014;343(6175):1154-1158.

[41] Bonilla-Aldana DK, Suarez JA, Franco-Paredes C, Vilcarromero S, Mattar S, Gomez-Marin JE, et al. Brazil burning! What is the potential impact of the Amazon wildfires on vector-borne and zoonotic emerging diseases? - A statement from an international experts meeting. Travel Med Infect Dis. 2019;31:101474.

[42] Rodriguez-Morales AJ, Paniz-Mondolfi AE, Faccini-Martínez ÁA, Henao-Martínez AF, Ruiz-Saenz J, Martinez-Gutierrez M, et al. The Constant Threat of Zoonotic and Vector-Borne Emerging Tropical Diseases: Living on the Edge. Frontiers in Tropical Diseases. 2021;2(3).

[43] Mohring F, Rawlinson TA, Draper SJ, Moon RW. Multiplication and Growth Inhibition Activity Assays for the Zoonotic Malaria Parasite, Plasmodium knowlesi. Bio Protoc. 2020;10(17):e3743.

[44] Cox-Singh J. Zoonotic malaria: Plasmodium knowlesi, an emerging pathogen. Curr Opin Infect Dis. 2012;25(5):530-536.

[45] Ramasamy R. Zoonotic malaria - global overview and research and policy needs. Front Public Health. 2014;2:123.

[46] Iseki H, Kawai S, Takahashi N, Hirai M, Tanabe K, Yokoyama N, et al. Evaluation of a loop-mediated isothermal amplification method as a tool for diagnosis of infection by the zoonotic simian malaria parasite Plasmodium knowlesi. J Clin Microbiol. 2010;48(7):2509-2514.

[47] Tan CH, Vythilingam I, Matusop A, Chan ST, Singh B. Bionomics of Anopheles latens in Kapit, Sarawak, Malaysian Borneo in relation to the transmission of zoonotic simian malaria parasite Plasmodium knowlesi. Malar J. 2008;7:52.

[48] Kawai S, Hirai M, Haruki K, Tanabe K, Chigusa Y. Cross-reactivity in rapid diagnostic tests between human malaria and zoonotic simian malaria parasite Plasmodium knowlesi infections. Parasitol Int. 2009;58(3): 300-302.

[49] Medeiros-Sousa AR, Laporta GZ, Coutinho RM, Mucci LF, Marrelli MT. A mathematical model for zoonotic transmission of malaria in the Atlantic Forest: Exploring the effects of variations in vector abundance and acrodendrophily. PLoS Negl Trop Dis. 2021;15(2):e0008736.

[50] Scott J. Proposed Integrated Control of Zoonotic Plasmodium knowlesi in Southeast Asia Using Themes of One Health. Trop Med Infect Dis. 2020;5(4).

[51] de Abreu FVS, Dos Santos E, Gomes MQ, Vargas WP, de Oliveira Passos PH, Nunes ESC, et al. Capture of Alouatta guariba clamitans for the surveillance of sylvatic yellow fever and zoonotic malaria: Which is the best strategy in the tropical Atlantic Forest? Am J Primatol. 2019;81(6):e23000.

[52] Abreu FVS, Santos ED, Mello ARL, Gomes LR, Alvarenga DAM, Gomes MQ, et al. Howler monkeys are the reservoir of malarial parasites causing zoonotic infections in the Atlantic forest of Rio de Janeiro. PLoS Negl Trop Dis. 2019;13(12):e0007906.

[53] de Alvarenga DAM, Culleton R, de Pina-Costa A, Rodrigues DF, Bianco C, Jr., Silva S, et al. An assay for the identification of Plasmodium simium infection for diagnosis of zoonotic malaria in the Brazilian Atlantic Forest. Sci Rep. 2018;8(1):86.

[54] Ferreira MU, Castro MC. Challenges for malaria elimination in Brazil. Malar J. 2016;15(1):284.

[55] Laporta GZ, Linton YM, Wilkerson RC, Bergo ES, Nagaki SS, Sant'Ana DC, et al. Malaria vectors in South America: current and future scenarios. Parasit Vectors. 2015;8:426.

[56] Gething PW, Smith DL, Patil AP, Tatem AJ, Snow RW, Hay SI. Climate change and the global malaria recession. Nature. 2010;465(7296):342-345.

[57] Martens P, Kovats RS, Nijhof S, de Vries P, Livermore MTJ, Bradley DJ, et al. Climate change and future populations at risk of malaria. Global Environmental Change. 1999;9:S89-S107.

[58] Parham PE, Michael E. Modeling the effects of weather and climate change on malaria transmission. Environ Health Perspect. 2010;118(5): 620-626.

[59] Caminade C, Kovats S, Rocklov J, Tompkins AM, Morse AP, Colon-Gonzalez FJ, et al. Impact of climate change on global malaria

distribution. Proc Natl Acad Sci U S A. 2014;111(9):3286-3291.

[60] Sinka ME, Rubio-Palis Y, Manguin S, Patil AP, Temperley WH, Gething PW, et al. The dominant Anopheles vectors of human malaria in the Americas: occurrence data, distribution maps and bionomic precis. Parasit Vectors. 2010;3:72.

[61] Midekisa A, Beyene B, Mihretie A, Bayabil E, Wimberly MC. Seasonal associations of climatic drivers and malaria in the highlands of Ethiopia. Parasit Vectors. 2015;8:339.

[62] Brugueras S, Fernandez-Martinez B, Martinez-de la Puente J, Figuerola J, Porro TM, Rius C, et al. Environmental drivers, climate change and emergent diseases transmitted by mosquitoes and their vectors in southern Europe: A systematic review. Environ Res. 2020;191:110038.

[63] Fischer L, Gultekin N, Kaelin MB, Fehr J, Schlagenhauf P. Rising temperature and its impact on receptivity to malaria transmission in Europe: A systematic review. Travel Med Infect Dis. 2020;36:101815.

[64] Mihailovic DT, Petric D, Petrovic T, Hrnjakovic-Cvjetkovic I, Djurdjevic V, Nikolic-Doric E, et al. Assessment of climate change impact on the malaria vector Anopheles hyrcanus, West Nile disease, and incidence of melanoma in the Vojvodina Province (Serbia) using data from a regional climate model. PLoS One. 2020;15(1):e0227679.

[65] Nissan H, Ukawuba I, Thomson M. Climate-proofing a malaria eradication strategy. Malar J. 2021;20(1):190.

[66] Verner G, Schutte S, Knop J, Sankoh O, Sauerborn R. Health in climate change research from 1990 to 2014: positive trend, but still underperforming. Glob Health Action. 2016;9:30723.

[67] Santalla E, Cordoba V, Blanco G. Greenhouse gas emissions from the waste sector in Argentina in business-as-usual and mitigation scenarios. J Air Waste Manag Assoc. 2013;63(8):909-917.

[68] Ceccarelli S, Rabinovich JE. Global Climate Change Effects on Venezuela's Vulnerability to Chagas Disease is Linked to the Geographic Distribution of Five Triatomine Species. J Med Entomol. 2015;52(6):1333-1343.

[69] Fe-Goncalves LM, Araujo JDA, Santos C, Val AL, Almeida-Val VMF. How will farmed populations of freshwater fish deal with the extreme climate scenario in 2100? Transcriptional responses of Colossoma macropomum from two Brazilian climate regions. J Therm Biol. 2020;89:102487.

[70] Weyant C, Brandeau ML, Burke M, Lobell DB, Bendavid E, Basu S. Anticipated burden and mitigation of carbon-dioxide-induced nutritional deficiencies and related diseases: A simulation modeling study. PLoS Med. 2018;15(7):e1002586.

[71] Hamilton SE, Lovette J. Ecuador's mangrove forest carbon stocks: a spatiotemporal analysis of living carbon holdings and their depletion since the advent of commercial aquaculture. PLoS One. 2015;10(3):e0118880.

[72] Piovezan-Borges AC, Valente-Neto F, Tadei WP, Hamada N, Roque FO. Simulated climate change, but not predation risk, accelerates Aedes aegypti emergence in a microcosm experiment in western Amazonia. PLoS One. 2020;15(10):e0241070.

[73] Fu R, Yin L, Li W, Arias PA, Dickinson RE, Huang L, et al. Increased dry-season length over southern Amazonia in recent decades and its implication for future climate

projection. Proc Natl Acad Sci U S A. 2013;110(45):18110-18115.

[74] Suárez JA, Carreño L, Paniz-Mondolfi AE, et al. Infectious diseases, social, economic and political crises, anthropogenic disasters and beyond: Venezuela 2019–implications for public health and travel medicine. Rev Panam Enf Infecc. 2018;1(2):73-93.

[75] PAHO. OPS insta a los países a seguir lucha contra malaria en tiempos de COVID-19, especialmente en comunidades vulnerables. https://www.paho.org/es/noticias/6-7-2020-ops-insta-paises-seguir-lucha-contra-malaria-tiempos-covid-19-especialmente 2021

Chapter 2

Point-of-Care Strategies Applied to Malaria Diagnosis

Alexandre Dias Tavares Costa, Anna Caroline Campos Aguiar, Angelina Moraes Silva and Dhelio Batista Pereira

Abstract

Rapid and specific diagnosis of malaria remains one of the main strategies to fight the disease. The diagnosis is made primarily by the simple and low-cost thick drop technique, considered the gold standard test. However, the requirement for good quality microscopes and well-trained personnel often lead to inaccurate diagnosis, especially in cases of mixed infections or low parasitemia. Although PCR-based tests can help in these situations, this technique requires large and sensitive equipments, being unsuitable for point of care (POC) settings. A myriad of POC diagnostic tests have being developed in the last years, relying on molecular methods but also on novel strategies. New platforms, miniaturization techniques, and multiplexing possibilities promise great potential to improve disease diagnostics through fast and accurate detection of cases, even at remote places. Here, we will address the main POC strategies developed for the diagnosis of malaria, highlighting their strengths and weakness as POC applications.

Keywords: point-of-care, diagnosis, malaria

1. Introduction

Malaria is one of the deadliest diseases of poverty. It is estimated that malaria causes 228 million illnesses and 405 thousands deaths each year. Among the sick, children aged under 5 years are the most vulnerable group affected by malaria; in 2018, they accounted for 67% (272 000) of all malaria deaths worldwide [1].

In many countries where malaria is endemic, a lack of access to adequate diagnostic services leads to poor health outcomes for fever patients, as well as poor surveillance of infections and outbreaks, and treatment monitoring [2].

To make matters worse, the appearance of antimalarial resistant parasites including artemisinin derivatives pose a major public health threat [3]. In addition, drugs such as the artemisinin-derivatives are more expensive, leading to an increased demand for patient evaluation by accurate diagnostic tests before treatment [4–6].

Therefore, it has grown in the last years a general agreement that new diagnostic tests are needed for remote areas in malaria-endemic countries. However, the new tests must show improved performance over existing techniques, so that adequate distribution of anti-malarial drugs can effectively target the disease and its outbreaks, contributing to the reduction of generation of drug-resistant parasite strains [7].

In malaria-endemic countries, the major hurdle for widespread access to malaria diagnostics is the limited health care infrastructure [8, 9]. According to the World Health Organization (WHO) guidelines, the useful diagnostic tool at the point of care (POC) is defined by some characteristics. It should be low cost, deliver sensitive and accurate results in as little time as possible, run on a portable instrument (ideally, should be instrument-free), require minimal external power, require minimal training before use, and not require refrigerated reagent storage and transportation. These guidelines are collectively known by the acronym ASSURED (affordable, sensitive, specific, user-friendly, rapid and robust, equipment-free, and deliverable to end-users) [10]. In addition to those requirements, an ideal POC malaria diagnostic device should determine which species is infecting the patient, to establish the level of parasitemia, and be able to detect mixed or low-level infections.

Current POC tests for malaria include the smear microscopy and immunochromatographic rapid tests (RDTs). However, more sensitive and specific techniques based on nucleic acid amplification tests (NAAT) have been praised as the best choice for a successful malaria POC diagnostic test. In this work, we will review the status of the diagnostic technologies that have been used for malaria detection at POC conditions, discussing their main advantages and disadvantages in the POC context.

2. Currently available POC tests

2.1 Smear microscopy

Microscopy remains the gold standard for malaria diagnosis in most endemic areas. This technique allows the identification of different malaria-causing parasites (*P. falciparum, P. vivax*, *P. malariae* and *P. ovale*), their various parasite stages, including gametocytes, and the quantification of parasite density to monitor response to treatment [11].

There are two variations of the microscopy technique, the thick drop and the blood smear, both use the Giemsa dye in their preparations and are performed with sample of peripheral blood. Thick droop is made by placing a few drops of blood on a glass slide, allowing the blood to dry, and then lysing the blood (usually with water) before staining. The blood smear is made from a thin layer of cells and are fixed with methanol before reading. The thick drop allows the identification of lower parasitemias, by concentrating the parasites. The blood smear technique is more sensitive in speciating the parasites, however it does not allow the identification of low parasitemias [12].

This technique has the great advantage of being cheap (costs approximately $ 0.20 per sample), fast (approximately 1 hour between collection and the result, if performed by a skilled laboratory technicians), and does not need sophisticated equipment. The number of patients tested by microscopic examination increased an increase of 165 million tests in 2010 [13] to more than 208 million testes in 2017[1]. The global total is dominated by India. The sensitivity of the optical microscopy technique using the thick drop method is50–500 parasites/μL, however, many factors may interfere with the results found in the thick drop technique, such as the quality of the microscope, the quality of the available staining reagents, and the skill of the technician. Several studies have shown that the sensitivity of the

[1] https://www.who.int/malaria/areas/diagnosis/microscopy/en/, accessed on February, 17th, 2021.

microscopy technique may be lower in several areas of transmission depending on the quality of the examination and the expertise of the microscopists, which can increase the number of false negative results [14, 15].

2.2 Rapid diagnostic tests (RDTs)

Rapid diagnostic test (RDT) is a quick diagnostic approach to detect malaria among malaria-suspected patients and rule out malaria among individuals without malaria. RDTs detect parasite-specific antigens in a drop of fresh blood through lateral flow immunochromatography using antibodies to detect one or several antigens [16] (**Figure 1**).

The RDTs detect a single species (either *P. falciparum* or *P. vivax*), some detect multiple species (*P. falciparum*, *P. vivax*, *P. malariae* and *P. ovale*) and some further distinguish between *P. falciparum* and non-*P. falciparum* infection, or between specific species. The most commonly used antibodies react to histidine-rich protein-2 (HRP2), aldolase and *Plasmodium* lactate dehydrogenase (pLDH). HRP-2 is a marker for *P. falciparum*, while pLDH antibodies can be specific for *P. falciparum*, or *P. vivax*. Aldolase antibodies are pan-specific, detecting all types of malaria parasite but not differentiating between them [17].

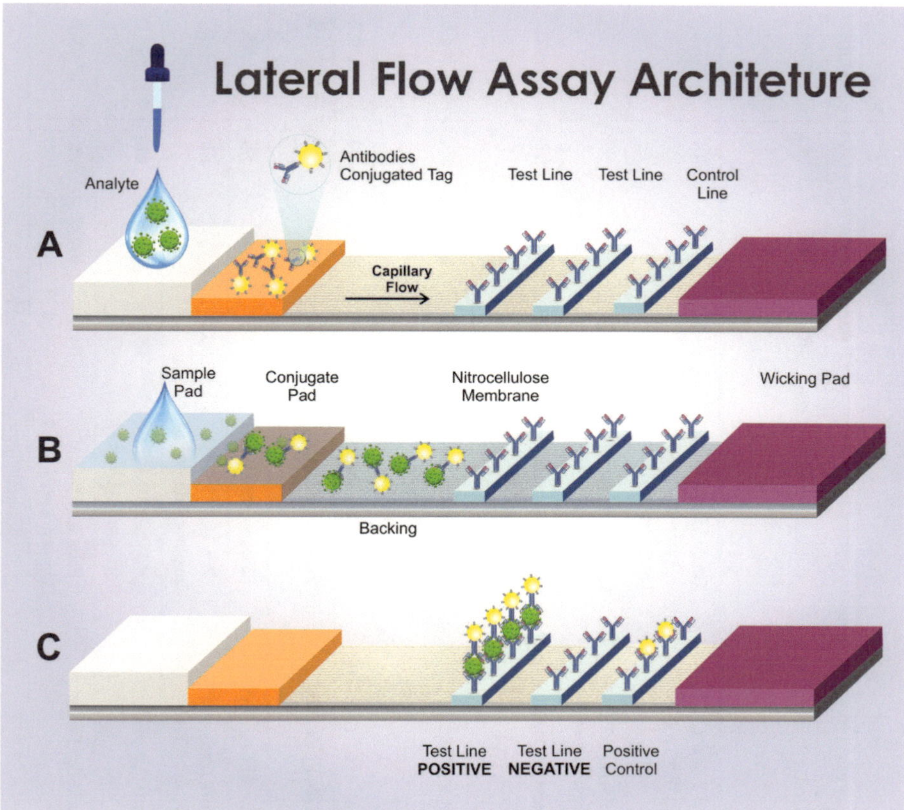

Figure 1.
Lateral flow assay architecture. Samples containing the analyte flow through the nitrocellulose membrane by capillary flow (panel A), carrying reporter antibodies (labeled with gold, latex or a fluorophore) until the mixture interacts with the test line (containing antibodies that bind the analyte of interest) and the control line (containing anti-IgG antibodies that bind to human IgG molecules) (panel B). If the control line shows a positive reaction, it is a valid test. If the test line shows a positive reaction, it is a positive sample for the specific analyte (panel C).

Product name	Manufacturer	Panel detection score				False positive rates (%)				Meets WHO performance criteria?
		200 parasites/μL		2000 parasites/μL		200 parasites/μL		2000 parasites/μL		
		Pf	Pv	Pf	Pv	Pf	Pv	Pf	Pv	
						non-Pf infection	Pf-infection	non-Pf infection	Pf-infection	
Paracheck Pf - Rapid Test for *P. falciparum* Malaria Device (Ver. 3)	Orchid Biomedical Systems – Tulip Diagnostics (P) Ltd	94.0	NA	100.0	NA	NA	1.4	NA	4.3	Yes
One Step test for Malaria Pf/Pan Ag MERISCREEN Malaria Pf/Pan Ag	Meril Diagnostics Pvt. Ltd	73.0	NA	99.0	NA	NA	0.7	NA	0.0	No
Parascreen - Rapid test for Malaria Pan/Pf	Zephyr Biomedicals – Tulip Diagnostics (P) Ltd	91.0	94.3	100.0	97.1	0.0	0.7	0.0	1.4	Yes
FalciVax - Rapid test for Malaria Pv/Pf	Zephyr Biomedicals – Tulip Diagnostics (P) Ltd.	95.0	100.0	100.0	100.0	0.8	0.0	0.0	0.0	Yes
STANDARD Q Malaria Pf/Pv Ag Tes	SD Biosensor, Inc	85.0	100.0	99.0	100.0	0.5	0.0	0.5	0.0	Yes
STANDARD Q Malaria Pf Pan Ag Test	SD Biosensor, Inc.	88.0	100.0	99.0	100.0	0.0	0.0	0.5	0.0	Yes
STANDARD Q Malaria Pf Ag Test	SD Biosensor, Inc.	87.0	NA	99.0	NA	NA	0.0	NA	0.0	Yes
First Response Malaria Antigen *P. falciparum* (HRP2) Card Test	Premier Medical Corporation Limited	95.0	NA	100.0	NA	NA	0.7	NA	0.0	Yes
First Response Malaria Ag. pLDH/ HRP2 Combo Card Test	Premier Medical Corporation Limited	85.0	73.0	100.0	100.0	0.3	0.0	0.0	0.0	No
First Response Malaria Ag. Pf/Pv Card Test	Premier Medical Corporation Limited	94.0	100.0	100.0	100.0	0.8	0.7	0.5	0.0	Yes

Product name	Manufacturer	Panel detection score				False positive rates (%)				Meets WHO performance criteria?
		200 parasites/μL		2000 parasites/μL		200 parasites/μL		2000 parasites/μL		
		Pf	Pv	Pf	Pv	Pf	Pv	Pf	Pv	
						non-Pf infection	Pf-infection	non-Pf infection	Pf-infection	
One Step test for Malaria Pf/Pv Ag MERISCREEN Malaria Pf/Pv Ag	Meril Diagnostics Pvt. Ltd	78.0	85.7	100.0	100.0	0.5	0.7	0.0	1.4	Yes
ParaHIT Ver. 1.0 Rapid Test for *P. falciparum* Malaria Device	ARKRAY Healthcare Pvt. Ltd	77.0	NA	100,0	NA	NA	0.0	NA	0.0	Yes

NA = not applied; Pf = Plasmodium falciparum; Pv = Plasmodium vivax.

Table 1.
Malaria RDT phase 2 performances in wild type clinical samples containing P. falciparum *and* P. vivax *at low (200) and high (2000) parasite density (parasites/μL) and clean-negative samples. Data modified from [18].*

	Microscopy	RDT	Nucleic Acid
Limit of detection (parasitemia)	50 parasites/μL	> 100 parasites/μL	0.5–5 parasites/μL
Time to perform	60 min	15–20 min	2 hours
Cost	$0.20	<$1 to $5	$1.50–$20
Need for technical training	Yes	No	Yes
Appropriate for remote field testing	Yes	Yes	Not yet

Some data were compiled from [29, 60].

Table 2.
Comparison of characteristics from currently commercially available malaria diagnostic methods.

The RDT test is highly sensitive and specific, it is easy to perform, simple to interpret and the results can be read in 15–30 min. These make it suitable for community-level health facilitates in rural areas and other endemic situations where equipment and professional microscopists are not accessible. However, they have a limited shelf life, and need to be kept dry and away from extremes of temperature. They may also fail to detect malaria in cases where there are low levels of parasites in the blood, and false positives are possible due to cross reactions or gametocytemia (infection with the sexual stage of the parasite only).

A brief comparison of WHO pre-qualified RDTs is presented in **Table 2.** WHO, in collaboration with Special Programme for Research and Training in Tropical Diseases (TDR), FIND, the United States Centers for Disease Control and Prevention (CDC) and other partners, established a protocol to measure the quality of malaria RDTs that are designed to diagnose *P. falciparum*-only through detection of histidine rich protein 2 (HRP2) and those designed to diagnose and distinguish *P. falciparum* and *P. vivax* or non-falciparum malaria. The protocol assesses the sensitivity and specificity of RDTs against specimen banks consisting of recombinant antigens, culture-derived parasites, wild-type parasites, and parasite-negative blood samples, as well as the stability of RDTs at various temperatures and usage conditions. The protocol also describes aspects of the RDTs that affect ease of use in the field, and methods for recording all information in specific databases. Up-to-data information on WHO pre-qualification policies and protocols can be found at WHO's website[2]. **Table 1** shows the malaria RDT performances in wild type *P. falciparum* and *P. vivax* clinical samples containing low (200 parasites /μL) and high (2000 parasites /μL) parasite density (parasites/μL) and clean-negative samples, an obligatory step of the WHO standardized tests [18]. The following criteria must be met for a product to be pre-qualified: (i) For the detection of *P. falciparum* in all transmission settings, the panel detection score should be at least 75% at 200 parasites/μL; (ii) For the detection of *P. vivax* in all transmission settings, the panel detection score should be at least 75% at 200 parasites/μL; (iii) The false positive rate should be less than 10%; (iv) The invalid rate should be less than 5%.

3. Nucleic acid amplification-based tests (NAAT)

NAAT have the potential to overcome several hurdles for malaria diagnostic at POC, more specifically related to the detection of low limits of infection, as well as the ability to discriminate the species and quantify the parasitemia.

[2] https://www.who.int/diagnostics_laboratory/evaluations/en/, accessed on February, 17th, 2021.

3.1 Polymerase chain reaction (PCR)

As the most known nucleic acid amplification technique, PCR has long been used for malaria diagnostic in laboratory settings. PCR-based malaria assays for laboratory use are found in many variations: conventional, nested, hydrolysis probe, digital, or high resolution melting [19–21].

As expected, there is a clear correlation between the level of PCR detection and the parasitemia of a given sample ([22] and **Figure 2**). The lower the parasitemia, the higher the detection cycle above the baseline/threshold (a value known as C_t). Conversely, the higher the parasitemia, the lower the C_t. **Figure 1** shows the detection of different amounts of parasites using two instruments: a lab-based and a portable, hand held thermocycler, the Q3-Plus [23, 24]. The linear regressions show that there is no difference in performance between both instruments using Spearman correlation, with r^2 ranging from 0.73 to 0.80, showing the viability of this portable platform for POC malaria diagnosis.

PCR is more sensitive than both microscopy and immunochromatographic tests. PCR has been found to be especially useful for identifying low-level infections often missed by other techniques, showing a detection limit in the range of 0.5–5 parasites per μL of sample. PCR can detect multiple targets in the same reaction without losing sensitivity and specificity and can be easily parallelized in high throughput instruments [23, 25–28]. The higher sensitivity is achieved by targeting multi copy genomic regions, such as 18S ribosomal RNA gene, which might be present in up to 1000 copies per genome and contains enough similarity across the genus *Plasmodium* and yet contains enough specificity to discriminate the species [23, 25–28].

PCR has been coupled with lateral flow strips to create a simple and easy-to-use detection method for the amplified products, called nucleic acid lateral flow immunoassay (NALFIA) [29, 30]. It combines the specificity of the PCR amplification with the simplicity of lateral flow strips, using DNA capture and recognition sequences and antibody-based colorimetric methods to visualize the targets on the nitrocellulose membrane. NALFIA has been evaluated under field condition

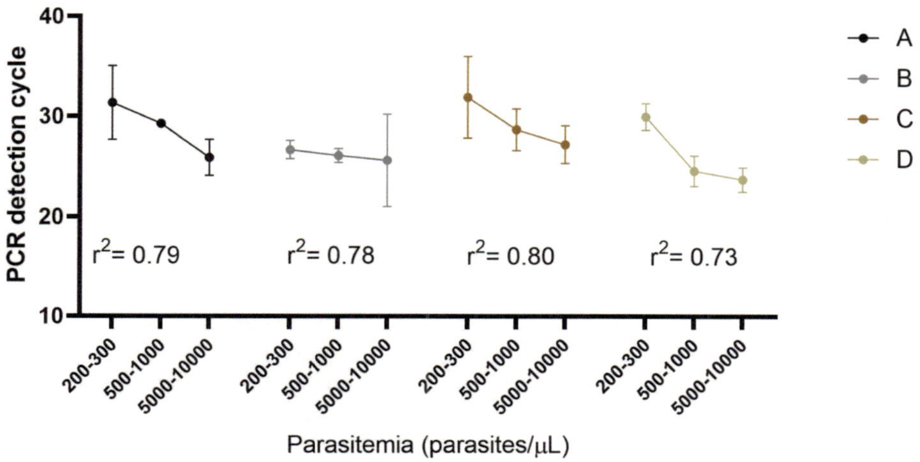

Figure 2.
Spearman correlation between PCR detection cycle and parasitemia estimated by optical microscopy. Detection of P. falciparum *or* P. vivax *DNA in human blood samples is plotted against the parasitemia estimated by optical microscopy. Samples were evaluated with two PCR instruments, the benchtop ABI7500 (applied Biosystems, Thermo fisher, USA) and the portable Q3-plus (ST microelectronics, Italy). Panels a and C show the detection of* P. falciparum *and* P. vivax *with the ABI7500. Panels B and D show the detection of* P. falciparum *and* P. vivax *with the Q3-plus.*

in Kenya, yielding results as sensitive and specific as laboratory PCR and a limit of detection of less than 3 parasites/μL [29].

However, in general, PCR reagents must be stored and transported at freezing temperatures (−20 °C), which is one of the main factors impairing its widespread use at POC settings all over the world and partially explaining why there are so many few available options for POC use for detection of infectious diseases. Some companies that have developed complete systems that use PCR, either conventional or nested, and melting curve analysis to detect targets of interest in POC conditions. However, neither has a solution targeted to malaria.

Much effort has been done to minimize or eliminate the requirement for freezing temperature for storage and transportation of PCR reagents. Even though some progress was indeed achieved, no commercial product is yet available. Rampazzo and colleagues [23] showed a ready-to-use qPCR that can be stored in the reaction vessel at room temperature for up to 28 days without losing performance. Iglesias and coworkers [31] showed similar results using a nested PCR for malaria detection, providing a comparison with microscopy and rapid diagnostic tests. Kamau and colleagues also reported a ready-to-use multiplex PCR for malaria detection [32]. Taylor and coworkers [33] developed a portable PCR instrument that performed 12 reactions in parallel, using lyophilized reagents and high resolution melting to detect and differentiate *Plasmodium* parasites, however with low sensitivity. Sun and colleagues [34] were able to pre-store the reagents in a portable device for rapid detection of *Campylobacter* sp. DNA. However, despite the availability of these technologies, we are unaware of a commercial product for malaria diagnosis that make use of them.

3.2 Isothermal amplification methods

Loop-mediated isothermal amplification (LAMP) is the most common isothermal amplification technique, although other methods have been developed in the last years. Other common isothermal methods, developed after the pioneering technique of the rolling circle amplification [35], are recombinase polymerase amplification (RPA), nucleic acid sequence-based amplification (NASBA), helicase-dependent amplification (HDA), strand displacement amplification (SDA), and even transcription mediated amplification (TMA) [36–42].

LAMP uses a complex set of four primers that bind to the region of interest and its boundaries and, after the initial amplification, create a secondary stem-and-loop structure that serves as a binding site constantly open for a new set of primers to anneal and keep the amplification happening [41, 43]. Amplification by LAMP involves two main repetitive steps of elongation by loop primers: the self-elongation step, where the template is elongated from the stem loop structure that was formed at the 3′ end, and the elongation step, where the formation of the new PCR product actually happens, polymerizing from the primers. That way, the end product is not a single band, but a series of concatamers of different sizes, all containing an amplified sequence of the target. Usually LAMP is performed at 55–65 °C by the enzyme Bst, from *Bacillus stearothermophilus*, and can use either RNA or DNA as templates. The requirement for a single stable temperature is a positive feature for a POC assay [41, 43].

Yamamura and colleagues have developed a rapid diagnostic solution for malaria by using DNA extraction through FTA paper, combined with a LAMP assay and melting curve analysis [44]. Although the solution was analyzed with real samples, the analyses were performed in the lab and not at the POC, so the protocol remains promising until tested in field conditions.

A complete technological solution able to extract DNA, amplify and detect specific DNA sequences from malaria parasites was published [43, 45]. The presented an origami device that vertically processed the sample coupled with a microfluidic lateral flow LAMP amplification and detection platform. The platform was able to detect the presence of the malaria parasite in 98% of infected individuals, with a better performance than standard POC tests, such as optical microscopy and commercial rapid immunochromatographic tests, which detected the parasite in 86 and 83% of the cases, respectively [43, 45].

A high throughput LAMP assay for malaria detection has been shown to work in field conditions, with a clinically relevant sensitivity and, importantly, low cost per analysis [46]. It needs to be evaluated on asymptomatic patients, but it remains one of the most promising candidates for a true POC test.

LAMP has also been coupled with a MiniION sequencer, being able to amplify a genomic target and then differentiate all five *Plasmodium* species. The procedure is sensitive enough to determine the C580Y mutation of *P. falciparum*, which confers protection against artemisinin and is an emerging threat for malaria eradication efforts. Although the procedure is relatively long because it is necessary to prepare the sequencing library, it is very versatile and shows great potential for POC settings [47, 48].

Detection of PCR-amplified products by lateral flow strips has been used for detection of malaria parasites in field samples [29]. In that work, DNA was extracted using a commercial kit. However, considering the difficulties of DNA extraction in the field, we believe that LAMP is the most suitable amplification technique to be conjugated with lateral flow strips as a feasible tool to be implemented in POC settings, and it should be further evaluated. Indeed, a meta-analysis of diagnostic accuracy of LAMP methods revealed that it is robust for diagnosing malaria, both in symptomatic and asymptomatic patients [49].

LAMP has also been used for detection of malaria parasites with a simple 1:1000 sample dilution, thus bypassing the hurdles of nucleic acid extraction in the field [50]. Although the protocol is fast and showed excellent detection limits, it has not been tested with real samples in field conditions, and therefore its positive features remain to be confirmed.

Nucleic acid sequence-based amplification (NASBA) is an isothermal reaction that continuously cycle between the reverse transcriptase activity that copies an RNA sequence into a cDNA, and the activity of a polymerase for subsequent amplification. NASBA generates a high number of copies of the target per cycle, usually reaching detectable concentrations of the product faster than other isothermal methods [42].

NASBA has been used to estimate the prevalence in asymptomatic migrants [51], to estimate gametocytes density [52] and has been shown to have significant correlation with quantitative PCR [53]. Because of its great potential for detecting low-level infections, NASBA has been proposed to be a good alternative to microscopy, especially in low prevalence areas [29, 37]. However, NASBA has not been tested in field conditions, so its performance remains to be evaluated.

4. Microfluidics and other new technologies

In recent year, biological research questions have become the center of convergence of several scientific disciplines, such as physics and engineering, joining the early partner chemistry.

Microfluidics is a general term for engineering techniques that leverage on physics forces at the micro scale to enable the miniaturization, simplification and automation of complicated analytical processes, while consuming less reagents, minimizing waste, and requiring less supporting instrumentation. Working at the microscale, microfluidic devices are portable, easy-to-use, self-contained, and low-cost diagnostic devices that allow the precise manipulation of minute amounts of liquids to be manipulated by miniaturized structures, such as micropumps, micromixers, microtweezers, and microvalves. Most attractive features of microfluidic technology for POC applications are the low volume of reagents required, faster reaction times, and compact/portable platforms [54, 55].

Microfluidics can be divided in conventional and paper-based assays. Conventional microfluidics focuses on miniaturizing regular laboratory protocols, with a special emphasis on integration of all necessary elements for the diagnostic reaction into stand-alone systems [54, 56]. In conventional microfluidic systems, liquid control can be exerted by acoustic, mechanical, magnetic, as well as capillary and centrifugal forces. Paper-based systems, on the other hand, rely mostly on the power of capillary forces, passively controlling liquid flow via hydrophilic and hydrophobic interactions. However, paper-based assays can integrate sample preparation and pre-concentration more easily than conventional microfluidic systems [56].

Mao and colleagues developed a portable multiplex microfluidic array system, which used LAMP to simultaneously amplify and detect malaria-related *Anopheles* and *Plasmodium* species. The system used a simple color change to discriminate positive from negative results [57].

Among the microfluidic devices, the centrifugal microfluidic device or lab-on-a-disc (LOAD) has advanced remarkably due to simple operation by rotation, allowing for total integration of protocol steps, and high-throughput capability. LOAD devices have been extensively used for molecular diagnostic assays [58]. Among many targets and applications, one stands out relative to our goals in this text. Choi and colleagues developed a platform consisting of a disposable centrifugal disc and a compact instrument able to perform real time PCR for malaria diagnosis with a relevant limit of detection [59]. Although this and other platforms showed great promise towards POC applications, they have not been tested in field conditions [58].

4.1 DNA-based capture molecules

Aptamers, also known as 'chemical antibodies', are short single-stranded oligonucleotides, either DNA- or RNA-based, obtained from synthetic libraries by a process called 'systematic evolution of ligands by exponential enrichment (SELEX)', that fold into distinct tertiary structures and are able to bind to the target with high affinity and specificity. Aptamer-coated surfaces, such as beads, sensors, or micro channels have been used to capture malaria parasites, which then can be detected by several techniques.

Fraser and colleagues developed a portable biosensor with a colorimetric approach to detect *P. falciparum* LDH in a device with three separate microfluidic chambers, obtaining high sensitivity and specificity [60]. Aptamers against other proteins, such as pGDH, PfEMP1, of HMGB1, have also been test in laboratory conditions but still largely remain as a promising approach for use in malaria-diagnosing POC assays [55].

4.2 Non-invasive samples and detection methods

Since blood collection is an invasive technique, other samples have been evaluated for their diagnostic capacity, in particular saliva and urine [61]. Although there has been some tests in the field using saliva for serological evaluation of samples with reasonable success, no nucleic acid amplification protocol has been used in conjunction with non-invasive samples in field application to help diagnose malaria [61]. In addition, PCR sensitivity in these samples is lower than other POC methods, impairing their current use as samples in molecular POC tests.

Infected or healthy red blood cells (RBCs) have different paramagnetic behaviors, likely due to the presence of hemozoin crystallites in iRBCs [62], and thus can be separated using magnetic fields, taking advantage of the miniaturization of magnetic resonance relaxometry (MRR) [63].

In fact, iRBCs can be enriched by a variety of methods, such as margination [64], dielectrophoresis [65], or magnetic methods [66] [67]. Margination is a separation method based on the deformability of RBCs, where microfluidic forces within the microchannels allow for the stiffer malaria iRBCs to segregate towards the device's sidewalls [62–64, 68]. Dielectrophoresis is a force exerted on any particle when it is subjected to a non-uniform electric field, and particle manipulation is dependent on physical properties of the medium and particle electrical properties, on particle size and shape as well as frequency of electric field [69]. In contrast to dielectrophoresis, microfluidic margination offers the convenience of not needing external electrical and magnetic fields for iRBCs separation. However, both dielectrophoresis as well as magnetic methods have been used for development of diagnostic methods for malaria infection [70]. Magnetic resonance relaxometry has also recently emerged as a very attractive technique to detect ring stage parasites, using a portable permanent magnet, with very encouraging results [62, 68]. However, although promising, dielectrophoresis, magnetic resonance, or margination have not been used in POC devices for malaria diagnosis.

Banoth and colleagues developed a portable device that measures optical absorbance at 405 nm of single RBCs flowing through microfluidic channels. Variation in optical absorbance is then used to discriminate infected from health RBCs from other cellular components present in few microliters of whole blood [71]. Nam and coworkers produced a device with microfluidic channels decorated with a magnetic wire where iRBCs can be separated from hRBCs due to the paramagnetic properties of hemozoin with very high efficiencies [72].

Some malaria diagnostic approaches try to avoid sample collection and processing altogether, such as infrared spectroscopy. Fourier transform infrared (FTIR) spectra are acquired directly from the biological sample without the need for any signal enhancer, such as dyes or reagents highlighting the targets of interest [73, 74]. The acquired FTIR spectra are representative of the molecular composition of the sample, and multivariate data analysis can be used to uncover changes in the FTIR spectra produced by cellular and biochemical changes induced by the presence of a specific pathogen [75, 76]. A work describing the use of this technique for malaria diagnosis employed Attenuated Total Reflection Fourier transform infrared (ATR-FTIR) to detect gametocytes at a level 100 times lower than microscopy-based testing [77]. Heraud and colleagues evaluated this technique using portable infrared spectrometers at four regional clinics in Thailand, comparing against laboratory-based qPCR. The analysis of 318 patients resulted in a high degree of sensitivity and specificity, supporting further testing in POC settings [78]. Recently, Mwanga and colleagues extended previous work [77] and provided the first demonstration that infrared spectroscopy could be coupled with supervised machine learning to accurately diagnose malaria in human dried blood spots [79]. Although more extensive field-testing must be performed, FTIR spectroscopy is indeed a promising method for point of care diagnostic of malaria.

5. The nucleic acid extraction problem

Sample preparation has always been a challenge for molecular assays as well as a bottleneck in translating complex molecular based tests to easy-to-use point of care products. Several prototype devices have been proposed and have shown good results in laboratory settings [80].

For nucleic acid testing, Govindarajan and colleagues reported a low cost μPAD for POC extraction of bacterial DNA from raw viscous samples using microfluidic origami. As demonstrated, *Escherichia coli* with a bacterial load as low as 33 CFU/mL was reliably extracted from pig mucin (simulating sputum) and subsequently detected [81].

The testing of clinical samples for nucleic acids has also been performed for infectious disease diagnosis in resource-limited environments, for example, to detect Ebola virus from extracted RNA or other infectious diseases [82, 83].

A complete technological solution able to extract DNA, amplify and detect specific DNA sequences from malaria parasites was published [43, 45].

Gan and colleagues developed a plastic microfluidic device that integrated a filter disc for DNA extraction from samples as distinct as whole blood, dried blood on various paper substrates, buccal swabs, saliva, and even cigarette ends. The device produced DNA suitable in quantity and quality for several downstream applications such as sequencing, SNP evaluation, and PCR [84].

Rodriguez and colleagues integrated nucleic acid extraction with isothermal amplification and detection by lateral flow on a foldable paper-based device able to detect RNA from Influenza A (H1N1) in less than one hour [85].

Kastania and coworkers present a polymeric microfluidic chip capable of purifying DNA through solid phase extraction that can be used as a stand-alone device or integrated in a lab-on-chip platform. The microfluidic channels were randomly roughened in the micro-nano scale with oxygen plasma, thereby creating high surface area as well as high density of carboxyl groups (–COOH). The –COOH groups together with an optimized buffer are able to bind DNA on the microchannel surface. DNA was the washed away by changing the solution biochemical properties. DNA extracted by this device was evaluated by conventional PCR, yielding satisfactory results [86].

These are just some examples. For an in-depth analysis of the issues of nucleic acid extraction possibilities and problems, the reader is directed to excellent reviews on the subject [80, 87–90].

Currently, magnetic beads and solid-phase extraction are the prime choices for nucleic acid extraction in POC devices, even though neither is yet ready for large-scale application [80, 91, 92]. Although both methods rely on the use of chaotropic agents for cell lysis and release the nucleic acids from structural proteins, washing steps are more efficient in beads-based methods in POC prototypes. However, some simplified protocols do not use beads or membranes and rely purely on both chemical and mechanical methods to denature cell membranes as well as scaffold proteins to release nucleic acids in adequate amounts and purity for diagnosis tests [80].

As shown above, despite extensive advances, no extraction method has made its way to the market of POC diagnostic solutions, and this is a major obstacle for nucleic acid-based assays. Although promising, integration of sample preparation, nucleic acid extraction, amplification and detection of genomic targets into microfluidic devices has not yet achieve the maturity to have impacts on the diagnosis of malaria in field settings. This is clear when one considers that FTA cards are primarily used for sample transportation from the field to the lab, instead as part of a complete kit combining their sample preparation and nucleic acid capabilities with the portability, not to mention sensitivity and specificity, of some of the techniques discussed in the prior sections of this work. We are not aware of such commercial kit.

A less-spoken but nonetheless quite important challenge of POC devices is waste disposal. Proper discard of biological waste generated by POC tests is a matter of concern, and open air burning might be the only option in some circumstances. However, the situation is more complex, since some chemical waste require special treatment before disposal, such as guanidine thiocyanate used in nucleic acid extraction protocols [93]. Developers need to take this issue in consideration when developing the assays and user-friendly tests.

6. Advantages and disadvantages for POC settings

An absolute requirement for identification and treatment of all parasite carriers, both symptomatic and asymptomatic, is inherent to all malaria elimination programs. Such identification implies that an active search for asymptomatic patients must be performed in POC conditions: since these patients will not look for medical attention, the medical team must find them. In addition, all techniques described in the present text have intrinsic advantages and disadvantages for application in POC settings, and thus each will fulfill a different aspect of the diagnostic needs, some better than others. **Table 2** presents a brief comparison between the different techniques used.

Microscopy, for example, requires few and inexpensive equipments, can be operated under virtually any environment conditions and within a few hours of collecting the blood, the microscopy test can provide valuable information. However, microscopy requires a very skilled professional for appropriate reading of the slides, which poses a problem due to the relative scarce availability. Furthermore, a review work found out that microscopy underestimates *P. falciparum* prevalence by 50% when compared to PCR, the gap being even more significant in low transmission areas [94, 95]. Likewise, Cheng and colleagues described that, on average, 69.5% of infections by *P. vivax* in areas of low transmission are detected only by PCR [94, 96]. Besides, microscopy results are only as reliable as the laboratories performing the tests. In non-endemic areas where the number of cases is low, the laboratorian does not perform this test regularly, and may not be maintaining optimal proficiency.

RDTs, on the other hand, do not require a skilled professional and also does not require expensive instruments. In fact, RDTs can be used with the naked eye, which makes it the perfect choice for remote and hard-to-reach areas. Although they identify *P. falciparum*, specifically, RDTs have no species-specific capacity to identify all five malaria species and cannot provide information on developmental stages. The RDTs rely on antibody detection of parasite antigens, which are constantly under selective pressure and evolve over time, resulting in tests with lower affinities and, consequently, lower sensitivity and specificity [97]. It is important to mention that false-positive results are associated with persistence of PfHRP2 in peripheral blood, cross reactivity against human rheumatoid factor, and other infectious diseases and false-negative results are associated with deletions of pfhrp2 and pfhrp3 genes [98].

PCR is very sensitive and specific, as well as a very robust and well understood technique. Although PCR is more sensitive and specific than microscopy or RDTs, it has limited use as a POC diagnostic tool because of its proneness to contamination, relative expensive reagents, delicate instruments, the need for a stable power source and skilled workers [99–101]. If a portable and robust PCR instrument is developed and is loaded with a malaria detecting reaction as it has been recently done [23, 33], then PCR might have a place in POC settings.

Compared to PCR, LAMP has the advantage of not requiring a complex and sensitive instrument, using less energy and time to achieve a sensitive target detection. However, LAMP is prone to contamination and production of false positive results from non-target amplifications, which decreases the specificity. If these technological hurdles are solved, LAMP is the most promising nucleic acid amplification technique for use in POC settings. NASBA, a sensitive and specific amplification technique, also does not require a complex thermocycler. However, it is high cost, prone to contamination and thus production of false positives, and requires a more extensive sample preparation than LAMP. Although equipment-free, NASBA is still far from POC applications.

Non-invasive methods such as infrared detection of hemozoin are very promising due to the good results in field tests and low cost of the instrument. Together with LAMP, it remains one of the most promising techniques for POC malaria diagnosis.

Finally, yet importantly, microfluidic techniques should collaborate with any nucleic acid amplification technique to make feasible a robust, sensitive and specific malaria POC diagnostic assay. Microfluidics have the capability of overcoming most of the obstacles of sample preparation and adequate amplification and detection of genomic targets. We believe that microfluidics will be in the center of a malaria POC diagnostic assay within a few years.

7. Costs and cost effectiveness

When one considers the production of the tests and its associated accessories such as required instruments (microscope, thermal cycler, thermal block, to name a few) in the cost analysis, microscopy is the cheapest in the long term, after the cost of the microscope is diluted over the years, and qPCR is the most expensive. The average cost for a microscopy slide test is in the range of \$0.20, while RDTs typically have a production cost of \$0.50 to \$2.00 per test, and nucleic acid amplification techniques harbor a production cost ranging from <\$1–\$5 for a LAMP assay up to \$10–\$20 per qPCR or NASBA assay (**Table 2**). Non-invasive methods have a negligible cost per assay, but its overall cost is expected to be as high as qPCR tests due to instrument costs [30, 61].

Costs associated with the different available tests must be considered not solely in terms of production costs. Cost evaluation models must also include variables such as DALY, patient's waiting time, cost acceptance (or 'willingness to pay') and, perhaps most importantly, adherence to the test result by patients, pharmacists, and health care providers, which is ultimately related to the perceived reliability of the test.

As discussed in the previous sections, microscopy and RDTs are the only current diagnostic tools adapted for use in resource-limited settings. Although samples can be transported to centralized laboratories to be evaluated by nucleic acid amplification techniques, turn-around time are typically too long in rural areas of developing countries, defeating the purpose of point of care testing.

Some works have explored cost effectiveness of available malaria diagnostic options for low-resource areas: presumptive, standard microscopy, and RDTs. Shillcut and colleagues used a decision tree model and probabilistic sensitivity analysis to evaluate costs and effects of RDT-positive patients and RDT-negative non-malaria febrile patients [5]. The authors found that the threshold level at which RDTs are more cost-effective than presumptive treatment is intrinsically related to the disease prevalence in the area. A health care provider can be 95% certain that RDTs are cost-effective relative to presumptive treatment at any prevalence below 62%, while there is a 95% certainty that RDTs are not cost-effective if the prevalence if higher than 90%. Microscopy would be cost-effective with 95% certainty relative to presumptive treatment if prevalence were below 41%, and would not be effective at prevalence rates above 83%. Finally, Shillcut and colleagues determined that RDTs are more than 85% likely to be cost-effective relative to microscopy at any level of disease prevalence [5]. Although the authors clearly show that RDTs are cost-effective, little is known about the impact of the facility of use and adherence to therapy that easy-to-use diagnostic tests might have on the patients [5, 102]. Similar results were observed in a deeper analysis using data from urban and rural areas of Nigeria [103], Kenya [104], and the Brazilian Extra-Amazon Region [105].

However, a recent study showed that patients are not always willing to pay for RDTs [106]. Since subsidies for artemisinin combination therapies (ACTs) already exist, it has been argued that similar subsidies could incentivize patients and health care providers to choose RDTs instead of presumptive treatment [107, 108]. Under that assumption, Bath and colleagues used a more complete decision tree and showed that subsidized RDTs could promote increased use of first-line antimalarials. Therefore, RDTs cost-effectiveness relative to microscopy or presumptive treatment would be true also in high prevalence areas, where a greater proportion of patients would benefit from increased first-line antimalarials use [108].

8. Conclusion

In summary, there are different methods can be employed for the diagnosis of human malaria. While microscopy remains the gold standard, being the mainstay of parasite-based diagnosis, its characteristics are inadequate for ensuring good sensitivity and specificity of malaria diagnosis in the field, adversely affecting health outcomes and optimal use of resources. An acceptable microscopy service is one that is both cost-effective and provides results that are consistently accurate and sufficiently timely to have a direct impact on treatment. This requires a comprehensive and functioning quality assurance program that is lacking in most malaria-endemic countries. RDT tests, which require little expertise to use and are quality-assured from the factory, are a good alternative for malaria diagnosis in remote areas. However, RDTs have no species-specific capacity to identify all five malaria species, and the parasite can present different mutations that hinder this diagnosis by increasing false-negative results. Nuclei acid-based tests, on the contrary, are specific, sensitive, and flexible to be adapted into a POC assay. Nucleic acid-based POC tests have the potential to reduce inappropriate use of anti malarials in endemic regions, bypassing the time and expertise required for microscopic analysis; however, they are more expensive and have not yet been truly adapted for use in remote areas. However, significant advances have been made to facilitate the use of POC methods, so we firmly believe that, within the coming years, interdisciplinary partnership will certainly blend innovative knowledge in biology, chemistry and physics to overcome the major hurdles impairing widespread use of nucleic acid POC tests.

Acknowledgements

The authors would like to express gratitude to Mr. Wagner Nagib de Souza Birbeire for the development of the scientific image in **Figure 1**.

Author details

Alexandre Dias Tavares Costa[1*], Anna Caroline Campos Aguiar[2], Angelina Moraes Silva[3] and Dhelio Batista Pereira[3]

1 Instituto Carlos Chagas (ICC), Fundação Oswaldo Cruz (Fiocruz), Curitiba, PR, Brazil

2 Universidade Federal de São Paulo (UNIFESP), Departamento de Biociências, Santos, SP, Brazil

3 Centro de Pesquisa em Medicina Tropical (CEPEM), Porto Velho, RO, Brasil

*Address all correspondence to: alexandre.costa@fiocruz.br

References

[1] Global Malaria Programme: WHO Global. World malaria report 2019. WHO Regional Office for Africa. 2019.

[2] WHO. World Malaria Report. World Health Organization. 2016. doi:10.4135/9781452276151.n221

[3] Uwimana A, Legrand E, Stokes BH, Ndikumana J-LM, Warsame M, Umulisa N, et al. Emergence and clonal expansion of in vitro artemisinin-resistant *Plasmodium falciparum* kelch13 R561H mutant parasites in Rwanda. Nat Med. 2020;26: 1602-1608. doi:10.1038/s41591-020-1005-2

[4] Das LK, Jambulingam P, Sadanandane C. Impact of community-based presumptive chloroquine treatment of fever cases on malaria morbidity and mortality in a tribal area in Orissa State, India. Malar J. 2008;7: 75. doi:10.1186/1475-2875-7-75

[5] Shillcutt S, Morel C, Goodman C, Coleman P, Bell D, Whitty C, et al. Cost-effectiveness of malaria diagnostic methods in sub-Saharan Africa in an era of combination therapy. Bull World Health Organ. 2008;86: 101-110. doi:10.2471/BLT.07.042259

[6] UNICEF, UNAIDS, World Health Organization, Médicins sans Frontières, Management Sciences for Health, Population Services International. Sources and Prices of Selected Products for the Prevention, Diagnosis and Treatment ofMalaria. Geneva: World Health Organization; 2004.

[7] Drakeley C, Reyburn H. Out with the old, in with the new: the utility of rapid diagnostic tests for malaria diagnosis in Africa. Trans R Soc Trop Med Hyg. 2009;103: 333-337. doi:10.1016/j.trstmh.2008.10.003

[8] Breman J, Alilio M, White N. Defining and Defeating the Intolerable Burden of Malaria III: Progress and Perspectives. Am Soc Trop Med Hyg. 2007;77.

[9] Snow RW, Guerra CA, Noor AM, Myint HY, Hay SI. The global distribution of clinical episodes of *Plasmodium falciparum* malaria. Nature. 2005;434: 214-217. doi:10.1038/nature03342

[10] Meeting MPAC. WHO technical consultation on research requirements to support policy recommendations on highly sensitive point-ofcare diagnostics for *P. falciparum* malaria. Geneva; 2018.

[11] Mathison BA, Pritt BS. Update on Malaria Diagnostics and Test Utilization. Kraft CS, editor. J Clin Microbiol. 2017;55: 2009-2017. doi:10.1128/JCM.02562-16

[12] World Health Organization. Basic malaria microscopy – Part I: Learner's guide. 2nd ed. Geneva, Switzerland: World Health Organization; 2010.

[13] WHO Global Malaria Programme. World Malaria Report 2010. Geneva, Switzerland; 2011.

[14] Berzosa P, de Lucio A, Romay-Barja M, Herrador Z, González V, García L, et al. Comparison of three diagnostic methods (microscopy, RDT, and PCR) for the detection of malaria parasites in representative samples from Equatorial Guinea. Malar J. 2018;17: 333. doi:10.1186/s12936-018-2481-4

[15] Thimasarn K, Miller RS, Maneechai N, Sattabongkot J, Soyseng V, Rachaphaew N, et al. Comparison of field and expert laboratory microscopy for active surveillance for asymptomatic *Plasmodium falciparum* and *Plasmodium vivax* in western Thailand. Am J Trop Med Hyg. 2002;67: 141-144. doi:10.4269/ajtmh.2002.67.141

[16] WHO. Malaria Rapid Diagnostic Test Performance - results of WHO product testing of malaria RDTs: Round 1 (2008). Malaria Rapid Diagnostic Test Performance - Summary results of WHO product testing of malaria RDTs: round 1-7 (2008-2016). Geneva, Switzerland; 2017.

[17] Ling X-X, Jin J-J, Zhu G-D, Wang W-M, Cao Y-Y, Yang M-M, et al. Cost-effectiveness analysis of malaria rapid diagnostic tests: a systematic review. Infect Dis Poverty. 2019;8: 104. doi:10.1186/s40249-019-0615-8

[18] WHO, FIND, CDC. Malaria rapid diagnostic test performance. Results of WHO product testing of malaria RDTs: round 8 (2016-2018). Geneva, Switzerland; 2018.

[19] Murillo E, Muskus C, Agudelo LA, Vélez ID, Ruiz-Lopez F. A new high-resolution melting analysis for the detection and identification of Plasmodium in human and Anopheles vectors of malaria. Sci Rep. 2019;9: 1674. doi:10.1038/s41598-018-36515-9

[20] Roth JM, Korevaar DA, Leeflang MMG, Mens PF. Molecular malaria diagnostics: A systematic review and meta-analysis. Crit Rev Clin Lab Sci. 2016;53: 87-105. doi:10.3109/10408363.2015.1084991

[21] Koepfli C, Nguitragool W, Hofmann NE, Robinson LJ, Ome-Kaius M, Sattabongkot J, et al. Sensitive and accurate quantification of human malaria parasites using droplet digital PCR (ddPCR). Sci Rep. 2016;6: 39183. doi:10.1038/srep39183

[22] Ballard E, Wang CYT, Hien TT, Tong NT, Marquart L, Pava Z, et al. A validation study of microscopy versus quantitative PCR for measuring *Plasmodium falciparum* parasitemia. Trop Med Health. 2019;47: 49. doi:10.1186/s41182-019-0176-3

[23] Rampazzo RCP, Graziani AC, Leite KK, Surdi JA, Biondo CA, Costa MLN, et al. Proof of Concept for a Portable Platform for Molecular Diagnosis of Tropical Diseases. J Mol Diagnostics. 2019;21: 839-851. doi:10.1016/j.jmoldx.2019.04.008

[24] Cereda M, Cocci A, Cucchi D, Raia L, Pirola D, Bruno L, et al. Q3: A Compact Device for Quick, High Precision qPCR. Sensors. 2018;18: 2583. doi:10.3390/s18082583

[25] Rougemont M, Saanen M Van, Sahli R, Hinrikson HP, Bille J, Jaton K. Detection of Four Plasmodium Species in Blood from Humans by 18S rRNA Gene Subunit-Based and Species-Specific Real-Time PCR Assays. 2004;42: 5636-5643. doi:10.1128/JCM.42.12.5636

[26] Kamau E, Alemayehu S, Feghali KC, Saunders D, Ockenhouse CF. Multiplex qPCR for Detection and Absolute Quantification of Malaria. PLoS One. 2013;8. doi:10.1371/journal.pone.0071539

[27] Alemayehu S, Feghali KC, Cowden J, Komisar J, Ockenhouse CF, Kamau E. Comparative evaluation of published real-time PCR assays for the detection of malaria following MIQE guidelines. Malar J. 2013;12: 277. doi:10.1186/1475-2875-12-277

[28] Kamau E, Tolbert LS, Kortepeter L, Pratt M, Nyakoe N, Muringo L, et al. Development of a highly sensitive genus-specific quantitative reverse transcriptase real-time PCR assay for detection and quantitation of plasmodium by amplifying RNA and DNA of the 18S rRNA genes. J Clin Microbiol. 2011;49: 2946-2953. doi:10.1128/JCM.00276-11

[29] Mens P, Spieker N, Omar S, Heijnen M, Schallig H, Kager PA. Is molecular biology the best alternative for diagnosis of malaria to microscopy?

A comparison between microscopy, antigen detection and molecular tests in rural Kenya and urban Tanzania. Trop Med Int Heal. 2006; 061127095204005-??? doi:10.1111/j.1365-3156.2006.01779.x

[30] Cordray MS, Richards-Kortum RR. Emerging nucleic acid-based tests for point-of-care detection of malaria. Am J Trop Med Hyg. 2012;87: 223-30. doi:10.4269/ajtmh.2012.11-0685

[31] Iglesias N, Subirats M, Trevisi P, Ramírez-Olivencia G, Castán P, Puente S, et al. Performance of a new gelled nested PCR test for the diagnosis of imported malaria: comparison with microscopy, rapid diagnostic test, and real-time PCR. Parasitol Res. 2014;113: 2587-91. doi:10.1007/s00436-014-3911-z

[32] Kamau E, Alemayehu S, Feghali KC, Juma DW, Blackstone GM, Marion WR, et al. Sample-ready multiplex qPCR assay for detection of malaria. Malar J. 2014;13: 158. doi:10.1186/1475-2875-13-158

[33] Taylor BJ, Howell A, Martin KA, Manage DP, Gordy W, Campbell SD, et al. A lab-on-chip for malaria diagnosis and surveillance. Malar J. 2014;13: 179. doi:10.1186/1475-2875-13-179

[34] Sun Y, Høgberg J, Christine T, Florian L, Monsalve LG, Rodriguez S, et al. Pre-storage of gelified reagents in a lab-on-a-foil system for rapid nucleic acid analysis. Lab Chip. 2013;13: 1509-14. doi:10.1039/c2lc41386h

[35] Ali MM, Li F, Zhang Z, Zhang K, Kang D-K, Ankrum JA, et al. Rolling circle amplification: a versatile tool for chemical biology, materials science and medicine. Chem Soc Rev. 2014;43: 3324-41. doi:10.1039/c3cs60439j

[36] Li J, Macdonald J, von Stetten F. Review: a comprehensive summary of a decade development of the recombinase polymerase amplification. Analyst. 2018;144: 31-67. doi:10.1039/c8an01621f

[37] Oriero EC, Jacobs J, Van Geertruyden J-P, Nwakanma D, D'Alessandro U. Molecular-based isothermal tests for field diagnosis of malaria and their potential contribution to malaria elimination. J Antimicrob Chemother. 2014;70: 2-13. doi:10.1093/jac/dku343

[38] Vincent M, Xu Y, Kong H. Helicase-dependent isothermal DNA amplification. EMBO Rep. 2004;5: 795-800. doi:10.1038/sj.embor.7400200

[39] Toley BJ, Covelli I, Belousov Y, Ramachandran S, Kline E, Scarr N, et al. Isothermal strand displacement amplification (iSDA): a rapid and sensitive method of nucleic acid amplification for point-of-care diagnosis. Analyst. 2015;140: 7540-9. doi:10.1039/c5an01632k

[40] Comanor L, Anderson F, Ghany M, Perrillo R, Heathcote EJ, Sherlock C, et al. Transcription-mediated amplification is more sensitive than conventional PCR-based assays for detecting residual serum HCV RNA at end of treatment. Am J Gastroenterol. 2001;96: 2968-72. doi:10.1111/j.1572-0241.2001.04669.x

[41] Becherer L, Borst N, Bakheit M, Frischmann S, Zengerle R, von Stetten F. Loop-mediated isothermal amplification (LAMP) – review and classification of methods for sequence-specific detection. Anal Methods. 2020;12: 717-746. doi:10.1039/C9AY02246E

[42] Compton J. Nucleic acid sequence-based amplification. Nature. 1991;350: 91-92. doi:10.1038/350091a0

[43] Reboud J, Xu G, Garrett A, Adriko M, Yang Z, Tukahebwa EM, et al. Paper-based microfluidics for DNA diagnostics of malaria in low resource underserved rural communities. Proc Natl Acad Sci. 2019;116: 4834-4842. doi:10.1073/pnas.1812296116

[44] Yamamura M, Makimura K, Ota Y. Evaluation of a new rapid molecular diagnostic system for *Plasmodium falciparum* combined with DNA filter paper, loop-mediated isothermal amplification, and melting curve analysis. Jpn J Infect Dis. 2009;62: 20-25.

[45] Xu G, Nolder D, Reboud J, Oguike MC, van Schalkwyk DA, Sutherland CJ, et al. Paper-Origami-Based Multiplexed Malaria Diagnostics from Whole Blood. Angew Chemie Int Ed. 2016;55: 15250-15253. doi:10.1002/anie.201606060

[46] Britton S, Cheng Q, Sutherland CJ, McCarthy JS. A simple, high-throughput, colourimetric, field applicable loop-mediated isothermal amplification (HtLAMP) assay for malaria elimination. Malar J. 2015;14: 335. doi:10.1186/s12936-015-0848-3

[47] Imai K, Tarumoto N, Misawa K, Runtuwene LR, Sakai J, Hayashida K, et al. A novel diagnostic method for malaria using loop-mediated isothermal amplification (LAMP) and MinION™ nanopore sequencer. BMC Infect Dis. 2017;17: 621. doi:10.1186/s12879-017-2718-9

[48] Imai K, Tarumoto N, Runtuwene LR, Sakai J, Hayashida K, Eshita Y, et al. An innovative diagnostic technology for the codon mutation C580Y in kelch13 of *Plasmodium falciparum* with MinION nanopore sequencer. Malar J. 2018;17: 217. doi:10.1186/s12936-018-2362-x

[49] Picot S, Cucherat M, Bienvenu A-L. Systematic review and meta-analysis of diagnostic accuracy of loop-mediated isothermal amplification (LAMP) methods compared with microscopy, polymerase chain reaction and rapid diagnostic tests for malaria diagnosis. Int J Infect Dis. 2020;98: 408-419. doi:10.1016/j.ijid.2020.07.009

[50] Modak SS, Barber CA, Geva E, Abrams WR, Malamud D, Ongagna YSY. Rapid Point-of-Care Isothermal Amplification Assay for the Detection of Malaria without Nucleic Acid Purification. Infect Dis Res Treat. 2016;9: IDRT.S32162. doi:10.4137/IDRT.S32162

[51] Marangi M, Di Tullio R, Mens PF, Martinelli D, Fazio V, Angarano G, et al. Prevalence of Plasmodium spp. in malaria asymptomatic African migrants assessed by nucleic acid sequence based amplification. Malar J. 2009;8: 12. doi:10.1186/1475-2875-8-12

[52] Pett H, Gonçalves BP, Dicko A, Nébié I, Tiono AB, Lanke K, et al. Comparison of molecular quantification of *Plasmodium falciparum* gametocytes by Pfs25 qRT-PCR and QT-NASBA in relation to mosquito infectivity. Malar J. 2016;15: 539. doi:10.1186/s12936-016-1584-z

[53] Schneider P, Wolters L, Schoone G, Schallig H, Sillekens P, Hermsen R, et al. Real-time nucleic acid sequence-based amplification is more convenient than real-time PCR for quantification of *Plasmodium falciparum*. J Clin Microbiol. 2005;43: 402-5. doi:10.1128/JCM.43.1.402-405.2005

[54] Pham NM, Karlen W, Beck H-P, Delamarche E. Malaria and the 'last' parasite: how can technology help? Malar J. 2018;17: 260. doi:10.1186/s12936-018-2408-0

[55] Gitta B, Kilian N. Diagnosis of Malaria Parasites Plasmodium spp. in Endemic Areas: Current Strategies for an Ancient Disease. BioEssays. 2020;42: 1-12. doi:10.1002/bies.201900138

[56] Naik P, Jaitpal S, Paul D. The Resurgence of Paperfluidics: A new technology for cell, DNA, and blood analysis. IEEE Nanotechnol Mag. 2020;14: 35-45. doi:10.1109/MNANO.2020.2966063

[57] Mao R, Ge G, Wang Z, Hao R, Zhang G, Yang Z, et al. A multiplex

microfluidic loop-mediated isothermal amplification array for detection of malaria-related parasites and vectors. Acta Trop. 2018;178: 86-92. doi:10.1016/j.actatropica.2017.10.025

[58] Nguyen H Van, Nguyen VD, Nguyen HQ, Chau THT, Lee EY, Seo TS. Nucleic acid diagnostics on the total integrated lab-on-a-disc for point-of-care testing. Biosens Bioelectron. 2019;141: 111466. doi:10.1016/j.bios.2019.111466

[59] Choi G, Prince T, Miao J, Cui L, Guan W. Sample-to-answer palm-sized nucleic acid testing device towards low-cost malaria mass screening. Biosens Bioelectron. 2018;115: 83-90. doi:10.1016/j.bios.2018.05.019

[60] Fraser LA, Kinghorn AB, Dirkzwager RM, Liang S, Cheung Y-W, Lim B, et al. A portable microfluidic Aptamer-Tethered Enzyme Capture (APTEC) biosensor for malaria diagnosis. Biosens Bioelectron. 2018;100: 591-596. doi:10.1016/j.bios.2017.10.001

[61] Mbanefo A, Kumar N. Evaluation of Malaria Diagnostic Methods as a Key for Successful Control and Elimination Programs. Trop Med Infect Dis. 2020;5: 102. doi:10.3390/tropicalmed5020102

[62] Peng WK, Kong TF, Ng CS, Chen L, Huang Y, Bhagat AAS, et al. Micromagnetic resonance relaxometry for rapid label-free malaria diagnosis. Nat Med. 2014;20: 1069-1073. doi:10.1038/nm.3622

[63] Fook Kong T, Ye W, Peng WK, Wei Hou H, Marcos, Preiser PR, et al. Enhancing malaria diagnosis through microfluidic cell enrichment and magnetic resonance relaxometry detection. Sci Rep. 2015;5: 11425. doi:10.1038/srep11425

[64] Hou HW, Bhagat AAS, Lin Chong AG, Mao P, Wei Tan KS, Han J, et al. Deformability based cell margination—A simple microfluidic design for malaria-infected erythrocyte separation. Lab Chip. 2010;10: 2605. doi:10.1039/c003873c

[65] Gascoyne P, Mahidol C, Ruchirawat M, Satayavivad J, Watcharasit P, Becker FF. Microsample preparation by dielectrophoresis: isolation of malaria. Lab Chip. 2002;2: 70. doi:10.1039/b110990c

[66] ZIMMERMAN PA, FUJIOKA H, THOMSON JM, ZBOROWSKI M, COLLINS WE. DIAGNOSIS OF MALARIA BY MAGNETIC DEPOSITION MICROSCOPY. Am J Trop Med Hyg. 2006;74: 568-572. doi:10.4269/ajtmh.2006.74.568

[67] Ribaut C, Berry A, Chevalley S, Reybier K, Morlais I, Parzy D, et al. Concentration and purification by magnetic separation of the erythrocytic stages of all human Plasmodium species. Malar J. 2008;7: 45. doi:10.1186/1475-2875-7-45

[68] Thamarath SS, Xiong A, Lin P-H, Preiser PR, Han J. Enhancing the sensitivity of micro magnetic resonance relaxometry detection of low parasitemia *Plasmodium falciparum* in human blood. Sci Rep. 2019;9: 2555. doi:10.1038/s41598-019-38805-2

[69] Jubery TZ, Srivastava SK, Dutta P. Dielectrophoretic separation of bioparticles in microdevices: a review. Electrophoresis. 2014;35: 691-713. doi:10.1002/elps.201300424

[70] Kasetsirikul S, Buranapong J, Srituravanich W, Kaewthamasorn M, Pimpin A. The development of malaria diagnostic techniques: a review of the approaches with focus on dielectrophoretic and magnetophoretic methods. Malar J. 2016;15: 358. doi:10.1186/s12936-016-1400-9

[71] Banoth E, Kasula VK, Gorthi SS. Portable optofluidic absorption flow

analyzer for quantitative malaria diagnosis from whole blood. Appl Opt. 2016;55: 8637. doi:10.1364/AO.55.008637

[72] Nam J, Huang H, Lim H, Lim C, Shin S. Magnetic Separation of Malaria-Infected Red Blood Cells in Various Developmental Stages. Anal Chem. 2013;85: 7316-7323. doi:10.1021/ac4012057

[73] Baker MJ, Trevisan J, Bassan P, Bhargava R, Butler HJ, Dorling KM, et al. Using Fourier transform IR spectroscopy to analyze biological materials. Nat Protoc. 2014;9: 1771-1791. doi:10.1038/nprot.2014.110

[74] Perez-Guaita D, Marzec KM, Hudson A, Evans C, Chernenko T, Matthäus C, et al. Parasites under the Spotlight: Applications of Vibrational Spectroscopy to Malaria Research. Chem Rev. 2018;118: 5330-5358. doi:10.1021/acs.chemrev.7b00661

[75] Diem M, Griffiths PR, Chalmers JM. Vibrational Spectroscopy for Medical Diagnosis. Wiley Anal. Weinheim, Germany: Wiley-VCH Verlag GmbH & Co; 2008.

[76] Brereton RG. Chemometrics for Pattern Recognition. West Sussex, United Kingdom: John Wiley & Sons, Ltd; 2009.

[77] Khoshmanesh A, Dixon MWA, Kenny S, Tilley L, McNaughton D, Wood BR. Detection and Quantification of Early-Stage Malaria Parasites in Laboratory Infected Erythrocytes by Attenuated Total Reflectance Infrared Spectroscopy and Multivariate Analysis. Anal Chem. 2014;86: 4379-4386. doi:10.1021/ac500199x

[78] Heraud P, Chatchawal P, Wongwattanakul M, Tippayawat P, Doerig C, Jearanaikoon P, et al. Infrared spectroscopy coupled to cloud-based data management as a tool to diagnose malaria: a pilot study in a malaria-endemic country. Malar J. 2019;18: 348. doi:10.1186/s12936-019-2945-1

[79] Mwanga EP, Minja EG, Mrimi E, Jiménez MG, Swai JK, Abbasi S, et al. Detection of malaria parasites in dried human blood spots using mid-infrared spectroscopy and logistic regression analysis. Malar J. 2019;18: 341. doi:10.1186/s12936-019-2982-9

[80] Ali N, Rampazzo RDCP, Costa ADT, Krieger MA. Current Nucleic Acid Extraction Methods and Their Implications to Point-of-Care Diagnostics. Biomed Res Int. 2017;2017. doi:10.1155/2017/9306564

[81] Govindarajan a. V., Ramachandran S, Vigil GD, Yager P, Böhringer KF. A low cost point-of-care viscous sample preparation device for molecular diagnosis in the developing world; An example of microfluidic origami. Lab Chip. 2012;12: 174-181. doi:10.1039/c1lc20622b

[82] Magro L, Escadafal C, Garneret P, Jacquelin B, Kwasiborski A, Manuguerra J-C, et al. Paper microfluidics for nucleic acid amplification testing (NAAT) of infectious diseases. Lab Chip. 2017;17: 2347-2371. doi:10.1039/C7LC00013H

[83] Magro L, Jacquelin B, Escadafal C, Garneret P, Kwasiborski A, Manuguerra J-C, et al. Paper-based RNA detection and multiplexed analysis for Ebola virus diagnostics. Sci Rep. 2017;7: 1347. doi:10.1038/s41598-017-00758-9

[84] Gan W, Zhuang B, Zhang P, Han J, Li C-XX, Liu P. A filter paper-based microdevice for low-cost, rapid, and automated DNA extraction and amplification from diverse sample types. Lab Chip. 2014;14: 3719-3728. doi:10.1039/c4lc00686k

[85] Rodriguez NM, Linnes JC, Fan A, Ellenson CK, Pollock NR, Klapperich CM. Paper-Based RNA

Extraction, in Situ Isothermal Amplification, and Lateral Flow Detection for Low-Cost, Rapid Diagnosis of Influenza A (H1N1) from Clinical Specimens. Anal Chem. 2015;87: 7872-7879. doi:10.1021/acs.analchem.5b01594

[86] Kastania AS, Tsougeni K, Papadakis G, Gizeli E, Kokkoris G, Tserepi A, et al. Plasma micro-nanotextured polymeric micromixer for DNA purification with high efficiency and dynamic range. Anal Chim Acta. 2016;942: 58-67. doi:10.1016/j.aca.2016.09.007

[87] Huang QS, Mei QB, Shi JL, Xu F, Gong Y, Yang H, et al. Advances in paper-based sample pretreatment for point-of-care testing. Crit Rev Biotechnol. 2016;37: 411-428. doi:10.3109/07388551.2016.1164664

[88] Foudeh AM, Fatanat Didar T, Veres T, Tabrizian M. Microfluidic designs and techniques using lab-on-a-chip devices for pathogen detection for point-of-care diagnostics. Lab Chip. 2012;12: 3249-66. doi:10.1039/c2lc40630f

[89] Cui F, Rhee M, Singh A, Tripathi A. Microfluidic Sample Preparation for Medical Diagnostics. Annu Rev Biomed Eng. 2015;17: 267-286. doi:10.1146/annurev-bioeng-071114-040538

[90] Ibrahim F, Thio T, Faisal T, Neuman M. The Application of Biomedical Engineering Techniques to the Diagnosis and Management of Tropical Diseases: A Review. Sensors. 2015;15: 6947-6995. doi:10.3390/s150306947

[91] Azimi SM, Nixon G, Ahern J, Balachandran W. A magnetic bead-based DNA extraction and purification microfluidic device. Microfluid Nanofluidics. 2011;11: 157-165. doi:10.1007/s10404-011-0782-9

[92] Kim J, Johnson M, Hill P, Gale BK. Microfluidic sample preparation: cell lysis and nucleic acid purification. Integr Biol (Camb). 2009;1: 574-86. doi:10.1039/b905844c

[93] Wang S, Lifson MA, Inci F, Liang L-G, Sheng Y-F, Demirci U. Advances in addressing technical challenges of point-of-care diagnostics in resource-limited settings. Expert Rev Mol Diagn. 2016;16: 449-59. doi:10.1586/14737159.2016.1142877

[94] Britton S, Cheng Q, McCarthy JS. Novel molecular diagnostic tools for malaria elimination: a review of options from the point of view of high-throughput and applicability in resource limited settings. Malar J. 2016;15: 88. doi:10.1186/s12936-016-1158-0

[95] Okell LC, Ghani AC, Lyons E, Drakeley CJ. Submicroscopic Infection in *Plasmodium falciparum* –Endemic Populations: A Systematic Review and Meta-Analysis. J Infect Dis. 2009;200: 1509-1517. doi:10.1086/644781

[96] Cheng Q, Cunningham J, Gatton ML. Systematic Review of Sub-microscopic *P. vivax* Infections: Prevalence and Determining Factors. Rodrigues MM, editor. PLoS Negl Trop Dis. 2015;9: e3413. doi:10.1371/journal.pntd.0003413

[97] World Health Organization. Malaria rapid diagnostic test performance: results of WHO product testing of malaria RDTs: round 5 (2013). Geneva, Switzerland; 2014.

[98] Cheng Q, Gatton ML, Barnwell J, Chiodini P, McCarthy J, Bell D, et al. *Plasmodium falciparum* parasites lacking histidine-rich protein 2 and 3: a review and recommendations for accurate reporting. Malar J. 2014;13: 283. doi:10.1186/1475-2875-13-283

[99] Kralik P, Ricchi M. A basic guide to real time PCR in microbial diagnostics:

Definitions, parameters, and everything. Front Microbiol. 2017;8: 1-9. doi:10.3389/fmicb.2017.00108

[100] Gonçalves-de-Albuquerque SDC, Pessoa E Silva R, de Morais RCS, Trajano-Silva LAM, Régis-da-Silva CG, Brandão-Filho SP, et al. Tracking false-negative results in molecular diagnosis: proposal of a triplex-PCR based method for leishmaniasis diagnosis. J Venom Anim Toxins Incl Trop Dis. 2014;20: 16. doi:10.1186/1678-9199-20-16

[101] Lorenz TC. Polymerase Chain Reaction: Basic Protocol Plus Troubleshooting and Optimization Strategies. J Vis Exp. 2012. doi:10.3791/3998

[102] Loubiere S, Moatti J-P. Economic evaluation of point-of-care diagnostic technologies for infectious diseases. Clin Microbiol Infect. 2010;16: 1070-1076. doi:10.1111/j.1469-0691.2010.03280.x

[103] Uzochukwu BS, Obikeze EN, Onwujekwe OE, Onoka CA, Griffiths UK. Cost-effectiveness analysis of rapid diagnostic test, microscopy and syndromic approach in the diagnosis of malaria in Nigeria: implications for scaling-up deployment of ACT. Malar J. 2009;8: 265. doi:10.1186/1475-2875-8-265

[104] Zurovac D, Larson BA, Skarbinski J, Slutsker L, Snow RW, Hamel MJ. Modeling the financial and clinical implications of malaria rapid diagnostic tests in the case-management of older children and adults in Kenya. Am J Trop Med Hyg. 2008;78: 884-91.

[105] de Oliveira MRF, Giozza SP, Peixoto HM, Romero GA. Cost-effectiveness of diagnostic for malaria in Extra-Amazon Region, Brazil. Malar J. 2012;11: 390. doi:10.1186/1475-2875-11-390

[106] Ezennia IJ, Nduka SO, Ekwunife OI. Cost benefit analysis of malaria rapid diagnostic test: the perspective of Nigerian community pharmacists. Malar J. 2017;16: 7. doi:10.1186/s12936-016-1648-0

[107] Hansen KS, Lesner TH, Østerdal LP. Optimal price subsidies for appropriate malaria testing and treatment behaviour. Malar J. 2016;15: 534. doi:10.1186/s12936-016-1582-1

[108] Bath D, Goodman C, Yeung S. Modelling the cost-effectiveness of introducing subsidised malaria rapid diagnostic tests in the private retail sector in sub-Saharan Africa. BMJ Glob Heal. 2020;5: e002138. doi:10.1136/bmjgh-2019-002138

Chapter 3

Prompt and Accurate Diagnosis, A Veritable Tool in Malaria Elimination Efforts

Chukwudi Michael Egbuche

Abstract

The concept of malaria elimination is to get rid of local transmission of malaria parasites in a defined geographical area. Among the measures required for malaria elimination is prompt and accurate diagnosis. Malaria diagnostic tools currently in use: clinical diagnosis, Malaria Rapid Diagnostic Tests (mRDT) and molecular diagnosis, have limitations. Clinical diagnosis can be used as first step in making prompt malaria diagnosis, but cannot confirm cases. Malaria RDTs satisfies the need for prompt diagnosis but has low accuracy in confirming cases. Accuracy of microscopy depends on making good blood films, and accurate film interpretation. Molecular diagnosis required for species-specific diagnosis of malaria parasites, and determination of genes that confers drug resistance to *Plasmodium* species is not available for routine use. As part of elimination efforts, there is development of mRDT kits that utilize urine or saliva instead of blood specimen, microscopy digital image recognition and different technologies for molecular diagnosis. So far, none of these diagnostic tools has satisfied the need for prompt and accurate diagnosis. It is therefore recommended that more than one diagnostic tool is needed for malaria elimination to be achieved in a given area. This will ensure early detection and treatment of cases, as well as prevent the re-establishment of transmission.

Keywords: malaria, elimination, malaria diagnosis, clinical diagnosis, rapid diagnostic tests, microscopy, molecular diagnosis

1. Introduction

Malaria in humans is a parasitic disease caused by four species of *Plasmodium*: *P. falciparum*, *P. vivax*, *P. ovale* and *P. malariae*; with increasing recognition of enzoonotic transmission of a simian species, *P. knowlesi*. In most cases, the malaria parasites are transmitted through the bite of infected female anopheline mosquitoes. The mosquitoes carry infective sporozoites of malaria parasite in their salivary glands, and they inoculate or transfer these sporozoites into the blood stream of humans during blood meals [1]. After inoculation, the individual(s) is /are said to be infected with malaria parasites. The disease, malaria begins once (i) the asexual parasite multiplies within the red blood cells and (ii) the host produces some immunological response against the parasites. On rare occasions, malaria parasite infection can be acquired by transfusion of blood from a malaria patient, also known as transfusion malaria; transmission of infection to foetus in uterus through the placenta, also known as congenital malaria and by the use of contaminated syringes particularly among drug addicts [2].

Malaria results in a wide range of outcomes and pathologies with severity of the disease ranging from asymptomatic infection to rapidly progressive fatal illness. Generally, malaria is characterized by many signs and symptoms: fever, chills, headache, nausea, vomiting, sweating, chest or abdominal pain, diarrhea and cough. Severe infection may result in serious complications such as severe anemia, algid malaria, spleenomegaly, cerebral malaria, black water fever, hypoglycaemia, complications in pregnancy, respiratory distress, metabolic acidosis, pulmonary oedema, concomitant pneumonia, shock and coma [3]. Death due to malaria can occur as a result of delay in diagnosis and treatment of infected individuals. Thus malaria has remained a major threat to public health despite decades of control and elimination efforts.

2. Diagnosis of malaria

Prompt and accurate diagnosis is important in malaria elimination efforts. This will help in early detection of malaria cases before complications set in. Also, malaria cases are separated from other diseases that present with the same symptoms as malaria especially in cases of co-infections (with diseases such as typhoid fever, HIV, hepatitis, Covid-19 e. t. c.). Incorrect diagnosis of malaria will not only waste resources, but also delays treatment thereby resulting in poor outcome of patients. It may also contribute to increasing resistance of malaria parasite to available anti-malaria drugs, there by frustrating malaria elimination efforts. To achieve malaria elimination, different diagnostic tools are required. The malaria diagnostic tools could be broadly classified as provisional or clinical diagnosis and parasite-based diagnosis. These diagnostic tools have been used over the years; nevertheless, they have their limitations.

3. The use of clinical diagnosis or provisional diagnosis to achieve malaria elimination

Clinical diagnosis is achieved based on signs and symptoms presented by a patient. This is because the release of malaria antigens, pigments and toxins give rise to a cascade of pathological events. The earliest symptoms: headache, fever, body pains and chills could be used in making prompt diagnosis for malaria parasite infection. [4] reported that 27.0% of mothers and caregivers practice home management of malaria because of the need for prompt diagnosis and treatment. The most commonly recognized and used symptom for clinical diagnosis is fever [5]. It has been used in making provisional diagnosis for malaria parasite infection in Nigeria and other malaria endemic regions. It gives prompt indication of malaria parasite infection in such area. A study in Nigeria reported 83.2% cases of malaria parasite infection among patients that presented with fever [6]. Another study in Southwestern Nigeria reported 66.8% cases of malaria parasite infection among febrile patients [7]. Even though these findings confirm that not all fever conditions can be attributed to malaria, but then a significant number of individuals would have been treated of malaria based on fever outcome. However, this may only be achievable in malaria endemic area because clinical diagnosis alone is not reliable and cannot be used to confirm malaria parasite infection. Its uncertainty and varied results makes it an inaccurate method for achieving malaria elimination. In malaria endemic areas, under reporting of malaria cases (with inclusion of non-cases (false positive cases) and exclusion of actual cases (false negative cases)) using clinical diagnosis alone is most likely. A typical example can be presented by using the data in the work of [6]. In that study, 350 patients were examined for malaria parasite infection and 200 (57.14%) cases were confirmed using microscopy. However, clinical diagnosis showed 149 (42.57%) cases; 124 (35.43%) actual cases, 25 (7.14%) false positive cases and 76 (21.71%) missed cases or false negative cases. In the work of [8], clinical diagnosis recorded 74.30% prevalence of malaria as against 95.33% recorded with microscopy. This makes it clear that in malaria endemic areas, one can only use clinical diagnosis as a first step in making prompt or early malaria diagnosis and not to confirm malaria cases. In non-endemic areas, over reporting of cases may occur because diseases other than malaria may be the cause of common clinical signs observed in that area. Clinical diagnosis is therefore recommended for use alongside a parasite based diagnostic method.

3.1 Limitations of using clinical diagnosis in malaria elimination

There are issues in the use of clinical diagnosis alone to achieve malaria elimination.

a. Using clinical diagnosis alone, asymptomatic cases are unreported especially in *P. vivax* and *P. ovale* malaria where high parasitaemia is a prerequisite for mild and severe disease [9]. It is also applicable with *P. malariae* infection that is rarely fatal and the blood stage of the parasite persists for up to 40 years. In a study, [6] reported 37.8% malaria prevalence among non-febrile patients. This is to show that there might be missed cases of malaria parasite infection in a given population if one relies on clinical diagnosis alone.

b. There are inconsistencies in the choice of symptom for clinical diagnosis. While some people may focus on fever alone, some other may focus on chills, stomach upset, vomiting, body ache and headache [5]. This brings about uncertainty with this diagnostic tool.

c. The symptoms of malaria are non-specific. This makes precise calculation of malaria burden difficult especially in co-morbidity states. This may result in either under treatment of malaria cases or over treatment of malaria cases; none of which is good for malaria elimination. For example, [10] reported a case of *Plasmodium vivax* malaria and COVID-19 co-infection in Qatar. He presented the difficulty in distinguishing COVID-19 from malaria because COVID-19 presents with a variety of clinical manifestations including, but not limited to, fever, cough, diarrhea, vomiting, headache, myalgia and fatigue. This case was identified during the time of COVID-19 pandemic and it was possible that some other cases like this existed but more attention was given to COVID – 19 at the expense of other diseases including malaria. This is a typical scenario that could lead to missed cases of malaria, and malaria positive individuals still remaining in the environment serve as a source of infection and reinfection of other susceptible.

   In the same way, malaria may be over reported and/or given more attention at the expense of other diseases in malaria endemic areas. In the work of [11], 155 participants tested for malaria and typhoid fever infection shows there were 64 (41.7%) cases of malaria and 60 (38.0%) cases of typhoid fever, with 40 (25.0%) cases that were mixed infection. If we look critically in that finding,

24 cases were malaria only whereas 20 cases were typhoid fever only. Then the total number of persons that would have been reported to have malaria based on clinical diagnosis alone is 84 (24 malaria only cases +20 typhoid fever only cases +40 cases of mixed infection). The implication will be excessive and indiscriminate use of antimalarial. When such happens, some strains of malaria parasites with genes that confer resistance to commonly used antimalarial will emerge and bring about treatment failure. This will definitely frustrate malaria elimination efforts because researchers will need to go back to the laboratory to develop another antimalarial that can take care of the emergent strain of malaria parasite. Of course, the researchers will not be able to develop a new product without identifying and characterizing the malaria parasite strain, using a parasite based diagnostic method.

4. The use of parasite-based diagnosis to achieve malaria elimination

Parasite based diagnosis is required to provide accurate result needed to achieve malaria elimination. The malaria case management guidelines released by WHO in 2009 recommended prompt parasitological confirmation of diagnosis either by microscopy or malaria rapid diagnostic test (RDT) in all patients with suspected malaria before treatment is administered [12]. The above statement supported the role of clinical or provisional diagnosis in making prompt and accurate diagnosis of malaria. Early indication of cases through clinical diagnosis (promptness) facilitates the use of parasite based diagnostic method (accuracy). On the other hand, malaria parasite infection has been reported among non-febrile individuals [6] and in line with making prompt diagnosis, frequent check-up or routine laboratory test using parasite based diagnostic method is required. This is to ensure that asymptomatic individuals are captured early enough before complications due to malaria set in. Parasite based diagnosis can also be achieved using molecular techniques.

5. The use of malaria rapid diagnostic test (mRDT) to achieve malaria elimination

The World Health Organization recommends the use of mRDTs as a good alternative method for malaria diagnosis. As such, it has become a primary tool for parasitological diagnosis or confirmation of malaria. Malaria Rapid Diagnostic Tests (mRDT) are immuno-chromatographic tests that target certain proteins produced by *Plasmodium* species. There are different brands of mRDT kits. They include: SD Bio Line®, Tell®, First Response®, Sky Tech®, optiMAL®, Care Stat®, Paracheck®, Marrow Care®, Binaxnow® Malaria, Fyodor® and so on. They come in different test formats: strips, cassette etc., for ease of use and safety. These mRDT kits detect specific antigens (proteins) produced by malaria parasites in the blood of infected individuals. To achieve malaria elimination, the commercial test kits are manufactured with different antigens targeted to suit the local malaria epidemiology of a given area [13]. Rapid Diagnostic Test (RDT) kits most widely used for malaria are based on the detection of the following target antigens of the parasite: Histidine-Rich Protein II (HRP2), *Plasmodium* Lactate Dehydrogenase (*P*LDH) and P-Aldolase [14]. Some of these antigens could be excreted in the urine or are found in the saliva of sick or infected individuals. Thus one may require any of blood, urine or saliva as specimen for conducting the test, depending on the mRDT brand in use. Nevertheless, blood has been the most widely used specimen because that is where the highest concentration of the malaria parasite antigens are found.

Most commonly used RDT devices have two bands (a control line and a test line) and are designed to detect *P. falciparum*. The test line targets either histidine-rich protein-2 (HRP-2) or *P. falciparum* specific parasite lactate dehydrogenase (*Pf*-pLDH), depending on the RDT brand. However, RDTs that distinguish *P. falciparum* from the three non - *P. falciparum* species are available. Such RDT device may have either three bands (a control line and two test lines) or four bands (a control line and three test lines). In the case of RDT test device with three bands, one test line targets *P. falciparum* specific antigen; the second test line targets antigens common to the four species, such as pan-*Plasmodium*-specific parasite lactate dehydrogenase (pan-pLDH) or aldolase. In the case of RDT test device with four bands, the third test line targets *Plasmodium vivax*-specific parasite lactate dehydrogenase (*Pv*-pLDH).

In general, HRP2-based mRDTs are more sensitive and stable than mRDTs based on other *Plasmodium* antigens, and so are the mRDTs of choice in most endemic countries where *P. falciparum* malaria predominates [15]. *Plasmodium* lactate dehydrogenase (*P*LDH) which is another antigen detected by mRDT has been less widely used but have higher specificity, mostly due to a much shorter time to become negative [16]. Emphasis on the malaria antigen (HRP2) being stable when excreted in urine, may have encouraged [17] to experiment using urine specimen to conduct malaria rapid diagnostic test with mRDT kit manufactured to use blood specimen. In that study, they found that mRDT using urine specimen could serve as a practical method for detection of malaria parasites even though the sensitivity is dependent on the level of parasitaemia. It was based on this, that Fyodor®, a non-invasive dipstick test that uses monoclonal antibody to target *P. falciparum* protein (Highly repetitive cognate poly histidine-rich protein2 (HRP2) excreted in urine was developed. Fyodor® has been reported to demonstrate nearly equivalent performance compared to available blood-based RDT for the diagnosis of malaria [6, 18, 19]. Fyodor® was found to be useful in malaria diagnosis with 76.9% sensitivity and 82.5% specificity, even when the parasitaemia level is as low as 260 parasites/µl of blood [6]. In addition to Fyodor®, [20] produced a prototype saliva-based RDT for *P. falciparum* gametocyte detection in carrier individuals. This is still in line with the efforts to advance malaria elimination strategies.

RDTs as diagnostic tools for malaria are simple to perform and provide quick result. It is a simple and fast way for health workers to test for malaria parasites in a patient's blood. It is easy to learn and people living in rural areas can access and use this form of test because it does not require electricity or any other special equipment. It is also simple to interpret the test result. Some (that require urine or saliva as specimens) are not invasive and so can be used closer to homes. Thus, it was developed for use in areas where the only realistic alternative is clinical diagnosis especially to tell if a feverish condition is caused by malaria parasite. This satisfies the need for prompt diagnosis in malaria elimination efforts. However, a major concern in the use of malaria RDTs is its low accuracy in reporting of malaria cases. In both malaria endemic and non-endemic areas, under reporting of malaria cases (with inclusion of non-cases (false positive cases) and exclusion of actual cases (false negative cases)) is likely. Using the same data in the work of [6], blood based mRDT reported 77 (22.0%) cases; 71 (20.29%) actual cases, 6 (1.71%) false positive cases and 129 (36.86%) missed cases or false negative cases. On the other hand, urine base mRDT reported 39 (11.14%) cases; 36 (10.29%) actual cases, 3 (0.86%) false positive cases and 164 (46.86%) missed cases or false negative cases. It could be deduced from the above that mRDT is more specific in reporting malaria cases than clinical diagnosis, even though its sensitivity seems low.

Using mRDT requires training of health workers on the importance of continuous quality control monitoring for the mRDT kits while they use them [21, 22].

The training should be carried out in connection with the brand of mRDT being used. The quality control can be achieved by checking its expiration date, storage conditions and using microscopy and/or PCR to assess the performance. In molecular epidemiology studies to assess the performance of mRDTs, RDT used strips or cassettes can be used as a source of DNA for molecular detection of malaria parasites [23].

5.1 Limitations of mRDTs in malaria elimination effort

Many factors may affect the performance of malaria RDTs in achieving malaria elimination. These include:

a. Number of different species of malaria parasites infecting a host: Some RDTs can detect only one species (*P. falciparum*) while others detect multiple species (*P. vivax*, *P. malariae* and *P. ovale*) of malaria parasites. Even with mRDTs that detect multiple species of malaria parasites, the species are poorly classified as *P. falciparum* and non *P. falciparum*.

b. This test does not also detect actual parasite, rather it detects parasite antigens; this makes it difficult to accurately identify the species of malaria parasites present or prevalent in a given locality. The RDTs indirectly tells whether a patient has malaria parasites are present or absent. Also, RDTs cannot be used to quantify malaria parasites that are present in the blood.

c. Level of parasitaemia: High level of parasitaemia is normally required for recording high level of sensitivity with mRDTs. This has been shown with the significant weak positive correlation between malaria parasite density of microscopy result and mRDT results as reported by [6]. It then makes the test limit of detection for RDTs low; as a result, false negative results occur. In the work of [7], 32.8% false negative results were recorded. The implication is that if such RDT is used alone for malaria diagnosis, approximately 33 in every 100 malaria cases will be missed and malaria elimination will be hard to achieve.

d. Variability in parasite antigenic structure: There is variability within the parasite antigen being detected by the mRDTs, which also leads to false negative results. While false-negative mRDT results have been attributed primarily to the tests' limit of detection, [24, 25] have confirmed that genetic variation of *P. falciparum* can also affect mRDT performance. The variability may be due to the (i) presence or absence of the target epitope, (ii) variation in the number of epitopes present in a particular parasite isolate [26]. Genetic diversity among malaria parasites may be particularly important for *Pf*HRP2-based RDTs, since the antigen consists of a number of alanine- and histidine - rich amino acid repeats [27] that vary in size among malaria parasite strains [28]. Comparison of the *Pf*HRP2 sequences from several parasite strains has shown differences in the number of tri- and hexa- peptide repeat units and rare amino acid variants [27, 29, 30]. An additional report showed that the amino acid sequence of *Pf*HRP2 in a Chinese isolate was different from that in South American (7G8) and Gambian (FCR3) isolates [31].

e. Persistence of the malaria antigens in the blood after treatment, thereby giving false positive results with mRDTs. False positive results occur because the mRDT devices can still detect the antigens of malaria parasites after the patient has been treated due to the persistence of HRP2 antigen in the blood for several days after infection. The device tests positive to infection when the patient is actually free from the parasite infection. For instance, [7] reported 4.4% cases of false positive result with HRP2-based mRDTs. This limits their specificity and usefulness in accurate reporting of malaria cases.

f. Problem of storage. Even though RDTs are recommended for use in places electricity is poor or not available, it can be damaged by heat and humidity when not stored properly (in a cool dry place at a temperature of 2 °C to 8 °C). [32] reported that exposure to high temperature can damage the nitrocellulose membrane of the RDT test device or denature the antibodies in the test membrane, thereby causing poor performance of RDTs in the tropics. The effect is mostly high level of false negative results which implies high number of unreported malaria cases.

6. The use of malaria microscopy to achieve malaria elimination

Malaria is commonly diagnosed using microscopy of stained blood films. Although the use of rapid diagnostics test for malaria diagnosis is on the increase, microscopy has remains the gold standard and as well serves as a reference standard in the evaluation of new tools for malaria diagnosis [33]. Venous blood or capillary blood can be used for malaria microscopy. This method involves the staining of thick and thin blood films on a clean grease free glass slide, to visualize the malaria parasite. Thick blood film is used for malaria parasite detection while the thin blood film is used for malaria parasite species identification. Commonly used stains for the preparation of blood films are Giemsa stain, Leishmann stain, Fields stains A and B. The standard procedure for preparation and examination of blood films for malaria parasite detection and species identification are contained in the documents by [33, 34]. A good binocular (compound or digital) microscope is required for accurate reading of the blood films.

In malaria endemic areas, routine microscopy is usually done using binocular light microscope. Microscopy is cheaper than the use of RDTs, considering the cost of consumables alone. Using microscopy, malaria parasite stages are seen and can also be counted. Microscopy has the advantage of providing a quantitative assessment of peripheral blood parasitaemia and parasite stages as well as information on the other blood components [35]. Thus it gives accurate diagnosis of malaria when properly done. Due to its conventional use it helps to reduce cases of wrong administration of anti-malaria drugs to patients exhibiting non-malaria fever as a symptom. In Tanzania, this diagnostic method has help to reduce the wrong administration of malaria drugs to patients with non-malaria fevers [36].

The use of microscopy in malaria diagnosis will require continuous training, practice and experience. There is also need for assessment and supervision of microscopists (slide readers) for quality control of their test results. This is because detection, identification and quantification of malaria parasites using microscopy will depend on making good blood films, having a good microscope and accurate film interpretation by the laboratory scientist/technician. For improved microscopy needed to achieve malaria elimination, there is development of microscopy digital image recognition using artificial intelligence [37–43]. The concept is that a standard blood film is prepared using Giemsa stain or field stain. After that, a digital microscope or imaging scanner is used to capture the image viewed under the microscope. The captured image is stored in a computer and is used as an input for the image-recognition algorithms that will extracts useful visual features to locate, identify and count the malaria parasites. This is with the view to achieve better microscopy result because of inherent human factors in blood film preparation and interpretation. When developed and certified, it will open new possibilities for automated recognition of malaria parasites in standard blood films and thus eliminate uncertainty about the quality of microscopic diagnoses worldwide.

6.1 Limitations of microscopy in malaria elimination

The challenges in the use of microscopy for malaria elimination are stated below:

a. Malaria microscopy requires specialized personnel for accurate detection and identification of malaria parasites. This is particularly important especially when the level of parasitaemia is low or in cases of mixed infection with different *Plasmodium* species. It's low sensitivity at low parasitaemia is a problem and can implicate the use of RDTs for false positive result.

b. Compared to mRDTs, this method is labour intensive and time consuming. Delay in its use may occur during blood film preparation or examination. In some cases, one may even have to prepare a new slide where poor staining or loss due to breaking of a slide occurs.

c. Variability in blood film preparation techniques and reading skills can account for inaccurate results. It may be due to slide differences because variation of parasite density within slides occurs even when prepared from a homogenous sample [44]. Accuracy of results obtained through microscopy also depends on individual technician performance in blood film preparation and examination, thereby making its standardization difficult.

d. Non accessibility of this method by rural areas due to lack of facilities is also a major issue. In malaria endemic countries where greater efforts are required for elimination, poor and high cost of electricity reduces the frequency of microscopy use for diagnosis. There could be a delay in providing results for patient especially when the blood films have to be made repeatedly.

e. Poor quality stains sold in the market can affect the quality of the thick and thin films, there by affecting the accuracy of the result.

f. The technology for automated microscopy using image-recognition algorithms has not been fully developed and certified. More so, the data base of the digital image to be analyzed is not yet robust to contain any distortion or unusual presentation of the malaria parasites in the blood films.

7. The use of molecular diagnosis to achieve malaria elimination

Molecular diagnosis of malaria is a laboratory techniques developed to detect and characterize the malaria parasites. It may not be used in routine diagnosis because of cost and time; but its use has increased the analytical sensitivity of assays for malaria parasites. In places where treatment failure occurs and drug resistance is suspected, molecular diagnosis is required. It is needed for species specific diagnosis of malaria parasites, determination of genes that confers drug resistance to the *Plasmodium* species and in selecting treatment options. For instance, there is growing concern on the antigen variability expressed by *P. falciparum* the most prevalent malaria parasite species in the Sub-Saharan Africa that accounted for 99.7% of estimated malaria cases in 2018 [45].

Molecular diagnostic tool has the ability to detect low level parasitaemia and allows accurate identification of malaria parasite species. It is therefore a confirmatory test used for the diagnosis of malaria when microscopy shows negative result. Molecular diagnosis can also detect mixed infection [46] and identify asymptomatic malaria carriers who may be targeted for treatment [47]. With molecular diagnosis, large number of specimens can be processed simultaneously using standard protocols and equipment [48]. In the general protocol, DNA of *Plasmodium* species is extracted using DNA extraction kit from a given manufacturer. The extracted DNA is subjected to selective amplification of the target gene. This can be achieved by using more than 65 primer sets with at least five molecular targets that can be used to test as many as five human *Plasmodium* species: *P. falciparum, P. ovale, P. malariae, P. vivax* and *P. knowlesi* [49]. After the DNA amplification, electrophoresis is run and the bands interpreted in order to know the result of the test [50]. This basically explains Polymerase Chain Reaction (conventional PCR, nested PCR, real-time PCR) and Restriction Fragment Length Polymorphism (RFLP) as diagnostic tools for malaria. Polymerase Chain Reaction (PCR) was used to confirm parasitaemia using *P. falciparum* Merozoite Surface Protein 2 (MSP2) as a marker while Restriction Fragment Length Polymorphism (RFLP) was used to identify *P. falciparum* Sulfadoxine – Pyrimethamine (SP) resistance molecular markers at codons 51, 59, 108, 164 of dihydrofolate reductase (dhfr), and codons 437, 540, 581 and 431 of dihydropteorate synthetase (dhps) genes [51]. Nested-Polymerase Chain Reaction (nPCR) was used to detect *P. falciparum* DNA in blood and saliva of febrile patients in Cameroon [52].

Other molecular diagnostic techniques includes: Loop – Mediated Isothermal Amplification (LAMP), Flow Cytometry (FC) assay techniques, Nucleic Acid Sequence Based Amplification (NASBA), Luminex Xmax Technology and so on. These techniques can greatly improve detection, species-specific identification and precise parasite count by using species-specific primers or probes [49]. Loop-Mediated Isothermal Amplification (LAMP) technique detected the conserved 18 s RNA gene of *P. falciparum, P. vivax, P. ovale, P. malaria* [46] and *P. knowlesi* [47]. Lamp has certain advantages compared to conventional PCR in the diagnosis of malaria because of its ability to perform the reaction and react without opening the tubes. It also has potential application for clinical diagnosis and surveillance of infectious diseases without the need for sophisticated equipment and skilled personnel in developing countries. Flow cytometric technique was developed to detect and quantify *P. falciparum* in the laboratories [53]. Flow cytometry was proposed as a malaria rapid diagnostic tool that counts the number of parasites and evaluate the malaria infected red blood cells [54]. FC is a very powerful tool in malaria research because it can use the nucleic acid content to identify various developmental stages of *P. falciparum* without being impaired by changes in the morphology of the parasite developmental stages [55]. Nucleic Acid Sequence Based Amplification (NASBA) is a homogenous, sensitive, isothermal and transcription based amplification system that uses three specific enzymes (Reverse transcriptase from avian myeloblastosis virus, T_7 RNA polymerase and Ribonuclease H) [56]; and do not require expensive thermal-cycling equipment [57]. Prevalence and density of *Plasmodium* gametocytes has been determine using quantitative NASBA (QT-NASBA) that has the ability to detect as low as 0.02–0.1 gametocytes per microliter of blood [58]; it is also used increasingly to detect both *P. falciparum* and *P. vivax* gametocytes [59]. Luminex Xmax Technology approach is very useful for the diagnosis of parasitic diseases and it is based on bead flow cytometry assay. It has been used to detect all the blood stage of the four human *Plasmodium* species [60]. Luminex Technology can improve the speed, the accuracy and reliability of other PCR methods because it eliminates the need for gel electrophoresis, and samples can be handled simultaneously and continuously through 96-well plate format from DNA extraction [61].

To enhance malaria elimination, molecular diagnosis should be used alongside microscopy in the quality control (QC) of mRDTs. With proper storage and handling of mRDTs, the QC may have two foci in determining sensitivity and specificity of mRDTs: (i) the ability of the test devices to detect malaria parasite if present in a blood specimen. Here, different drops of blood from the same specimen are used to perform the two tests respectively. (ii) the ability of the test devices to detect malaria parasite if present in the same drop of blood collected from a specimen. Microscopy alone can be used to achieve item (i) and not item (ii), since the same drop of blood used for microscopy cannot be used for mRDT. One can pick a drop of blood for Microscopy and it contains malaria parasite and another drop picked for mRDT from the same specimen may not contain malaria parasite antigen; and vice versa. Even, two slides prepared from the same blood specimen may not have the same microscopy readings. This is an issue relating to non-homogenous distribution of malaria parasites and the probability of picking malaria parasite in a drop of blood from a given blood specimen. Non-homogenous distribution of malaria parasites in the blood also affects PCR as much as microscopy and mRDTs. Nevertheless, PCR is a more robust tool for QC of mRDTs since it can achieve items (i) and (ii). To achieve item (ii), already used Rapid Diagnostic Test cassettes or strips are sources of DNA to detect malaria parasite by PCR [23]. Using the same cassette or strip, one can score the mRDT device based on what it picks from the specimen, rather than scoring it from another blood sample of the same specimen as is the case with microscopy. This approach is good for the overall quality control of mRDTs i. e. control for sensitivity, specificity, expiration, storage and handling.

7.1 Limitations in the use of molecular diagnosis for malaria elimination

a. Molecular diagnosis is still confined to few and special laboratories, thus it is not available for routine use.

b. PCR molecular assays are not feasible for field settings as it can be contaminated easily there by affecting the accuracy of the test result.

c. PCR also requires post amplification protocols like electrophoresis and it takes 3–4 hours in order to know the result [50]. Even the real-time PCR (with reduced risk of contamination) developed to replace the conventional nested and semi-nested PCR is difficulty and time consuming [62]. In other words, it does not give prompt diagnosis.

8. Conclusion

A significant challenge in the global malaria elimination effort is inadequacy of the tools needed for prompt and accurate diagnosis. In asymptomatic condition, clinical diagnosis lacks both promptness and accuracy. In symptomatic condition, clinical diagnosis provides prompt indication of malaria but still lacks accuracy. Following routine or frequent check-up in asymptomatic condition, Microscopy and RDTs which are the most widely used parasite based diagnostic tools techniques provides more prompt and accurate result than clinical diagnosis. In symptomatic condition, Microscopy and RDTs provides accuracy to complement the promptness of clinical diagnosis. Between the two, RDT provides more prompt diagnosis than microscopy whereas microscopy provides more accurate result than RDT. Molecular diagnosis is not prompt, but has higher level of accuracy needed to detect, identify and characterize malaria parasite.

No one diagnostic tool has satisfied the need for prompt and accurate diagnosis. For malaria elimination to be achieved, serious attention should be given to the performances of the diagnostic tools. Where one tool fails, another one should be used to complement, rather than replace it. Clinical diagnosis is the basis for suspected malaria cases, even though routine check-up is highly encouraged. Confirmation of cases should be done using parasite based diagnostic tools. There is also need for scale up on the quality of parasite-based diagnostic methods in use. It is therefore recommended that more than one diagnostic tool is needed for malaria elimination to be achieved in a given area.

Author details

Chukwudi Michael Egbuche
Department of Parasitology and Entomology, Faculty of Biosciences, Nnamdi Azikiwe University Awka, Nigeria

*Address all correspondence to: cm.egbuche@unizik.edu.ng

References

[1] Najera JA, Hempel J. The burden of Malaria. CTD/Mal/ 96.10. 2006; pp. 35.

[2] Arora DR, Arora B. Sporozoa. Medical Paraitology. 2005; 5: 67-80.

[3] Weatherall DJ, Miller, LH, Brauch DI, Marsh K, Doumbo OK, Casals-Pascuala C, Robert DJ. Malaria and red cells. Haematology. 2002; 415 (6872): 673-679.

[4] Obiukwu, MO, Egbuche CM, Okonkwo NJ, Chukwuma IF, Ezugbo-Nwobi IK, Umeanaeto PU. Malaria: Home Management Practices of Caregivers in Onitsha North LGA, Anambra State of Nigeria. Natural and Applied Science Journal. 2011; 12(2): 190-192

[5] Iwueze MO, Ezugbo-Nwobi IK, Umeanaeto PU, Egbuche CM, and Anaso CI. Knowledge, Attitude and Management Practices on Malaria: A Case Study of Amansea, Awka North Local Government Area of Anambra State, Nigeria. The Bioscientist. 2013; 1(1): 32-38.

[6] Egbuche CM, Ukonze CB, Udofia IJ, Okafor T, Okoye KC, Chukwuzoba OA, Obasi CJ. Comparative assessment of urine based RDT in malaria diagnosis during febrile and non-febrile conditions. Nigerian Journal of Parasitology. 2019; 40(1): 37-45.

[7] Oyeyemi OT, Ogunlade AF, Oyewole IO. Comparative Assessment of Microscopy and Rapid Diagnostic Test (RDT) as Malaria Diagnostic Tools. Research Journal of Parasitology. 2015; 10 (3): 120-126.

[8] Moyeh MN, Ali IM, Njimoh DL, Nji AM, Netongo PM, Evehe MS, Atogho-Tiedeu B,Ghogomu SM, Mbacham WF. Comparison of the accuracy of four malaria diagnostic methods in a high transmission setting in coastal Cameroon. Journal of Parasitology Research. 2019; pp 8.

[9] Miller LH, Baruk DI, Marsh K, Doumbo OK. The pathogenic basis of malaria. Nature. 2002; 415: 673-679.

[10] Sardar S, Sharma R, Alyamani TYM, Aboukamar M. COVID-19 and *Plasmodium vivax* malaria co-infection. ID Cases. 2020; *21*: e00879.

[11] Onyido AE, Okafor AC, Chikezie FM, Egbuche CM, Umeanaeto PU, Okafor EN, Ezihe EK, Iwueze MO, Ogbonna CU, Anumba JU. Coinfection of typhoid and malaria fevers among the inhabitants of a sub-urban community in the south eastern Nigeria. Nature and Science. 2015; 13(12): 47-56.

[12] Schellenberg D, Willey B, Grobusch MP. Improved Patient Care with better Malaria Diagnosis. Therapy; 2010; 7(1): 7-10.

[13] Bell DJ, Wongsrichanalai C, Barwell JW. Ensuring quality and access for malaria diagnosis, how can it be achieved? National Revised Microbiology. 2006; 4: 7-20.

[14] Ugah UI , Alo MN, Owolabi JO, Okata-Nwali OD, Ekejindu IM. Evaluation of the utility value of three diagnostic methods in the detection of malaria parasites in endemic area. Malaria Journal. 2017; 16:189.

[15] Coldiron ME, Assao B, Langendorf C, Sayinzoga-Makombe N, Ciglenecki I, de la Tour R, Piriou E, Yarima BM, Mumina A, Guindo O, Page A, Grais RF. Clinical diagnostic evaluation of HRP2 and pLDH-based rapid diagnostic tests for malaria in an area receiving seasonal malaria chemoprevention in Niger. Malaria Journal. 2019; 18(1): 443.

[16] World Health Organization. Malaria rapid diagnostic test performance: results for WHO product testing of malaria RDTs: round 6 (2014-15). Geneva, Switzerland: WHO. 2015

[17] Samal AG, Behera PK, Mohanty AK, Satpathi S, Kumar A, Panda RR, Minz AM, Mohanty S, Samal A, Van Der Pluijm RW. The sensitivity and specificity of a urine based Rapid Diagnostic Test for the diagnosis of *Plasmodium falciparum* in a malaria endemic area in Odisha, India. Pathogens and Global Health. 2017; 111(7): 383-387.

[18] Oyibo WA, Ezeigwe N, Ntadom G, Oladosu OO, Rainwater-Loveth K, Meara, WO, Okpokoro E, Brieger E. Multicenter Pivotal Clinical Trial of Urine Malaria Test for Rapid Diagnosis of *Plasmodium falciparum* malaria. Journal of Clinical Microbiology. 2016; 55: 253-263.

[19] Godwin AA, Sulieman MM, Panda SM. Diagnosis efficiency of urine malaria test kit for the diagnosis of malaria for febrile patients in Gombe, Nigeria. Nigerian Journal of Parasitology. 2018; 39(1): 14-18.

[20] Tao D, McGill B, Hamerly T, Kobayashi T, Khare P, Dziedzic A, Leski T, Holtz A, Shull B, Jedlicka AE, Walzer A, Slowey PD, Slowey CC, Nsango SE, Stenger DA, Chaponda M, Mulenga M, Jacobsen KH, Sullivan DJ, Ryan SJ, Ansumana R, Moss WJ, Morlais I, Dinglasan RR. A saliva-based rapid test to quantify the infectious subclinical malaria parasite reservoir. Science Translational Medicine. 2019; 11(473): eaan4479.

[21] Maltha J, Gillet P, Jacobs J. Malaria rapid diagnostic tests in endemic settings. Chronic Microbial infection. 2013; 19: 399-407.

[22] Joel CM, Dean GJP. Malaria rapid diagnostic tests: challenges and Prospects. Journal of Medical Microbiology. 2013; 62: 1491-1505.

[23] Engwa GA, Achundoh OA, Mbacham WF. Rapid Diagnostic Test Cassette: A Source of DNA for Malaria Diagnosis by PCR and a Quality Control Tool for the Test Performance. Academic Journal of Interdisciplinary Studies. 2013; 2(13): 69-75.

[24] Berhane A, Anderson K, Mihreteab S, Gresty K, Rogier E, Mohamed S, Hagos F, Embaye G, Chinorumba A, Zehaie A, Dowd S, Waters NC, . Gatton ML, Udhayakumar V, Cheng Q, Cunningham J. *major* threat to malaria control programs by *Plasmodium falciparum* lacking histidine-rich protein 2, Eritrea. Emerging Infectious Diseases 2018; 24:462-470.

[25] World Health Organization. False-negative RDT results and implications of new reports of *P. falciparum* histidine-rich protein 2/3 gene deletions. Geneva, Switzerland: WHO, 2017.

[26] Baker J, McCarthy J, Gatton M, Kyle DE, Belizario V, Luchavez J, Bell D, Cheng Q: Genetic Diversity of *Plasmodium falciparum* Histidine-Rich Protein 2 (PfHRP2) and Its Effect on the Performance of PfHRP2-Based Rapid Diagnostic Tests. Journal of Infectious Diseases. 2005; 192: 870-877.

[27] Wellems TE, Howard RJ. Homologous genes encode two distinct histidine rich proteins in a cloned isolate of *Plasmodium falciparum*. Proceedings of the National Academy of Sciences of the United States of America. 1986; 83(16), 6065-6069.

[28] Rock EP, Marsh K, Saul AJ, Wellems TE, Taylor DW, Maloy WL, Howard RJ. Comparative analysis of the *Plasmodium falciparum* histidine-rich proteins HRP-I, HRP-II and HRP-III in malaria parasites of diverse origin. Parasitology. 1987; 95 (Part 2), 209-227.

[29] Knapp B, Shaw A, Hundt E, Enders B, Kupper HA. (1988). A histidin alanine rich recombinant antigen protects *Aotus* monkeys from *P. falciparum* infection. Behring Institute Mitteilungen. 1988; 82:349-359.

[30] Pologe LG, Ravetch JV. Large deletions result from breakage and healing of *P. falciparum* chromosomes. Cell. 1988; *55*: 869-874.

[31] Xiao J, Li M, Bi H, Wang P, Li Y. Cloning and sequence analysis of histidine-rich protein-II gene fragment of *Plasmodium falciparum Yunnan* strain (Chinese) Zhongguo Ji Sheng Chong Xue Yu Ji Sheng Chong Bing Za Zhi. **1999**; 17:143-145.

[32] Chiodini PL, Bowers K, Jorgensen P, Barnwell JW and Grady KK *et al*., The heat stability of *Plasmodium* lactate dehydrogenase-based and histidine-rich protein 2-based malaria rapid diagnostic tests. Trans. Royal Society of Tropical Medicine and Hygiene; 2007; 101: 331-337.

[33] WHO. Basic malaria microscopy. 2nd ed. Geneva: World Health Organization; 2010.

[34] Cheesbrough M. Parasitological tests. District laboratory practice in tropical countries; Part 1. University press, Cambridge. 2009; 5: 178-306.

[35] World Health Organization. Cross – checking malaria slide results. Malaria microscopy quality assurance manual. 2016; 10: 66-79

[36] Ngasala B, Mubi M, Warsame M, Petzold MG, Massele AY, Gustafsson LL, Tomson G, Premji Z, Bjorkman A. Impact of training in clinical and microscopy diagnosis of childhood malaria on anti-malaria drug prescription and health outcome at primary health care level in Tanzania: a randomized control trial. Malaria Journal. 2008; 7: 199.

[37] Uguen C, Rabodonirina M, De Pina JJ, Vigier JP, Martet G, Maret M, Peyron F. ParaSight-F rapid manual diagnostic test of *Plasmodium falciparum* infection. Bulletin of World Health Organization. 1995; 73: 643-649.

[38] Ross NE, Pritchard CJ, Rubin DM, Dusé AG. Automated image processing method for the diagnosis and classification of malaria on thin blood smears. Medical and Biological Engineering and Computing. 2006; 44: 427-436.

[39] Gillet P, Bosselaers K, Cnops L, Bottieau E, Van Esbroeck M, Jacobs J. Evaluation of the SD FK70 malaria Ag *Plasmodium vivax* rapid diagnostic test in a non-endemic setting. Malaria Journal. 2009; 8: 129.

[40] Tek FB, Dempster AG, Kale I. Computer vision for microscopy diagnosis of malaria. Malaria Journal. 2009; 8:153.

[41] Prescott WR, Jordan RG, Grobusch MP, Chinchilli VM, Kleinschmidt I, Borovsky J, Plaskow M, Torrez M, Mico M, Schwabe C. Performance of a malaria microscopy image analysis slide reading device. Malaria Journal. 2012; 11: 155.

[42] Vink JP, Laubscher M, Vlutters R, Silamut K, Maude RJ, Hasan MU, Haan GDE. An automatic vision-based malaria diagnosis system. Journal of Microscopy. 2013; 250:166-178.

[43] Torres K, Bachman CM, Delahunt CB, Baldeon JA, Alava F, Vilela DG, Proux S, Mehanian C, McGuire SK, Thompson CM, Ostbye T, Hu L, Jaiswal MS, Hunt VM, Bell D. Automated microscopy for routine malaria diagnosis: a field comparison on Giemsa-stained blood films in Peru. Malaria Journal. 2018; 17: 339

[44] Alexander N, Schellenberg D, Ngasala B, Petzold M, Drakeley C,

Sutherland C. Assessing agreement between malaria slide density readings. Malaria Journal. 2010; 9: 4.

[45] WHO. World malaria report. Available at https://www.who.int/publications/i/item/world-malaria-report-2019 (accessed October16, 2020).

[46] Tangpukdee N, Duangdee C, Wilairatana P, Krudsood S. Malaria diagnosis: A brief review. Korean Journal of Parasitology. 2009; 47(2): 93-102.

[47] Oriero EC, Jacobs J, Geetruyden JV, Nwakanma D, Alessandro U. Molecular based isothermal tests for field diagnosis of malaria and their potential contribution to malaria elimination. Journal of Antimicrobial and chemotherapy. 2014; 70: 2-13.

[48] Steketee N, Incardona S, Chy S, Duval L, Ekala M. Towards High Throughput Molecular detection of *Plasmodium* : new approaches and molecular markers. Malaria Journal; 2009; 8: 86.

[49] Murphy SC, Shott JP, Parikh S, Etter P, Prescott WR, Stewart VA. Review Article: Malaria Diagnostics in clinical trials. American Journal of Tropical Medicine and Hygiene. 2013; 89(5) : 824-839.

[50] Dhama K, Kharthik K, Chakraborty S, Tiwari R, Kapoor S. Loop –mediated Isothermal Amplification of DNA (LAMP) : A new diagnostic tool lights the world of diagnosis of animal and human pathogens; A Review. Pakistan Journal of Biological Sciences. 2014; 17(2): 151-166.

[51] Achu CE, Nwaorgu OC, Egbuche CM, Ezeagwuna DA, Ajibaye O, Aribodor DN. Frequency of Merozoite Surface Protein 2 (MSP2) Allelic Families and Sulphadoxine-Pyrimethamine (SP) Resistance Markers among Asymptomatic Pregnant Women in Delta State, Nigeria. *American* Journal of Biosciences. 2020; 8(1): 6-14.

[52] Mfuh KO, Yunga ST, Esemu LF, Bekindaka ON, Yonga J, Djontu JC, Mbakop CD, Taylor DW, Nerurkar VR, and Leke RGF. Detection of *Plasmodium falciparum* DNA in saliva samples stored at room temperature: potential for a non-invasive saliva-based diagnostic test for malaria. Malaria Journal. 2017; 16: 434.

[53] Grimberg BT, Erickson JJ, Sramkoski RM, Jacobberger JW, Zimmerman PA. Monitoring *Plasmodium falciparum* growth and development by UV flow cytometry using an optimized Hoechst-Thiazole orange staining strategy. Cytometry A. 2008; 73: 546-554

[54] Jang JW, Kim JY, Yoon J, Yoon SY, Cho CH, Han ET, An SSA, Lim CS. Flow Cytometric Enumeration of Parasitemia in Cultures of *Plasmodium falciparum* Stainedwith SYBR Green I and CD235A. Research Article. 2014; https://doi.org/10.1155/2014/536723

[55] Chevalley S, Coste A, Lopez A, Pipy B, Valentin A. "Flow cytometry for the evaluation of anti-plasmodial activity of drugs on *Plasmodium falciparum* gametocytes," Malaria Journal. 2010; 9(1): 49

[56] Fakruddin MD, Mazumdar RM, Chowdhury A, Mannan KSB. Nucleic Acid Sequence Based Amplification (NASBA) - Prospects and applications. International Journal of Life Sciences and Pharma Research. 2012; 2(1): L106 – L121.

[57] Oriero EC, Jacobs J, Geetruyden JV, Nwakanma D, Alessandro U. Molecular based isothermal tests for field diagnosis of malaria and their potential contribution to malaria elimination. Journal of Antimicroboial and chemotherapy. 2015; 70: 2-13.

[58] Bousema T, Okell L, Shekalaghe S, Griffin JT, Omar S, Sawa P, Sutherland C, Sauerwein R, Ghani AC, Drakeley C. Revisiting the circulation time of *Plasmodium falciparum* gametocytes: molecular detection methods to estimate the duration of gametocyte carriage and the effect of gametocytocidal drugs. Malaria Journal. 2010; 9(1): 136.

[59] Wampler R, Mwingira F, Javati S, Robinson L, Betuela I, Siba P, Beck H-P, Mueller I, Felger I. Strategies for the detection of Plasmodium Species Gametocytes. Plos One. 2013; 8(9): e76316

[60] McNamara DT, Kasehagen LJ, Grimberg B, Cole-Tobian J, Collins WE, Zimmerman PA. Diagnosing infection levels of four human malaria parasite species by a polymerase chain reaction/ ligase detection reaction fluorescent microsphere based Assay. The American Journal of Tropical Medicine and Hygiene. 2006; 74(3): 413-421.

[61] Ndao M. Diagnosis of Parasitic Diseases: Old and New Approaches. Interdisciplinary perspectives on infectious Diseases. 2009; 2009: 278246

[62] Ahmed KS, Ahmed S, Mushahid N, Anwer M, Saeed S. Comparison of Real time Polymerase Chain Reaction with microscopy and Antigen Detection Assay for the diagnosis of Malaria. Journal of the college of physician and surgeon Pakistan. 2013; 23 (11): 787-792.

Section 2

Epidemiology and Surveillance

Chapter 4

Malaria Elimination: The Role and Value of Sero-Surveillance

Kingsley Badu, Amma Aboagyewa Larbi and Kwadwo Boampong

Abstract

As countries move from intense malaria transmission to low transmission there will be a demand for more sensitive tools and approaches in tracking malaria transmission dynamics. Surveillance tools that are sensitive in tracking real time infectious bites as well as infectious reservoir will be preferred to counting number of cases in the hospital or parasite prevalence. The acquisition and maintenance of anti-malarial antibodies is a direct function of parasite exposure, seroprevalence rates has been used as an efficient tool in assessing malaria endemicity and confirming malaria elimination. Plasmodium antibodies are explicit biomarkers that can be utilised to track parasite exposure over more extensive time spans than microscopy, rapid diagnostic testing or molecular testing and the conventional entomological inoculation rate. Seroprevalence studies can therefore help monitor the impact of malaria control interventions, especially when the parasite occurrence is low. As a result, antibody responses to Anopheles salivary proteins or Plasmodium species may potentially offer reliable information of recent or past exposure; recognise short-term or gradual changes in exposure to Plasmodium infection or to estimate individual-level exposure to infection. This book chapter will present about four studies we have conducted across eastern and western Africa on the efficiency of salivary gland proteins and antimalarial antibodies in tracking malaria transmission intensity. We hope that these could be used as surveillance tools in malaria elimination efforts.

Keywords: malaria elimination, sero-surveilance, antibody response, MSP1 malaria surveilance, seroepidemiology

1. Introduction

1.1 Malaria elimination

Since the inception of initiatives such as the Roll Back Malaria and the creation of the United Nations Millennium Development Goals (MDGs) on combating HIV/AIDS, malaria, and other diseases in September 2000, unprecedented progress has been made in the fight against malaria. Malaria vector control interventions such as indoor residual spraying (IRS), the provision of insecticide-treated bed nets (ITNs) and the use of artemisinin-based combination therapy for the prompt treatment of clinical malaria cases has led to a decrease in the number of malaria morbidity and mortality rates in many endemic areas in the world [1]. Globally, the rate of new malaria infections and deaths decreased by 41% and 62% respectively between 2000 and 2015

[2]. Despite the many interventions, malaria remains a major public health concern in many African countries. According to the World health Organisation (WHO), an estimated 229 million malaria cases were recorded in 2019 with 409,000 deaths [3]. Increasing insecticide resistance and behavioural changes by vectors that transmit malaria parasites as well as drug-resistant parasites threaten the progress made so far.

The advances made in malaria control in many countries have in effect led to the disease becoming more varied, leading to a new challenge of understanding the disposition of lingering transmissions in certain populations [4]. The remedy to this conundrum is a rigorous surveillance system with the ability to measure spatial and temporal variations in malaria transmission accurately and efficiently. The Global technical strategy for malaria 2016–2030 provides a comprehensive framework to guide countries in their efforts to accelerate progress towards malaria elimination [5, 6]. The strategy sets the target of reducing global malaria incidence and mortality rates by at least 90% by 2030 [6]. This technical strategy recognises the critical role that surveillance plays in malaria elimination.

Malaria surveillance metrics used over the years to measure transmission include both entomological and parasitological metrics such as parasite prevalence, clinical cases and serological measurements which rely on host antibody responses to both the vector and parasite antigens [4, 7].

2. The significance of malaria surveillance

Malaria surveillance deals with continually and systematically collecting malaria specific data, analysing and interpreting such data [6]. This could be essential in the planning, implementation and evaluation of public health practice. As part of the Global Technical Strategy for Malaria 2016–2030, WHO has urged endemic countries and those that have achieved elimination to strengthen their disease surveillance in order to identify any reinfection, reemergence or resistance. Malaria surveillance also makes available data to help all transmission settings make appropriate decisions regarding malaria control strategies, priorities and resource allocation. In order to achieve malaria elimination globally, surveillance is crucial because it will provide accurate data at any point in time regarding the state of a particular country in connection with malaria.

3. Challenges to malaria surveillance

The continuous and systematic collection, analysis and interpretation of malaria-specific data and the use of such data in the planning, implementation and evaluation of public health practice is paramount in the quest to eradicate malaria. Surveillance programmes can enable resource-poor malaria-endemic countries to prioritise populations that are most in need, re-strategize in cases where interventions have not resulted in decrease in cases and appropriately respond to pockets of outbreak cases without wasting resources. Malaria surveillance programmes should therefore seek to identify the most affected populations, trends in incidence and mortalities as well as the overall impact of control measures [5].

In many countries, malaria surveillance systems remain inadequate to support the goal of elimination [8]. The intensity of malaria transmission is closely linked to the epidemiology of the disease. Transmission intensity is often measured using the parasite prevalence metric, which measures the proportion of the population with detectable parasites in the blood in a given locale. The entomological inoculation rate, malaria-positive fraction, incidence rate and deaths are other metrics used to measure malaria transmission intensity [9]. The 2020 world Malaria Report rightly recognised the weak surveillance systems in moderate to high malaria transmission countries that rely solely on parasite prevalence or clinical case reporting for surveillance [3]. This greatly affects the quality of data for epidemiological studies. Improving the scope and quality of surveillance is critical to malaria elimination.

Many malaria endemic countries use clinical case reports for surveillance due to its ease and affordability. However, clinical case reporting has some limitations such as the inability to measure asymptomatic infections as well as infections among transient populations who contribute to transmission [10, 11]. Parasite prevalence surveys are also useful in malaria surveillance, however, in cases of low transmission, large sample sizes are required before useful prevalence data can be obtained. Other seldomly used metrics such as entomological inoculation rate is very labor intensive and costly to implement in malaria endemic populations on routine basis, making it less useful [12]. It is therefore critical that countries adopt surveillance metrics such as serum anti-malarial antibody based seroprevalence surveys that can effectively measure both high and low transmission as well as the temporal and spatial variations in malaria transmission. Such a metric can complement the already existing clinical case reporting and parasite prevalence surveys.

Seroprevalence is a surveillance metric used to measure the antibody markers that are elicited by host cells in response to vectors and parasites. Measuring the proportion of the population who are seropositive for malaria could inform the rate of malaria transmission over time and space [13, 14].

4. Markers of malaria exposure

Measurement of serum anti-malarial antibodies is a useful marker of malaria exposure that indicates long-term transmission potential especially if such measurements are done over a period of time. This is mainly because anti-malarial antibodies develop after repeated exposures and can persist for months to years after infection [7, 14]. In very low transmission settings, where parasite prevalence and entomological inoculation rate (EIR) are insensitive, serological measures offer a way of accurately assessing endemicity and identifying focal areas of transmission supporting the potential for elimination [7]. Evaluating serological evidence of malaria exposure in the human population provides insight into malaria endemicity. Seroconversion rates are related to the force of infection of malaria as reflected through the immune responses of exposed individuals. Thus, the seroconversion rates provide measures of malaria exposure that compare with the malaria transmission intensity [14]. Different antibodies can be used in malaria intensity studies depending on the life span of that protein and how well it is produced in low or high endemic regions as a direct response to exposure.

IgG response to whole saliva extracts of *Anopheles gambiae* has been observed as a marker of exposure to *Anopheles gambiae* bite, and consequently, high anti-saliva IgG levels is a predictive indicator of malaria morbidity [15]. One protein that is being explored is the salivary gland protein and its peptide P1. The *Anopheles gambiae* salivary gland gSG6 protein and derived P1 peptide are specific to *An. gambiae* and elicit specific antibody response in the human host. It is said to have the potential to represent a general epidemiological marker of exposure of the main Afro-tropical malaria vectorial system, *Anopheles arabiensis* and *Anopheles funestus* up to 99% and 80% respectively [15].

Other malaria antibodies that are used in most malaria antibody studies include circumsporozoite protein (CSP), apical merozoite antigen-1 (AMA1), merozoite surface proteins 1 and 3 (MSP -1, MSP-3) [16, 17].

5. Seroprevalence as malaria transmission metric for surveillance

Changes in vector exposure, parasite infections in humans and human immunity can alter the metrics of malaria transmission. Thus, the malaria transmission metric used to determine transmission intensity should depend on the intrinsic variability of the metric across space and time [18]. These variations that might go undetected by parasite prevalence can be identified with the use of seroprevalence data, antibody density and seroconversion rates. In the era where transmission intensity of malaria is decreasing it becomes particularly difficult to use popular methods like the entomological inoculation rate (EIR). Thus, the use of other serological tools based on antibody responses to parasite and vector antigens are potentially valuable for robust transmission measurement.

Serosurveillance offers an approximation of the antibody levels elicited against an infectious disease. Many developed countries have well established national serosurveillance programs for different infectious diseases [19]. Serosurveillance of malaria offers the advantage of making known active transmission in cases that would otherwise be deemed as interrupted transmission [20]. A case example was observed in Ghana where the parasite prevalence was well below 5% throughout the year, whereas an equivalent seroprevalence of mosquito salivary protein gSG6-P1 and *Plasmodium falciparum* merozoite surface protein $MSP1_{19}$ were above 40% (**Figure 1**) [21]. A similar observation was made in a study in Somalia where the prevalences of $MSP1_{19}$ were 17.9% and 19.3% in the wet and dry seasons respectively when no parasites had previously been observed [20]. A prevalence of 10% and 50% were observed for parasite and $MSP1_{19}$ respectively in the uphill dwellers of the Western Kenyan highlands, emphasising robustness of serological markers in tracking temporal changes in vector exposure, especially in younger populations [17]. Human immune response to *Anopheles* salivary gSG6-P1 varies in relation to exposure to mosquitoes. Measuring human-mosquito contact using gSG6-P1 has therefore been shown to be very reliable.

Seroconversion rates (SCR) which is a function of age and exposure have been estimated using $MSP1_{19}$ age-specific seroprevalence. This has been used to measure the transmission intensity of malaria and has been shown to correlate with EIR measurements [7, 22]. Age-specific seroprevalence of $MSP1_{19}$ can distinguish between transmission intensities in low versus high malaria transmission areas or periods (**Figure 2**). When transmission intensity is below 5%, parasite prevalence is an inefficient metric for establishing changes in transmission or evaluating the impact of interventions [23].

Seroprevalence helps to overcome the challenge of subpatent malaria since microscopy and rapid diagnostic test (RDT) used to measure parasite prevalence

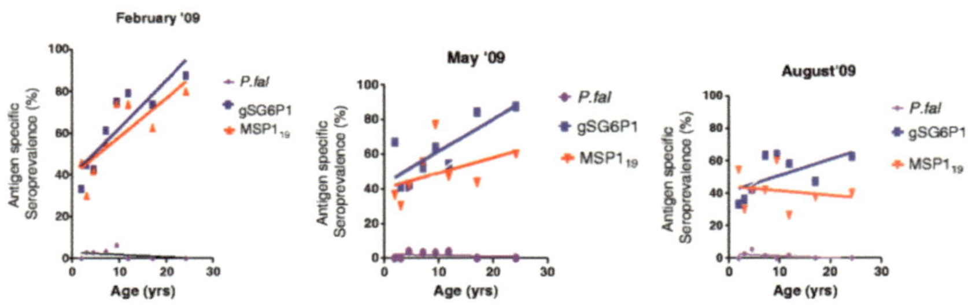

Figure 1.
Relationship between malaria parasite prevalence and antigen specific seroprevalence (adapted from Badu et al. 2015) [21].

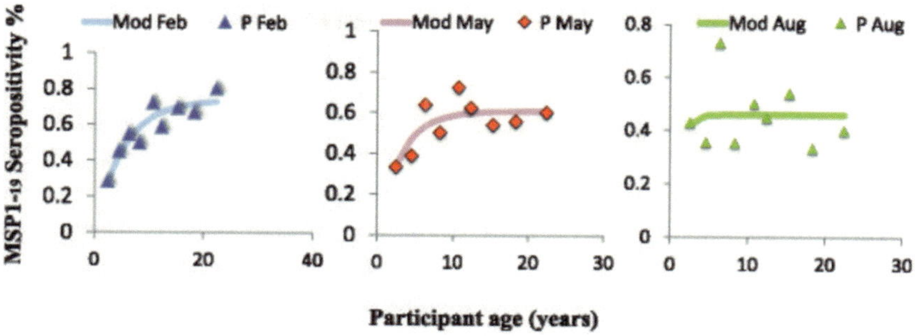

Figure 2.
Seroconversion rate of MSP1$_{19}$ (adapted from Badu et al. 2015 [21].

are less accurate where parasite load is less than 250 parasites per μl [24]. The profound effect of antimalarial drug intake on parasite density is also not accounted for in parasite prevalence measurements. With changing parasite load in the blood in the course of an infection, the accuracy of parasite prevalence is often unreliable [24].

A study has also indicated that to assess malaria endemicity at varying altitudes, the most suitable immunological marker to use is MSP -119 [7]. It has been demonstrated in our studies in Kenya that the prevalence of MSP-1 19 antibody in residents at the valley bottom was almost two-fold higher than that of the uphill residents with median total IgG titers indicating a 13-fold difference between the uphill and valley bottom residents suggesting a higher intensity of malaria

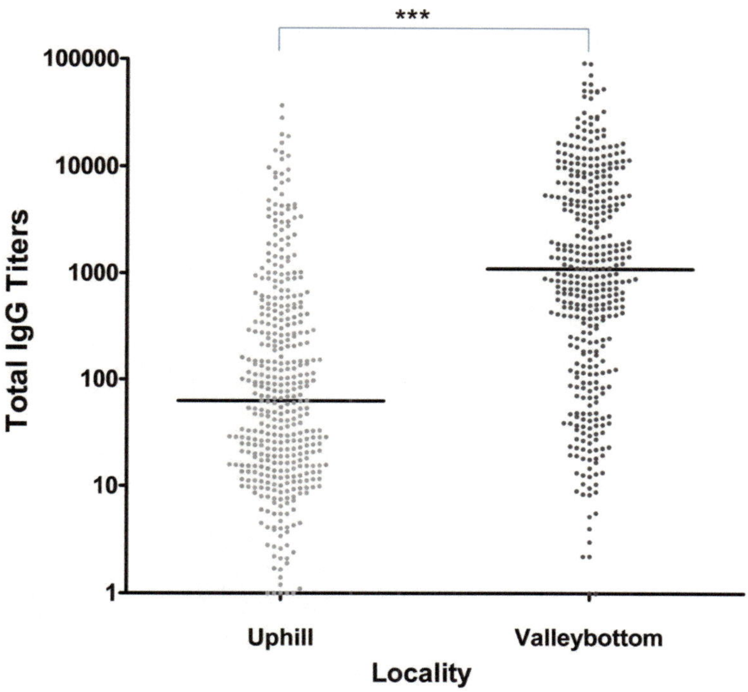

Figure 3.
*Differences in IgG titers among different localities. ***indicates the significance test by Mann-Whitney test, P value < 0.001 (Uphill n = 401, Valley n = 394). Source: Badu et al. [16].*

transmission in the valley area than the uphill area [17]. This was corroborated by a related study which revealed that in 82% of all malaria mosquitoes in the highland aggregated in <300 m area the valley bottom (Guof et al. 2004), [18] This clearly demonstrates that seroprevalence reflects cumulative exposure and thus, is less affected by seasonality or unstable transmission due to the longer duration of the specific antibody response. Age-specific seroprevalence was also used to estimate seroconversion rates (SCR) as a measure of malaria transmission intensity. Age seroprevalence curves of the study showed that in low transmission settings, development of antibodies is slow and is mainly exhibited by the adult population, whereas in a high transmission area, much of the population will be seropositive even at a younger age. **Figures 3** and **4** and **Table 1** below show the findings of this experiment.

Another study showed differences in gSG6-P1 specific seroprevalence and antibody levels depending on your location. The study observed differences in parasite prevalence and gSG6-P1 levels across different transmission settings. Thus, salivary gland gSG6-P1 could be effective in differentiating between vector densities. Again, the study showed that the risk of exposure to malaria parasite is higher in individuals presenting with anti -gSG6 P1 antibody and that gSG6-P1 seroprevalence is not cumulative [17].

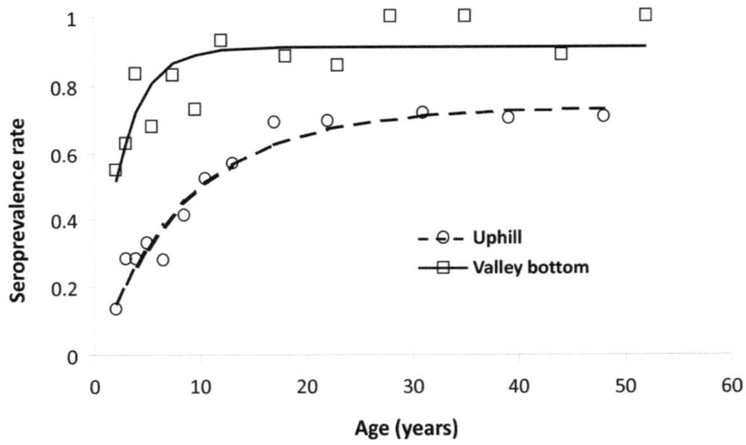

Figure 4.
Kinetics of the age-dependent antibody prevalence at different altitudes. Phill model: Pt = 0.73(1-e-0.11t), R2 = 0.95, P<0.001; valley bottom model: Pt = 0.91(1-e-0.39t), R2 = 067, P<0.001. Source: Badu et al. [16].

Parasite prevalence			
MSP-1_{19} seroprevalence			
Locality (n)	***Odds Ratio***	***95% CI***	***P value***
Uphill (401)	2.798	[1.018, 7.693]	0.046
Valley (394)	3.167	[1.196, 8.386]	0.020
Total Uphill and Valley (795)	4.282	[2.200, 8.330]	< 0.001

Table 1.
Showing the association between MSP-119 seroprevalence with plasmodium parasite prevalence at the different localities. Source: Badu et al. *(2012).*

We utilise a very simple reversible catalytic conversion model which estimates the rate of seroconversion from seronegative to seropositive and vice versa with respect to specific study sites. This we fit with standard maximum likelihood and which assumes a binomial error distribution [7, 16].

Thus seropositive are the percentage individuals whose antibody titers of specific malaria antigens are above the threshold of unexposed or naive individuals (Defined as three standard deviations above the value determine for the negative controls).

Reversible catalytic conversion models uses the average yearly rate of conversion to seropositive, λ, and the average yearly rate of reversion from seropositive to seronegative, ρ [7], The equation is thus fitted for each study site (uphill dwellers and that of valley bottom dwellers). Thus Pt is the proportion of individuals aged t that are seropositive

$$P_t = \frac{\lambda}{\lambda + \rho}(1 - \exp(-(\lambda + \rho)t))$$

Where λ is the respective site rate of seroconversion, and ρ is the site specific rate of reversion to seronegative [7, 16].

Box 1.
Reversible catalytic conversion model.

Age trends of gSG6-P1 is influenced by the differences in the transmission intensity and thus, children had higher responses to whole salivary gSG6 proteins while adults had diminished Antibody responses, suggesting desensitisation of the immune response to the salivary proteins. From all the above, gSG6-P1 measurement shows transient exposure (or seasonal) in a hypoendemic population and would be more useful even under low malaria transmission period as envisaged in the pre-elimination and elimination phase of malaria [17].

In a comprehensive study conducted in two malaria endemic western Kenyan highland areas, 107 proteins of *P. falciparum* that elicited antibody responses were identified. Many of these immunogenic proteins had been previously identified in other studies. Hsp70, ETRAMP10.2, MSP1, and conserved *Plasmodium* protein PF3D7. These were the most frequently recognised proteins among the sera groups studied [25]. Expectedly, more proteins were identified in sera from valley bottom than sera from hilltop residence. When comparing the breadth of antibody response to these proteins, the study observed that there was no difference between

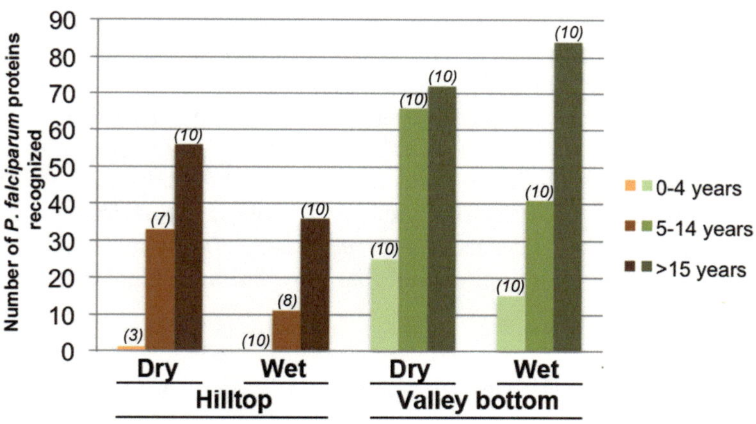

Figure 5.
Breadth of antibody binding to immunogenic P. falciparum *proteins by study sera groups. The number of proteins considered immunogenic by the study sera (Y axis) is plotted against sera cohorts stratified by age (0–4, 5–14 and > 15 years old), season (wet and dry) and site (hilltop and valley bottom) of sample collection (X axis). The number of serum samples tested in each sera group is provided in parenthesis above the corresponding bar (adapted from Baum et al. 2013) [25].*

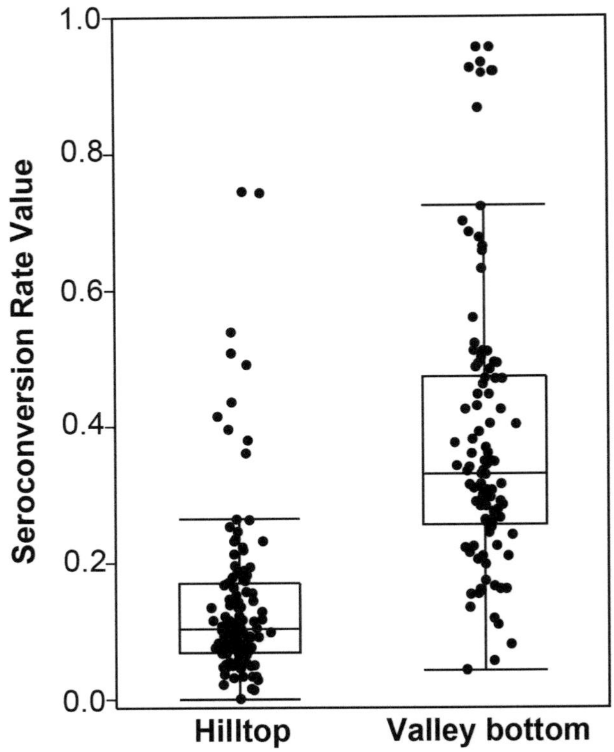

Figure 6.
Whisker box plot of seroconversion rate (SCR) values of immunogenic polypeptides of P. falciparum *for the hilltop and valley bottom sites. The SCR of 98 immunogenic polypeptides for which paired values were calculated (Y axis) is plotted against the site of serum sample collection (X axis). The lower and upper edges of the box indicate the first and the third quartiles, the line in the middle represents the median. The 1.5X interquartile range is indicated by the vertical line outside the boxes. Outlying values are indicated by dots outside boxes (adapted from Baum et al. 2013) [25].*

immunogenic proteins identified during the wet or dry season among valley bottom residents. However, seasonal variation in protein was observed in hilltop sera. Between donors below 5 years and those above 5 years, difference between antibody response was observed (**Figure 5**). This aligns with surveillance studies that used clinical cases or parasite prevalence metrics [16, 26].

The study also noted that seroconversion rates differed between hilltop and valley bottom donors, with lower SCR values recorded for hilltop than in the valley bottom (**Figure 6**). Overall, the antigens identified in the study can be used as protein candidates to sero-survey the intensity of malaria transmission across stable and unstable transmission areas and compared different age stratifications to give an overview of the effect of temporal and spatial variations on malaria transmission.

6. Sero-surveilance as for the confirmation of elimination

The development and utilisation of serological tools, especially, the antibody response to specific malaria antigens has a great potential to support malaria elimination agenda. A recent study [14] has identified about five priority areas in which this approached could be utilised to support the malaria elimination agenda. Among these, the confirmation of malaria elimination can be a practical benefit. "Certification of malaria elimination is the official recognition by WHO of a country's malaria-free status". WHO may grant this recognition to a country only when it can prove beyond reasonable doubt, that the indigenous malaria transmission of all human parasites has been interrupted across the whole country for at least three consecutive years. Not only that but the country also has "a fully functional surveillance and response system that can prevent re-establishment of local transmission" [27]. Practically, antibodies to malaria antigens are sensitive biomarkers of population-level malaria exposure and can be used among other things to confirm malaria elimination, and monitor re-emergence of malaria [28]. Specific anti malaria antibodies such as $MSP1_{19}$ and AMA that tend to accumulate in the population can be used to confirm malaria elimination in children born in the last three years. When antibody response in children born in the last three years are undetectable across all subnational sentinel sites, this will be a good indication of the confirmation of the malaria elimination.

7. Sero-surveilance for monitoring recent exposure and the impact of interventions

Reliable serological markers of recent malaria exposure could dramatically improve current surveillance methods by allowing for accurate estimates of infection incidence from limited data. According to Greenhouse et al. [14], Sero-surveilance could be implemented in two scenarios settings: 1) when new tools are being deployed for the first time; and 2) regularly to evaluate the success of such tools during implementation.

For the purpose of regular evaluation of intervention tools antibodies with relatively short half life will be more useful. Yman et al. 2016, studied We IgG antibody responses to over one hundred 111 *malaria antigens* in a longitudinal cohort of travellers who did not have a second express following heir initial exposure. They identified five serological markers (GAMA, MSP1, MSPDBL1 C- and N-terminal, and PfSEA1) which could detect exposure within the previous 3-months with >80% sensitivity and specificity. Others (Kerkhof et al. 2016) have studied through several cross-sectional studies among 8439 participants have demonstrated that *Plasmodium falciparum*, antibodies against LSA3.RE, GLURP and Pf.GLURP.R2 are capable of detecting exposure range of 6–8 months. The quest for standard antigenes or peptides as well as standard technologies that will ensure smooth implementation and comparable results across the world is a subject of intense research currently ongoing.

8. Conclusion

Currently, the utility of sero-surveilance in the support of malaria elimination (measuring transmission intensity, assessing the impact evaluation, confirmation of elimination and prevention of re-introduction) have moved beyond the prove of principle. However, full implementation is hampered by the current requirement for expensive high-throughput technologies for specimen storage and functioning assays, which are largely not available in many malaria-endemic communities. Therefore, governments and research programs should critically analyse the value being added by antibody tests before considering using it to complement other metrics [14, 28].

In their current state, sero-surveillance tools can only be performed by technicians who are well trained on the use of antibody detecting equipment. However, surveillance studies are often carried out by field workers who might lack the adequate knowledge and training needed to perform antibody tests. As such, it is very important that antibody detecting tools are easy to use, with test results being easy to interpret [14, 29]. This will ensure the generation of data that can easily be analysed to translate to action implementation.

The integration of seroprevalence as a malaria surveillance metric in endemic communities will require the understanding of stakeholders in malaria control and eradication at the local, national, and global level. This involves engaging and sensitising local communities, governmental and non-governmental organisations, research bodies and donor agencies on the need for sero-surveillance as a function of malaria exposure.

Author details

Kingsley Badu[1]*, Amma Aboagyewa Larbi[2] and Kwadwo Boampong[1]

1 Department of Theoretical and Applied Biology, Kwame Nkrumah University of Science and Technology, Kumasi, Ghana

2 Department of Biochemistry and Biotechnology, Kwame Nkrumah University of Science and Technology, Kumasi, Ghana

*Address all correspondence to: kingsbadu@gmail.com

References

[1] Bhatt, S., Weiss, D., Cameron, E. et al. The effect of malaria control on Plasmodium falciparum in Africa between 2000 and 2015. Nature 526, 207–211 (2015). https://doi.org/10.1038/nature15535

[2] Eliminating malaria. Geneva: World Health Organization; 2016. Available at: http://www.who.int/malaria/publications/atoz/ eliminating malaria/en/, accessed 28 April 2017.

[3] World malaria report 2020: 20 years of global progress and challenges. Geneva: World Health Organization; 2020. Licence: CC BY-NC-SA 3.0 IGO.

[4] Reiner RC, Le Menach A, Kunene S, et al.: Mapping residual transmission for malaria elimination. eLife. 2015; 4: pii: e09520.

[5] Global technical strategy for malaria 2016–2030. Geneva: World Health Organization; 2015 (http://www.who.int/malaria/areas/global_ technical_ strategy/en).

[6] WHO, 2018. Malaria surveillance, monitoring & evaluation: a reference manual. Geneva: World Health Organization; 2018. Licence: CC BY-NC-SA 3.0 IGO.

[7] Drakeley CJ, Corran PH, Coleman PG, Tongren JE, Mcdonald SLR, Malima R, et al. Estimating medium- and long-term trends in malaria transmission by using serological markers of malaria exposure. Proc Natl Acad Sci U S A. 2005;102:5108–5113.

[8] The malERA Consultative Group on Health Systems and Operational Research. A research agenda for malaria eradication: health systems and operational research. PLoS Med. 2011;8:e1000397.

[9] Irene N. Nkumama, Wendy P. O'Meara, Faith H.A. Osier, (2017). Changes in Malaria Epidemiology in Africa and New Challenges for Elimination. Trends in Parasitology, Volume 33, Issue 2, 2017. Pages 128–140, ISSN 1471–4922. https://doi.org/10.1016/j.pt.2016.11.006.

[10] Tadesse FG, Slater HC, Chali W, et al.: The Relative Contribution of Symptomatic and Asymptomatic Plasmodium vivax and Plasmodium falciparum Infections to the Infectious Reservoir in a Low-Endemic Setting in Ethiopia. Clin Infect Dis. 2018; 66(12): 1883–1891.

[11] Sáenz FE, Arévalo-Cortés A, Valenzuela G, et al.: Malaria epidemiology in low-endemicity areas of the northern coast of Ecuador: high prevalence of asymptomatic infections. Malar J. 2017; 16(1): 300.

[12] Okell LC, Ghani AC, Lyons E, et al.: Submicroscopic infection in Plasmodium falciparum-endemic populations: a systematic review and meta-analysis. J Infect Dis. 2009; 200 (10): 1509–1517.

[13] Wilson, S. E., Deeks, S. L., Hatchette, T. F., & Crowcroft, N. S. (2012). The role of seroepidemiology in the comprehensive surveillance of vaccine-preventable diseases. CMAJ: Canadian Medical Association journal = journal de l'Association medicale canadienne, 184(1), E70–E76. https://doi.org/10.1503/cmaj.110506

[14] Greenhouse B, Daily J, Guinovart C et al. Priority use cases for antibody-detecting assays of recent malaria exposure as tools to achieve and sustain malaria elimination [version 1; peer review: 5 approved] Gates Open Research 2019, 3:131 (https://doi.org/10.12688/gatesopenres.12897.1)

[15] Sagna, A. B., Sarr, J. B., Gaayeb, L., Drame, P. M., Ndiath, M. O., Senghor,

S., Sow, C. S., Poinsignon, A., Seck, M., Hermann, E., Schacht, A. M., Faye, N., Sokhna, C., Remoue, F., & Riveau, G. (2013). GSG6-P1 salivary biomarker discriminates micro-geographical heterogeneity of human exposure to Anopheles bites in low and seasonal malaria areas. Parasites and Vectors, 6 (1). https://doi.org/10.1186/1756-3305-6-68.

[16] Badu, K., Afrane, Y. A., Larbi, J., Stewart, V. A., Waitumbi, J., Angov, E., Ong'echa, J. M., Perkins, D. J., Zhou, G., Githeko, A., & Yan, G. (2012). Marked variation in MSP-1 19antibody responses to malaria in western Kenyan highlands. BMC Infectious Diseases, 12 (1), 50. https://doi.org/10.1186/1471-2334-12-50.

[17] Badu, K., Siangla, J., Larbi, J., Lawson, B. W., Afrane, Y., Ong'Echa, J., Remoue, F., Zhou, G., Githeko, A. K., & Yan, G. (2012). Variation in exposure to Anopheles gambiae salivary gland peptide (gSG6-P1) across different malaria transmission settings in the western Kenya highlands. Malaria Journal, 11(May 2014). https://doi.org/10.1186/1475-2875-11-318.

[18] Guofa Zhou, Noboru Minakawa, Andrew Githeko, Guiyun Yan, Spatial Distribution Patterns of Malaria Vectors and Sample Size Determination in Spatially Heterogeneous Environments: A Case Study in the West Kenyan Highland , *Journal of Medical Entomology*, Volume 41, Issue 6, 1 November 2004, Pages 1001–1009, h ttps://doi.org/10.1603/0022-2585-41.6.1001

[19] Charlwood, J. D., Smith, T., Lyimo, E., Kitua, A. Y., Masanja, H., Booth, M., Alonso, P. L. & Tanner, M. (1998) Am. J. Trop. Med. Hyg. 59, 243–251. [Pub Med] [Google Scholar]

[20] Tusting LS, Bousema T, Smith DL, Drakeley C. Measuring changes in plasmodium falciparum transmission: precision, accuracy and costs of metrics. Adv Parasitol. 2014;84:151–208. doi:10.1016/B978-0-12-800099-1.00003-X.

[21] Krsak M, Henao-Martínez AF, Franco-Paredes C. COVID-19: Way Forward With Serosurveillance Without Overemphasizing Neutralizing Antibodies. Viral Immunol. 2020 Nov 11. doi: 10.1089/vim.2020.0246. Epub ahead of print. PMID: 33181055.

[22] Bousema T, Youssef RM, Cook J, Cox J, Alegana VA, Amran J, et al. Serologic markers for detecting malaria in areas of low endemicity. Emerg Infect Dis. 2010;16:392–399. doi:10.3201/eid1603.090732.

[23] Badu et al. Parasites & Vectors (2015). Serological evidence of vector and parasite exposure in Southern Ghana: the dynamics of malaria transmission intensi8:251. DOI 10.1186/s13071-015-0861-y.

[24] Corran P, Coleman P, Riley E, Drakeley C. Serology: a robust indicator of malaria transmission intensity? Trends Parasitol. 2007;23:575–582. doi: 10.1016/j.pt. 2007. 08. 023.

[25] Drame PM, Poinsignon A, Besnard P, Cornelie S, Le MJ, Toto JL, et al. Human antibody responses to the Anopheles salivary gSG6-P1 peptide: a novel tool for evaluating the efficacy of ITNs in malaria vector control. PLoS One. 2010;5(12):e15596. doi:10.1371/journal.pone.0015596.

[26] Wongsrichanalai C, Barcus MJ, Muth S, Sutamihardja A, Wernsdorfer WH. A review of malaria diagnostic tools: microscopy and rapid diagnostic test (RDT). Am J Trop Med Hyg. 2007;77 Suppl 6:119–127.

[27] A framework for malaria elimination. Geneva: World Health Organization; 2017. Licence: CC BY-NC-SA 3.0 IGO.

[28] Elliott SR, Fowkes FJ, Richards JS, et al.: Research priorities for the development and implementation of serological tools for malaria surveillance. F1000Prime Rep. 2014; 6: 100.

[29] Baum E, Badu K, Molina DM, Liang X, Felgner PL, et al. (2013) Protein Microarray Analysis of Antibody Responses to Plasmodium falciparum in Western Kenyan Highland Sites with Differing Transmission Levels. PLoS ONE 8(12): e82246. doi:10.1371/journal.pone.0082246.

Chapter 5

The Role of Adaptive Surveillance as a Core Intervention to Achieve Malaria Elimination

Arantxa Roca-Feltrer, Ann-Sophie Stratil and James K. Tibenderana

Abstract

Adaptive surveillance systems are essential for national programmes to achieve their malaria elimination goals. Core principles of surveillance systems including accurate diagnosis and reporting of malaria cases, integration of health data across administrative levels and the need to link data to a response are well defined by international guidelines. Nevertheless, while the requirements of surveillance systems along the transmission continuum are clearly documented, the operationalization remains challenging for national programmes. Firstly, because the multi-level increase of surveillance efforts demanding real-time and case-based data as well as the capacity of the health force to trigger locally customized responses, is resource intensive and requires substantial investment. Secondly, because there is a gap in international alignment on best tools and practices on how to operationally implement these requirements. Recently, several initiatives have started to address this gap in international coordination, aiming to establish the operational guidance for elimination programmes to successfully implement adaptive surveillance systems.

Keywords: malaria elimination, adaptive surveillance, case investigation, digital systems, responsiveness

1. Introduction

The Global Technical Strategy for Malaria 2016–2030, published by the World Health Organization (WHO) in 2015, emphasizes surveillance as a core intervention for accelerating progress towards malaria elimination across endemic settings [1]. The successful and optimal implementation of other malaria interventions, including early detection and treatment and vector control measures, depend on the effectiveness of countries surveillance systems. Surveillance systems comprise all steps from the recording and reporting of data to data analysis and presentation, interpretation and evaluation and finally the dissemination and use of information [2]. The functioning of these systems depend on a competent and adequately resourced health force that adheres to surveillance requirements outlined national strategic plans, ensures high data quality throughout the system, and has the capacity to translate data into action while enabling rapid adaptations to respond to evolving contextual factors. Effective malaria surveillance systems allow national programmes to continuously monitor and evaluate the progress of their programmes, detect and respond to outbreaks in time, and identify gaps in service delivery and intervention coverage in order to (re-)allocate resources in line with the programmatic needs.

We argue that the ability of surveillance systems to adapt to changing circumstances is a crucial element to resilient and effective systems that can support the achievement of national elimination targets. Changing circumstances may include changes to in-country transmission dynamics, e.g. moving from control to elimination settings or implementing context-specific surveillance approaches that respond to in-country heterogeneous malaria transmissions. These may also include external factors that may impact on malaria trends by altering specific malaria surveillance indicators (e.g. due to disruptions to access to care as observed during the COVID-19 pandemic) which require careful and ongoing interpretation of generated data in such rapidly changing environments. This has been shown to be an especially important factor during the COVID-19 pandemic where programmes are now required to understand the influence of COVID-19 on malaria indicators in order to correctly interpret observed malaria trends and take appropriate actions [3].

Despite the importance of strong surveillance systems, national programmes continue to experience challenges in the operational implementation of their surveillance systems particularly at the lowest levels. A landscaping exercise of surveillance systems from elimination countries in 2015–2016 reported that "surveillance systems in 2015–2016 [were] insufficient to support planning and implementing of targeted interventions and to measure progress towards malaria elimination" [4]. While progress has been made since then, countries continue to experience challenges in implementing adaptive surveillance systems.

In the following sections, we outline the importance of adaptive surveillance as a core intervention to malaria elimination. First, we describe the key elements of a functioning adaptive surveillance system capable of responding to all needs across the malaria transmission continuum. Then, we focus on the implications for surveillance system when transitioning from control to elimination settings. Lastly, we describe remaining challenges and rising opportunities in establishing resilient and effective surveillance system across countries to accelerate the elimination of malaria.

2. What are the key elements of a functioning adaptive surveillance system capable of responding to all needs across the malaria transmission continuum?

A malaria surveillance system is considered functional and responsive when it can produce evidence-based information (from quality data) that is routinely used for planning and decision making. To provide guidance on the principles and requirements for a strong malaria surveillance system, a reference manual was published by WHO in 2018 [2]. These principles are essential for guiding the establishment of a malaria surveillance system's core competencies, operationalizing surveillance systems in malaria endemic countries remains challenging. Outlines the following key principles of the design and establishment of malaria surveillance systems (**Table 1**).

It is worth noting that countries that have eliminated malaria—or have nearly done so—have documented significant improvements in their surveillance systems that made them possible to deploy a range of interventions and adapt them to needs over time. This ability to develop an adaptive responsive surveillance and information systems has been consistently reported as a key components of elimination programmes [5, 6]. Adaptive surveillance and information systems mean that

#	Principles	Description
1	Accurate parasitological diagnosis of a malaria case	Considered the foundation of a malaria surveillance system. Diagnoses should be made with either quality-assured malaria microscopy or rapid diagnostic tests (RDTs).
2	Integration	All major components of a malaria surveillance system should be integrated into broader health management information systems (HMIS). The HMIS system should, in turn, be responsive to the promptness and granularity of data required for effective malaria surveillance.
3	Responsiveness to country needs and country heterogeneity (malaria surveillance as a continuum)	National SOPs for surveillance should be based on a country's needs and on WHO recommendations and be able to address the heterogeneity of malaria within a country's boundaries. The Global Technical Strategy for Malaria 2016–2030 introduced the concept of a continuum, whereby progress towards malaria elimination is considered to be a continuous process rather than a set of independent stages. [1]
4	Functional capacity to analyze, use and act on data	Regardless of the malaria burden, front-line staff involved in the detection, recording and reporting of cases should also be the first users of data. Necessary investments in surveillance and system transition, including in human resources, should be made to respond to the anticipated reduction in disease burden and be alert after interruption of transmission.
5	Surveillance data must be linked to a response	All surveillance data must be linked to a decision at some level of the health system, even if the decision results in no immediate change in interventions.
6	Multisectorial approach	In all transmission settings, a concerted effort must be made to include cases detected in other sectors (e.g. in private and other nongovernmental health care facilities), as well as those detected in public health facilities.
7	Enable innovations to accelerate efforts	Like most other health interventions, surveillance is likely to benefit from innovation and advances in technology.
8	Be able to track rapid changes of malaria epidemiological factors	Good understanding of the biology and behavioral ecology of vector species is essential for making programmatic decisions and monitoring and evaluating vector control interventions, including quality assurance.
9	Allow for continuous improvements	Surveillance systems should be assessed routinely to ensure their accuracy, reliability, completeness, precision, timeliness and integrity. The assessment should also include the appropriateness of actions taken as a consequence of the results of surveillance

Table 1.
Key principles of a malaria surveillance system (adapted from [2]).

they undergo through continuous improvement cycles that are triggered through the evolving country specific malaria epidemiological factors as well as changing external factors, ultimately leading to a resilient and robust system capable of responding to all malaria transmission contexts and reach malaria elimination. The next section details the specific implications of adaptive surveillance systems when transitioning across the continuum of malaria transmission intensities.

Only when health information systems (HIS) lead to public health decision-making, can surveillance systems be considered functional. For National Malaria Control Programmes, a good malaria information system (MIS) permits decisions on resource allocation to be done on and informed and unbiased way. A key step to understand MIS performance is to assess the quality of data, the use of information made by decision makers and the enabling organizational, technical and behavioral factors that influence MIS performance. System performance is measured through the quality of data produced and the effective use that is given to information produced [7]. Data quality can be assessed through it composite indicators: completeness, timeliness and accuracy and should be conducted at different levels of the system (community, health facility and district). Use of information is assessed through the production, sharing and discussion of relevant reports that guide programmatic activity implementation. Technical, organizational and behavioral components should also be routinely assessed at all levels as they constitute an integral part of the surveillance system.

Establishing and institutionalizing a data demand and data use culture is one of the most challenging components to effectively operationalize at country level as it requires significant investments for resourcing long-term organizational capacity across all administrative levels to implement actionable responses using existing health information systems and based on the surveillance intelligence produced. The following sections outline the key adaptations, challenges and opportunities that malaria surveillance systems face to respond to all levels of malaria transmission in the move towards elimination.

3. What are implications of transitioning from control to elimination?

Delivering on the key principles outlined in the previous section can be challenging for national programmes transitioning towards elimination. Surveillance systems in elimination and control settings are designed to achieve their respective goals, i.e. control and elimination of malaria. While in control setting, the goal is to provide data insights to guide interventions at scale, e.g. mass net distributions, in elimination settings, the focus shifts to quickly trigger locally targeted responses to every single case. These goals require different granularity levels in terms of temporal and case (investigation) resolution. We use the term resolution here to describe the level of needed data granularity. While periodic reporting is sufficient in control settings, surveillance systems in elimination settings strive for real-time reporting to trigger immediate responses, i.e. they strive for high temporal resolution. Similarly, in control settings, caseload is usually investigated at higher administrative levels leading to a response at national, province or district level, while in elimination settings, every single case needs to be investigated to trigger targeted local responses, i.e. elimination settings require high case-level resolution [8, 9]. **Figure 1** depicts the levels of temporal and case resolution needed along the transmission continuum.

When transitioning from control to elimination settings, national programmes need to continuously adapt their surveillance systems in order to cater to these new requirements and trigger appropriate responses. As the term transmission continuum suggests, transitioning from one phase to the next happens gradually and in specific geographical areas within countries (hence increasing the heterogeneity of the malaria transmission in that country) [10]. It is therefore advisable to strengthen and adapt surveillance components gradually and timely to ensure they are functioning when the elimination phase is reached.

In elimination settings, notification of every very case within 24 h, to trigger timely case investigation (often within 3 days), enabling a timely investigation of transmission foci (often within 7 days) [2]. This case-based surveillance approach has been named the "1–3-7 approach" and was launched in China in 2012 and has since been adapted to other country contexts, including Cambodia and Myanmar [11–13]. This approach demands the redesign of reporting structures to deliver on these timely reporting and response requirements. A priority is ensuring quality data reporting from both public and private service. It is a known challenge to

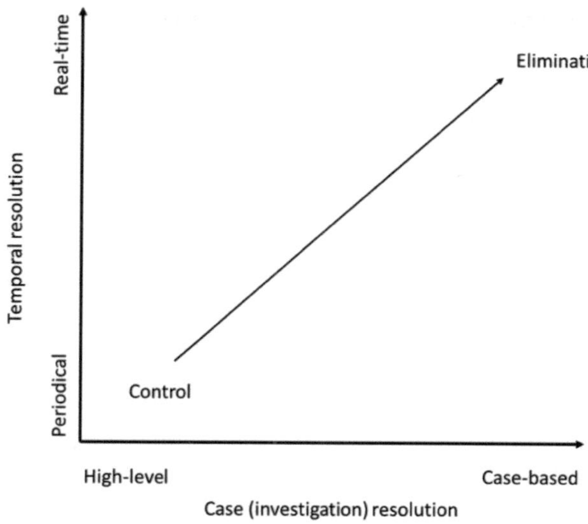

Figure 1.
Changes in surveillance system requirements along transmission continuum (adapted from [9]).

successfully integrate data from the private sector into the national surveillance system [14]. To achieve this, there is an increasing need to establish digital data collection to ensure rapid and complete case reporting from all health system levels, including the private sector [9, 15]. Many countries have developed digitalized reporting systems. One example is Mozambique, a country with high transmission heterogeneity, where, since 2016, community health workers are equipped with smartphones carrying an app through which they can report every patient consultation – including malaria cases. This facilitates the notification of community cases to higher administrative levels that carry out case investigations [16].

Additional to this temporal component of early case notification and investigations, surveillance system need to increase the case resolution to inform customized and locally targeted responses. This includes case investigations, focus investigation and the development of related data collection tools. Programmes also need to expand their case detection approaches to not only detect symptomatic cases actively seeking care with health providers (passive case detection), but also detect asymptomatic cases and populations that might not be easily reached through existing health system structures (active case detection) [2]. Active case detection requires more investment from existing health staff to go out to test remote populations and/or new personnel who carry these additional responsibilities. Sri Lanka's elimination strategy developed a specific approach were active case detection was carried out by mobile malaria clinics targeting remote areas with no immediate access to alternative health system structures [17]. More recently, Cambodia, where remaining malaria cases cluster along international borders and hard-to-reach forests, followed this example with a similar approach. The national programme has introduced the role of mobile malaria workers who go on outreach activities and actively approach forest workers including mobile and migrant populations, the population group most at risk of malaria infection. This approach has proven to be successful, with Cambodia aiming for *P. falciparum* malaria elimination by 2023 [18–20].

Once high-resolution data is available, national programmes need to generate insights through data analysis [9]. Previously, this required input from expert data analysts limiting the extent to which national programme could actually produce the necessary outputs to guide decision making. More recently, analytical outputs can be made available more easily through digitalized automated solutions. Data analysis in elimination setting should facilitate the identification of specific populations at risk, and should allow the micro-stratification of risk areas based on individual case data. Timely analysis of individual-level case data is crucial to improve early warning systems and establish robust alert systems to prevent epidemics and control foci. At this point, visualizing trends and risks via appropriate tools including charts and maps is essential.

Following data visualization and interpretation, the final and arguably most important step is linking data to action. The health force needs to be trained to interpret these high-resolution outputs and trigger targeted responses. Functioning communication flows between different administrative levels, decision-makers and other stakeholders are the enabling environment needed to link surveillance data to action. A case study mention "a well-coordinated surveillance system with excellent vertical and horizontal communication" as a key component that lead to the successful malaria elimination in Sri Lanka [17].

Lastly, it is critical that all these components are facilitated via an integrated platform with clear procedures for data recording, reporting, visualization and use. Systems should be built around central data storage and management system to ensure smooth integration of malaria indicators and data sources into routine HIS [9]. New digital solutions can facilitate this. The project Visualize No Malaria that has been implemented in Zambia since 2015 has exemplified an approach where a range of new digital tools facilitated linkages between exiting routine and non-routine database, automated data workflows, and create customized data visualizations to generate one integrated surveillance system [21]. Experiences from Cambodia outline the process and challenges of shifting from an offline information system towards an integrated web-based surveillance system for malaria elimination [22]. New digital solutions also help make surveillance systems more resilient to changes in external circumstances by allowing simple adaptations that were previously difficult to implement. External circumstances like the COVID-19 pandemic require rapid adaptations of surveillance systems [3, 23]. In a before mentioned project in Mozambique where community health workers submit data through a smartphone app, the underlying digital platform was adapted in response to the COVID-19 pandemic. Now, the app includes education modules related to COVID-19, and data entry forms for COVID-19 symptom tracking (some symptoms like fever overlap with malaria symptoms). This enabled the Ministry of Health to rapidly gather essential insights on COVID-19 knowledge gaps among community health workers and will strengthen malaria surveillance by providing insights into how community health workers handle the similarity of malaria and COVID-19 symptoms [24, 25].

These increased demands of the surveillance system require resources to create functioning data systems, procure appropriate testing (e.g. malaria species-sensitive tests that are able to differentiate between *P. falciparum* and *P. vivax* malaria to allow species-specific responses where required), develop new guidelines and build the capacity of the health force to fulfill these new/additional requirements. Due to these intensified focus on surveillance, the proportional spending on the surveillance component of malaria programmes increases and case studies show that programme expenses to achieve malaria elimination can even be greater than the expenses during the control phase, while international supporting funding of the health system decreases [26, 27]. This may put a specific strain on national programmes catering to the needs of multiple transmission strata at the same time. However, as surveillance systems become more resilient, resources and personnel can progressively shifts tasks and embed additional roles and responsibilities to optimize resources and expertise. Thailand for example has identified the need to integrate malaria services into the general health service system rather than continuing to implement a vertical malaria programme. Building capacity and mobilizing resources at all health system levels will support the achievement of the country's malaria elimination goal by 2024 [28].

4. What are the current gaps in surveillance systems of elimination countries and how to overcome?

One of the remaining challenges for many eliminating countries is the limited capacity of their surveillance systems to monitor and track interventions against *Plasmodium vivax* and monitor vivax relapses. In countries were both *Plasmodium falciparum* and *Plasmodium vivax* are present, malaria interventions have led to steady declines of falciparum malaria, resulting in an increase of the relative contribution of vivax malaria (among all infections). As opposed to *P. falciparum* infection, which does not have latency (dormant stages), treatment of *P. vivax* malaria poses a particular challenge to elimination efforts due to its potential to cause periodic relapses [29, 30]. A fit for purpose surveillance system in these countries should not only be able to monitor the delivery of tailored *P. falciparum* interventions, but also track the implementation of approaches to safely deliver appropriate treatment to *P. vivax* cases.

While the requirements of surveillance systems along the transmission continuum are clearly documented through comprehensive guidance documents outlined in previous sections, the operationalization of this guidance remains challenging for national programmes. Even though many countries are successful in establishing functioning systems on the path to elimination, as shown in previous sections [6], they mostly rely on a learning by doing approach. There remains a gap in coordinating and standardizing efforts among the wider surveillance community. In December 2020, the Malaria Policy Advisory Committee within WHO has acknowledged this "lack of coordination and standardization of tools to monitor the quality of malaria surveillance and to understand its strengths and weaknesses" [31]. Recently, several initiatives have started to address this gap, aiming to establish the operational guidance and best practices for surveillance systems of malaria elimination programmes. The WHO has recently developed a surveillance assessment toolkit which will be published in the first quarter of 2021 [31]. This toolkit will frame a systematic approach on how to measure the performance of malaria surveillance systems which will harmonize the way national programmes assess the quality of their surveillance systems and identify needs for improvement The WHO has further announced the set-up of a Malaria Strategic Information Reference Group (MSIRG). The MSIRG will focus on five main areas: Guidance, digital solutions, surveillance assessments and system strengthening, programme reviews and subnational tailoring of interventions and burden estimation. The RBM Surveillance, Monitoring and Reference Group (SMERG) is a global platform to foster communication on malaria surveillance, monitoring and evaluation and convenes members to coordinate related activities. The SMERG is currently in the process of establishing a Committee dedicated to Surveillance Practice and Data Quality (SP&DQ Committee) with the key objectives to improve the visibility of surveillance and data quality improvement initiatives and to strengthen global coordination on surveillance-related efforts. The two groups (MSIRG and SMERG) will work closely together to ensure synergic efforts between their recent initiatives [32].

These recent initiatives will lay the groundwork for more efficient international alignment of surveillance efforts and improved harmonization of systems in the future.

5. Conclusions

A strong surveillance system is critical to implementing an efficient and effective malaria program to monitor disease trends and optimize targeting of interventions to accelerate progress towards malaria elimination. For countries to strengthen and sustain the practice of using data for decision-making and accelerate efforts towards malaria elimination, dynamic and adaptive surveillance systems are needed. To accelerate efforts towards malaria elimination, surveillance systems must be able to respond to the dynamic and evolving external socio-ecological patterns (as recently experienced through the COVID-19 pandemic) guided by lessons learned on resilience and adaptive management in order to effectively operate at national and subnational levels. Several global initiatives to document these best practices are on the way and will provide international alignment of surveillance efforts and improved harmonization of systems in the future.

Author details

Arantxa Roca-Feltrer*, Ann-Sophie Stratil and James K. Tibenderana
Malaria Consortium, London, United Kingdom

*Address all correspondence to: a.roca@malariaconsortium.org

References

[1] World Health Organization. Global Technical Strategy for Malaria 2016-2030. 2015.

[2] World Health Organization. Malaria Surveillance, Monitoring and Evaluation: A Reference Manual. 2018.

[3] RBM Partnership to End Malaria - Surveillance Monitoring and Evaluation Reference Group. Monitoring and evaluation of malaria-related routine data during the COVID-19 pandemic 2020. Available from: https://endmalaria.org/sites/default/files/Monitoring%20and%20evaluation%20of%20malaria-related%20routine%20data%20during%20the%20COVID-19%20pandemic_August2020.pdf. [Accessed 6 December 2020].

[4] Lourenco C, Tatem AJ, Atkinson PM, Cohen JM, Pindolia D, Bhavnani D, et al. Strengthening surveillance systems for malaria elimination: a global landscaping of system performance, 2015-2017. Malar J. 2019;18:315.

[5] World Health Organization, Roll Back Malaria Partnership, PATH. Eliminating malaria: learning from the past, looking ahead (Progress & impact series, n. 8) ISBN: 9789241502504. 2011. Available from: https://apps.who.int/iris/bitstream/handle/10665/79937/9789241502504_eng.pdf;jsessionid=92E5273ADCB33FEB4CB841E0790F0EE1?sequence=1. [Accessed 21 January 2021].

[6] World Health Organization. Malaria - Elimination case studies 2012. Available from: https://www.who.int/malaria/areas/elimination/casestudies/en/. [Accessed 27 January 2021].

[7] MEASURE Evaluation. Performance of Routine Information System Management (PRISM) Toolkit: PRISM Tools 2019. Available from: https://www.measureevaluation.org/resources/publications/tl-18-12/. [Accessed 27 January 2021].

[8] Bridges DJ, Winters AM, Hamer DH. Malaria elimination: surveillance and response. Pathog Glob Health. 2012;106:224-31.

[9] Ohrt C, Roberts KW, Sturrock HJW, Wegbreit J, Lee BY, Gosling RD. Information systems to support surveillance for malaria elimination. Am J Trop Med Hyg. 2015;93:145-52.

[10] World Health Organization. A framework for malaria elimination. 2017.

[11] Kheang ST, Sovannaroth S, Barat LM, Dysoley L, Kapella BK, Po L, et al. Malaria elimination using the 1-3-7 approach: lessons from Sampov Loun, Cambodia. BMC Public Health. 2020;20:544.

[12] Aung PP, Thein ZW, Hein ZNM, Aung KT, Mon NO, Linn NYY, et al. Challenges in early phase of implementing the 1-3-7 surveillance and response approach in malaria elimination setting: A field study from Myanmar. Infect Dis Poverty. 2020;9:18.

[13] Lu G, Liu Y, Beiersmann C, Feng Y, Cao J, Muller O. Challenges in and lessons learned during the implementation of the 1-3-7 malaria surveillance and response strategy in China: a qualitative study. Infect Dis Poverty. 2016;5:94.

[14] Mercado CE, Ekapirat N, Dondorp AM, Maude RJ. An assessment of national surveillance systems for malaria elimination in the Asia Pacific. Malar J. 2017;16:127.

[15] Bennett A, Avancena ALV, Wegbreit J, Cotter C, Roberts K, Gosling R. Engaging the private sector in malaria surveillance: a review of

strategies and recommendations for elimination settings. Malar J. 2017;16:252.

[16] Malaria Consortium. upSCALE: Strengthening mobile health in Mozambique 2019. Available from: https://www.malariaconsortium.org/resources/publications/1287/upscale-strengthening-mobile-health-in-mozambique. [Accessed 21 January 2021].

[17] World Health Organization. Malaria-Free Sri Lanka 2016. Available from: http://origin.searo.who.int/srilanka/areas/malaria/malaria-free-sri-lanka.pdf. [Accessed 2020-12-07].

[18] Kingdom of Cambodia. Cambodia Malaria Elimination Action Framework 2021-2025. 2020.

[19] Lek D, Callery JJ, Nguon C, Debackere M, Sovannaroth S, Tripura R, et al. Tools to accelerate falciparum malaria elimination in Cambodia: a meeting report. Malar J. 2020;19:151.

[20] Stratil AS, Vernaeve L, Lopes S, Bourny Y, Mannion K, Hamade P, et al. Eliminating *Plasmodium falciparum* malaria: results from tailoring active case detection approaches to remote populations in forested border areas in north-eastern Cambodia. Malar J. 2021;20:108.

[21] Health Data Science Exchange. Data analytics for malaria elimination in Zambia 2015. Available from: https://datascienceforhealth.org/visualize-no-malaria. [Accessed 21 January 2021].

[22] Fu C, Lopes S, Mellor S, Aryal S, Sovannaroth S, Roca-Feltrer A. Experiences From Developing and Upgrading a Web-Based Surveillance System for Malaria Elimination in Cambodia. JMIR Public Health Surveill. 2017;3:e30.

[23] World Health Organization. Tailoring malaria interventions in the COVID-19 response. 2020.

[24] Feldman M, Krylova VL, Farrow P, Donovan L, Zandamela E, Rebelo J, et al. Community health worker knowledge, attitudes and practices towards COVID-19: Learnings from an online cross-sectional survey using a digital health platform, UpSCALE, in Mozambique 2020. Available from: https://www.malariaconsortium.org/resources/publications/1401/community-health-worker-knowledge-attitudes-and-practices-towards-covid-19-learnings-from-an-online-cross-sectional-survey-using-a-digital-health-platform-upscale-in-mozambique. [Accessed 21 January 2021].

[25] Kevin Baker. Rapid support of the COVID-19 response at community level in Mozambique through adapting the existing upSCALE digital health platform and telemedicine. 2020 Global Digital Health Forum; 7 December 2020; 2020. Available from: https://www.malariaconsortium.org/resources/publications/1406/rapid-support-of-the-covid-19-response-at-community-level-in-mozambique-through-adapting-the-existing-upscale-digital-health-platform-and-telemedicine. [Accessed:

[26] Haakenstad A, Harle AC, Tsakalos G, Micah AE, Tao T, Anjomshoa M, et al. Tracking spending on malaria by source in 106 countries, 2000-16: an economic modelling study. Lancet Infect Dis. 2019;19:703-16.

[27] Sabot O, Cohen JM, Hsiang MS, Kahn JG, Basu S, Tang L, et al. Costs and financial feasibility of malaria elimination. Lancet. 2010;376:1604-15.

[28] Ministry of Public Health Thailand. Guide to Malaria Elimination For Thailand's Local Administrative Organizations and the Health

Network 2019. Available from: http://malaria.ddc.moph.go.th/downloadfiles/Guide%20to%20Malaria%20Elimination%20for%20Thailand%20LAO_EN.pdf. [Accessed 21 January 2021].

[29] Baird JK, Valecha N, Duparc S, White NJ, Price RN. Diagnosis and Treatment of *Plasmodium vivax* Malaria. Am J Trop Med Hyg. 2016;95:35-51.

[30] Olliaro PL, Barnwell JW, Barry A, Mendis K, Mueller I, Reeder JC, et al. Implications of *Plasmodium vivax* Biology for Control, Elimination, and Research. Am J Trop Med Hyg. 2016;95:4-14.

[31] World Health Organization. Overview of the Malaria Surveillance Toolkit 2020. Available from: https://www.who.int/docs/default-source/malaria/mpac-documentation/mpac-december2020-session1-surveillance-toolkit-update.pdf?sfvrsn=f3091836_9. [Accessed 21 January 2021].

[32] RBM Partnership to End Malaria - Surveillance Monitoring and Evaluation Reference Group. Informative session on SP&DQ Committee. 27 January 2021; Virtual.

Chapter 6

Increased Trends of *P. vivax* in Sub-Saharan Africa: What Does it Mean for Malaria Elimination?

Mary Aigbiremo Oboh, Mamadou Ndiath, Olumide Ajibola, Kolapo Oyebola and Alfred Amambua-Ngwa

Abstract

Plasmodium vivax being the most geographically spread *Plasmodium* species is considered sparsely distributed in sub-Saharan Africa (sSA) while *P. falciparum* is the most prevalent species in this region. Thus, control strategies in sSA have been disproportionately targeted towards falciparum malaria. Nevertheless, with the use of more sensitive malaria diagnostic platforms, there are more reports of *P. vivax* and other non-falciparum malaria in sSA. In addition, *P. vivax* is presumed benign, however there are new findings of severe cases recorded from *P. vivax* single or mixed infection with other *Plasmodium* species. Besides, the extended dormant period (lasting for weeks or months) is a challenge for achieving effective cure for vivax infections. Although, chloroquine has been proscribed for treatment *P. falciparum*, it still remains the drug of choice for *P. vivax* in most Asian countries where it is predominant. In sSA, artemisinin combination-based therapies (ACTs) are used for treatment of falciparum malaria and, it is probable that the use of ACT could be enhancing adaptive selection for *P. vivax* in the face of its increasing prevalence in the population. Hence, understanding epidemiological and biological factors, and data that could be contributing to the observed steady increase in *P. vivax* prevalence in sSA is important. In this chapter, we discuss the mechanisms for invasion of red blood cells, trends in increasing prevalence of vivax malaria, diagnostic tools, and the public health implications of *P. vivax* and *P. falciparum* co-endemicity in Africa.

Keywords: *Plasmodium vivax*, *Plasmodium falciparum*, sub-Saharan African, Malaria elimination, Duffy negative antigen

1. Introduction

In sub-Saharan Africa (sSA), *Plasmodium falciparum* is responsible for most of the human malaria infection and less frequently, malaria could be due to *P. ovale*, *P. malariae* and *P. vivax* [1]. Significant gains observed in massive reduction in global malaria cases and mortalities in the early 2000s have been largely due to strategic malaria interventions [1]. Nevertheless, signals of reversal in gains are beginning to emerge in most African countries [1]. This stall in progress has been attributed to increased prevalence of non-falciparum malaria parasites on one hand and the development of resistance by both the parasite and vector to drugs and insecticides respectively [2–4]. Thus, refocusing control strategies to include all circulating species of *Plasmodium* in sSA aimed at reducing the burden of these non-falciparum parasites will greatly contribute to malaria control progress.

P. vivax is particularly interesting as regards its mechanism of invasion, reproduction, virulence and development. Understanding the biology of vivax parasites is crucial for developing strategies aimed at controlling malaria. Regrettably, vivax malaria poses a huge challenge for in vitro analysis to adapt in cell culture, in order to shed more light on invasion patterns, virulence, growth, and reproduction. For example, *P. vivax* has high predisposition for immature red blood cells-RBCs (reticulocytes) which is not readily available [5]. Another drawback as regards vivax control is the use of primaquine (PQ) to achieve hypnozoites clearance, which causes haemolytic anaemia in glucose 6 phosphate dehydrogenase (G6PD) deficient individuals [6, 7]. In sSA with very limited resources for ascertaining the G6PD status of individuals, this presents a practical challenge as individuals are either treated without their G6PD status known or remain untreated. The implication of the latter is the prolonged carriage of hypnozoites capable of relapsing weeks or months later. It has also been found that individuals with specific cytochrome P450 gene polymorphic alleles such as the CYP2D6 do not efficiently metabolise PQ and eventually miss out in the clearance of dormant liver parasites [8].

Overcoming vivax resistance to chloroquine [9], which is also a major drawback in vivax control is looking promising, with a single dose of tafenoquine seemingly independent of CYP2D6-impairement is effective in the prevention of vivax relapse [10, 11].

Evolution is shaping the biological interaction between vivax parasites and the human host [12, 13]. For instance, there is new evidence counteracting the former notion of *P. vivax* emergence in Asia from vivax-like macaque parasites [14, 15]. Recent evolutionary genomic analyses have postulated that vivax most probably originated in Africa [16]. Selection for Duffy-negative mutations could have been due to the high circulation of *P. vivax* in ancient Africans [12] which led to the eventual disappearance of vivax malaria in most parts of Africa [17]. There is need to carry out a comprehensive characterisation of the Duffy-independent vivax strains in West [18, 19] and East Africa [20] in order to understand the genetic similarities and phylogeny between the strains and, relationship with emerging zoonotic non-human primate (NHP) malaria.

Although, non-human primates (NHPs) and human vivax species are considered non-interbreedable (allopatric) [12], it is possible that recombination events between vivax parasites of apes and human lineages have occurred to favour the adaptation of currently circulating vivax strains [21]. This hypothesis is being supported by binding studies of recombinant orthologues; reticulocyte binding protein 2- RBP2 and RBP3, to gorillas, humans and chimpanzees erythrocytes' that displayed no evidence of host specificity to invasions of red cells [12]. Moreover, there has been detection of ape-like *P. vivax* in a European returnee from Africa [21], while human *P. vivax* has been identified in monkeys from the wild in South America [22]. To infer genetic epidemiology of *P. vivax* and relationship with other closely related species, population genetic studies is necessary. This has been employed in *P. falciparum* to demonstrate the origin, complexity, evolutionary history, changes in population size and relatedness between parasite populations.

2. Mechanism of invasion of *P. vivax* malaria to Duffy antigen receptor on red blood cells

Duffy antigen receptor for chemokines (DARC) gene is the fourth erythrocyte gene associated with resistance to *Plasmodium* species [23]. Polymorphisms in other genes associated with malaria are specifically accompanied by severity or protection against falciparum malaria. DARC confers protection against vivax malaria [24]. DARC has a 36–46 kDa glycoprotein major sub-unit and is made up of 338 amino acids (AAs) that is organised into seven transmembrane domain [25] with an extra-cellular epitope at the N-terminal that mediates *P. vivax* invasion of RBCs. DARC, a non-specific receptor is expressed on erythrocytes and employed by *P. vivax* merozoites in invasion of RBCs [26]. It is located on the long arm of chromosome 1 (1.q22–1.q23) and possesses two exons [27]. A mutation from a thymine to a cytosine at the GATA-box upstream of the promoter region (33rd position) results in the non-expression of DARC on RBCs, giving rise to the *FYO** allele also known as the Duffy negative phenotype [28].

The *FYO** allele is prevalent in sSA as well as in African-Americans but rare in other racial groups lacking black admixtures [27]. For instance, all 1000 individuals screened in a study in the Gambia were Duffy negative [29]; likewise more than 80% of the participants of a study carried out in northern Nigeria were Duffy-negative [30]. Similarly, another report among pregnant women in Nigeria confirmed a 9:1 Duffy negative to positive ratio [31]. Thus, the null expression of the Duffy gene and reduced prevalence of *P. vivax* in sSA suggests an interplay of adaptive features being employed by RBC overtime. Consequently, the rare observation of *FYA* and *FYB* alleles in this part of the world [32, 33] substantiates the argument of the selective adaptation of the Duffy gene on RBC and its exertion in sSA.

There are several reports of vivax malaria in hitherto low risk regions [34–37] in sSA. The first *Plasmodium* invasion molecules identified was the Duffy binding proteins (DBP) otherwise referred to as, erythrocyte-binding-like (EBL) proteins. These proteins are characteristically homogenous in their cysteine-rich Duffy-binding-like (DBL) domains. The EBL protein of *P. falciparum* and *P. knowlesi* are able to use different receptors in invading the RBC due to variation in EBL gene numbers [38]. Therefore, it is likely that, *P. vivax* having phylogenetic similarity to *P. knowlesi* might have developed diverse EBL proteins also capable of binding to other receptors in the RBCs [2]. The high genome diversity in *P. vivax* [39, 40] provides a plausible explanation that supports and augments its capability of developing alternative invasion pathways through other receptors [41]. An alternate hypothesis is that, *P. vivax* is more endemic in north Africa as well as the Afro-Asiatic populations found in Sudan, Somalia [42, 43] and Ethiopia [20, 44] where there are higher populations of Duffy positive individuals. In this case, the Duffy positive carriers are reservoirs of infection to Duffy negative individuals. Despite the two assumptions, the precise route of transmission of *P. vivax* to/from Africa has not been fully established.

3. Increasing trends of *P. vivax* in sub-Saharan Africa and potential selection for Duffy-negative individuals

Previous reports on vivax epidemiology are now under scrutiny due to the use of more sensitive detection tools [37, 45–51]. *P. vivax* has been detected in south-eastern Senegal: a region sharing border with Mali, Guinea Conakry and The Gambia. In addition, the detection of *Anopheles* vector capable of transmitting vivax in Kenya [52], as well as identification of vivax in mosquito in a study carried out in Angola and Equatorial Guinea [35] points to active transmission of vivax malaria in this sub-region. In a case report, a pregnant Nigerian residing in Italy visited Nigeria briefly and was diagnosed with vivax infection [53], with no further investigation as to the source of infection. Whether these infections were transmitted from Duffy positive individuals serving as reservoir to the negative individuals was not determined.

Although DBP1 possess unique sequences and are highly polymorphic [53], as revealed from correlation analysis of DBP1 mutations, they do not explain the ability of *P. vivax* to infect Duffy-null Africans [54]. The high haplotype diversity of DBP1 and its flanking region in Ethiopia is predictive of multiple independent emergence of vivax variants that were not purged from the population [55]. Therefore, genome-wide comparative studies of Duffy-dependent and emerging Duffy-independent strains are critical for understanding the different forms of adaptive responses, fitness and selection operating in the parasites. The occurrence of DBP1 gene amplification in Ethiopia [55], Madagascar [56] and Cambodia [57] is implicative of adaptation to blood stage infection in the host. A substantial knowledge of the patterns of genetic variation in different geographic scales as well as genetic differences between populations permits inference of population relatedness or structural variation [58].

4. Strategies for *P. vivax* diagnosis in Africa in the era of malaria elimination

Diagnosis of *P. vivax* has relied primarily on two approaches; light microscopy and rapid diagnostic tests (non-molecular). However, modern tools (molecular based tests) such as PCR tests have been demonstrated to be useful, but has suffered widespread utilisation in African countries due to lack of expensive equipment and trained personnel to carry these complex assays.

4.1 Light microscopy (LM)

The World Health Organisation's gold standard for *P. vivax* testing is the detection of parasites in Giemsa stained blood smears by light microscopy [59]. In detecting parasitemia from blood, thick smears are more sensitive, while thin smears allow for clearer visualisation of the morphology of the parasites for accurate speciation and calculation of parasite density. It is recommended that 3 sets of thick and thin smears should be collected for analysing *P. vivax* suspected blood smears. Light microscopy has a number of benefits in African health laboratories such as low cost of operation, and ease of deployment on the field. However, in Africa, the main constraint in accurate microscopy diagnosis is the lack of trained microscopists, and epileptic power supply in most parts of the continent. One of the main challenges in microscopic diagnosis of *P. vivax* is the presence of fewer number of parasites circulating in the blood compared to *P. falciparum* infections making it more likely to report false negatives. The preference of *P. vivax* for reticulocytes which accounts for less than 1% of the fraction of erythrocytes in circulation explains the reason for lower parasite densities compared to *P. falciparum*. In addition, clinical immunity to *P. vivax* infections occur earlier and the immune response is effective in the control of parasitemia [60].

4.2 Malaria rapid diagnostic tests (mRDTs)

The use of mRDTs has become very popular and critical to controlling malaria in Africa. Malaria RDTs provide results within 15 to 20 minutes, do not require special training to interpret results and special storage facilities. The use of mRDTs has contributed significantly to reducing the burden of malaria and is the most commonly used approach in rural laboratory settings with a sensitivity as high as 99% for *P. falciparum*. Malaria RDTs that test for *P. vivax* detect the P.vivax - pLDH antigen specific to *P. vivax*, or pan-pLDH or aldolase antigens common to all *Plasmodium* species. The sensitivity of mRDTs in detecting *P. vivax,* is lower [61–63] when compared to those for falciparum malaria. Moreover, cross reactions with other disease conditions, presence of certain immunological factors and gametocytaemia can result in false positives. They also have a limited shelf life (~24 months) and need to be kept dry and away from extreme temperatures (> 40°C). Malaria RDTs are very reliable at high parasitemia, while at lower parasitemia chances of false negatives increase [64]. A combination of RDTs with light microscopy would significantly improve *P. vivax* diagnosis in Africa.

4.3 Polymerase chain reaction (PCR)

LM has been the gold standard for malaria diagnosis, but with substantial progress in malaria control, interventions have begun to consider asymptomatic carriers as well. Hence, there is increase interests in the utilisation of molecular tools for detection of sub-microscopic infections. Molecular techniques allow investigation of 5–10 μL whole blood, which increases test sensitivity when compared to 0.025–0.0625 μL whole blood) used for LM [59].

PCR based tests such as conventional PCR and real time PCR have been used to detect *P. vivax* mostly in laboratory settings as part of research projects and not usually as routine clinical based tests. PCR based tests detect *P. vivax* with high sensitivities in diagnosing asymptomatic people particularly in samples with low parasitemia. Molecular based tests have a lower detection limit than both mRDTs and LM. The type of input material (DNA, RNA or whole blood) target gene, species detected, primer/probe composition and concentration, amplification technique (PCR or isothermal), read-out (gel electrophoresis, fluorescence detection, lateral flow) and whether it is qualitative or quantitative impact on the sensitivity of molecular detection tests. The standard molecular marker for *Plasmodium* species differentiation detection is the 18S rRNA genes [65]. In the reference genomes of *P. vivax* (Sal1 and P01), there are 3 distinct copies of 18S rRNA that are expressed at different stages [66]. Some of the Pv18S rRNA assays in use target only one of the three copies by qPCR [67]. Pv18S rRNA assays have also been used to target PV18S rRNA transcripts in addition to the genes [67, 68]. The detection of *P. vivax* in clinical samples can also be improved by targeting high multi-copy genes in PCR assays which provides improved sensitivity over low-copy Pv18S rRNA approaches. Targeting multicopy genes allows pooling samples in community surveys in areas with low parasite prevalence or in elimination settings. Pooling will also bring down costs of assays without compromising on the sensitivity. An example of a multi-copy gene that has been tested for *P. vivax* diagnosis is the non-coding subtelomeric repeat sequence Pvr 47 which has 14 copies in the *P. vivax* Sal1 reference genome. The Pvr47 single step PCR was almost as sensitive as the *P. vivax* 18S rRNA nested PCR [69]. Other targets such as vir/pir multigene family with high copy numbers similar to the var. gene family in *P. falciparum* have also been tested with limited success [70, 71]. Other molecular assays for *P. vivax* have also targeted the mitochondrial DNA in a one-step PCR reaction, loop mediated isothermal amplification or qPCR targeting cytochrome C oxidase I (*cox1*) [72–74], genus-specific PCR followed by targeting vivax specific non-coding regions between cytochrome B gene and *cox1* [75].

Loop-mediated isothermal amplification (LAMP) assays amplify single or multi-copy molecular markers in an isothermal reaction. This technique is useful at point of care settings in the field because of ease of implementation and limited infrastructure requirement. LAMP is also useful in detecting submicroscopic infections with high sensitivity [76, 77].

5. Public health implications of *P. vivax* and *P. falciparum* co-endemicity

Co-infections of *P. vivax* and *P. falciparum* are often unrecognised in sSA, likely due to the predominance of *P. falciparum* as the major infecting species in most parts of the continent and the dogma that *P. vivax* was absent in sSA [78, 79]. With several lines of evidence, it is now being appreciated that *P. vivax* prevalence in sSA might actually be much higher than presumed [80–82]. Detection of mixed species infection with *Plasmodium* vivax, are also missed as most health care facilities use mRDTs specific for *P. falciparum* and usually do not have skilled man-power and resources to analyse all species that might be present by microscopy. In health facilities that use microscopy, misdiagnosis of co-infections of *P. falciparum* and *P. vivax* as *P. vivax* mono-infection, will lead to wrong treatment which could increase antimalarial resistance or *P. falciparum* parasitemia, leading to severe malaria. There are conflicting reports on the impact of co-infections of *P. falciparum* and *P. vivax*, some studies reported a decrease in disease severity through cross species immunity [83], while others have suggested an increased morbidity in children [84]. A recent meta-analysis also demonstrated a high prevalence of severe mixed malaria compared to *P. falciparum* mono-infection in the studies included in the meta-analysis [85]. This finding has serious implications on malaria public health control efforts and further reiterates the reason why malaria remains a leading cause of morbidity and mortality globally. Also, this emphasises the importance of improved diagnostic tools and the use of species-specific mRDTs in combination with routine microscopy or PCR where present for continuous surveillance. The possibility of mixed infections resulting in a significantly higher risk of developing severe malaria than patients with *P. falciparum* mono-infections is a grave public health risk, considering that mixed infections are underreported in sSA [86, 87]. This could be one of the reasons why treatment failure from ACT use and antimalarial drug resistance is on gradual increase on the continent. Taken together, it is important that clinical laboratories recognise the likelihood of other non-falciparum species especially vivax in their setting, considering the movement of persons (due to trade within the continent) that could carry parasites from one location to the other. Therefore, improved capacity for detection of suspected cases of mixed infections through a combination of species specific mRDTs together with microscopy is crucial for accurate treatment.

6. Conclusion

Duffy negativity is no longer a guaranteed barrier against *P. vivax* invasion, and the transmission of Duffy-independent adapted-vivax parasites will interrupt malaria control. National malaria elimination programmes should prioritise *P vivax* surveillance. Focus should also be on *P. vivax* biology especially as it concerns erythrocyte invasion in order to improve control strategies. Fine-scale epidemiological mapping is also required to elucidate the evolutionary dynamics of erythrocyte invasion by *P. vivax*.

Acknowledgements

The authors appreciate all their colleagues who provided valuable suggestions on this manuscript especially Dr. Eniyou C. Oriero.

Conflict of interest

All authors declare that they have no competing interest.

Author details

Mary Aigbiremo Oboh[1*], Mamadou Ndiath[1], Olumide Ajibola[1,2], Kolapo Oyebola[3] and Alfred Amambua-Ngwa[1]

1 Medical Research Council Unit The Gambia, at The London School of Hygiene and Tropical Medicine, Fajara, Banjul, The Gambia

2 First Technical University Ibadan, Nigeria

3 National Institute of Health, USA

*Address all correspondence to: moboh@mrc.gm

References

[1] WHO. World Malaria Report. 2018.

[2] Rosenberg R. Plasmodium vivax in Africa : hidden in plain sight ? Trends Parasitol. 2007;23:193-196.

[3] Daniels RF, Deme AB, Gomis JF, Dieye B, Durfee K, Thwing JI, et al. Evidence of non-Plasmodium falciparum malaria infection in Kédougou, Sénégal. Malar J. 2017;16:9.

[4] Diallo MA, Badiane AS, Diongue K, Deme A, Lucchi NW, Gaye M, et al. Non-falciparum malaria in Dakar: A confirmed case of Plasmodium ovale wallikeri infection. Malar J. 2016;15:429.

[5] Malleret B, Li A, Zhang R, Tan KSW, Suwanarusk R, Claser C, et al. Plasmodium vivax : restricted tropism and rapid remodeling of CD71-positive reticulocytes. Blood. 2015;125:1314-1325.

[6] Baird JK, Rieckmann KH. Can primaquine therapy for vivax malaria be improved? Trends Parasitol. 2003;19:115-120.

[7] Baird JK, Hoffman SL. Primaquine Therapy for Malaria. Clin Infect Dis. 2004;39:1336-1345.

[8] Bennett JW, Pybus BS, Yadava A, Tosh D, Sousa JC, McCarthy WF, et al. Primaquine Failure and Cytochrome P-450 2D6 in Plasmodium vivax Malaria. N Engl J Med. 2013;369:1381-1382.

[9] Mekonnen SK, Aseffa A, Medhin G, Berhe N, Velavan TP. Re-evaluation of microscopy confirmed Plasmodium falciparum and Plasmodium vivax malaria by nested PCR detection in southern Ethiopia. Malar J. 2014;13:48. doi:10.1186/1475-2875-13-48.

[10] Lacerda MVG, Llanos-Cuentas A, Krudsood S, Lon C, Saunders DL, Mohammed R, et al. Single-dose tafenoquine to prevent relapse of plasmodium vivax malaria. N Engl J Med. 2019;380:215-228.

[11] St Jean PL, Xue Z, Carter N, Koh GCKW, Duparc S, Taylor M, et al. Tafenoquine treatment of Plasmodium vivax malaria: Suggestive evidence that CYP2D6 reduced metabolism is not associated with relapse in the Phase 2b DETECTIVE trial. Malar J. 2016;15:97.

[12] Loy DE, Plenderleith LJ, Sundararaman SA, Liu W, Gruszczyk J, Chen Y-J, et al. Evolutionary history of human *Plasmodium vivax* revealed by genome-wide analyses of related ape parasites. Proc Natl Acad Sci. 2018;:1-10. doi:10.1073/pnas.1810053115.

[13] Hamblin MT, Thompson EE, Di Rienzo A. Complex Signatures of Natural Selection at the Duffy Blood Group Locus. Am J Hum Genet. 2002;70:369-383. doi:10.1086/338628.

[14] Mu J, Joy DA, Duan J, Huang Y, Carlton J, Walker J, et al. Host switch leads to emergence of Plasmodium vivax malaria in humans. Mol Biol Evol. 2005;22:1686-1693.

[15] Cornejo OE, Escalante AA. The origin and age of Plasmodium vivax Omar. Trends Parasitol. 2006;22:558-563.

[16] Liu W, Li Y, Shaw KS, Learn GH, Plenderleith LJ, Malenke JA, et al. African origin of the malaria parasite Plasmodium vivax. Nat Commun. 2014;5:e3346.

[17] Niang M, Diop F, Niang O, Sadio BD, Sow A, Faye O, et al. Unexpected high circulation of Plasmodium vivax in asymptomatic children from Kédougou, southeastern Senegal. Malar J. 2017;16:497. doi:10.1186/s12936-017-2146-8.

[18] Wurtz N, Mint Lekweiry K, Bogreau H, Pradines B, Rogier C, Ould Mohamed Salem Boukhary A, et al. Vivax malaria in Mauritania includes infection of a Duffy-negative individual. Malar J. 2011;10:336.

[19] Fru-Cho J, Bumah V V., Safeukui I, Nkuo-Akenji T, Titanji VPK, Haldar K. Molecular typing reveals substantial Plasmodium vivax infection in asymptomatic adults in a rural area of Cameroon. Malar J. 2014;13:170.

[20] Lo E, Yewhalaw D, Zhong D, Zemene E, Degefa T, Tushune K, et al. Molecular epidemiology of Plasmodium vivax and Plasmodium falciparum malaria among duffy-positive and Duffy-negative populations in Ethiopia. Malar J. 2015;14:84.

[21] Prugnolle F, Rougeron V, Becquart P, Berry A, Makanga B, Rahola N, et al. Diversity, host switching and evolution of plasmodium vivax infecting african great apes. Proc Natl Acad Sci U S A. 2013;110:8123-8128.

[22] Buery JC, Rodrigues PT, Natal L, Salla LC, Loss AC, Vicente CR, et al. Mitochondrial genome of Plasmodium vivax/simium detected in an endemic region for malaria in the Atlantic Forest of Espírito Santo state, Brazil: Do mosquitoes, simians and humans harbour the same parasite? Malar J. 2017;16:437.

[23] Miller LH, Mason SJ, Clyde DF, McGinniss MH. The Resistance Factor to Plasmodium vivax in Blacks. N Engl J Med. 1976;295:302-304. doi:10.1056/NEJM197608052950602.

[24] Livingstone FB. The Duffy blood groups, vivax malaria, and malaria selection in human populations: a review. Hum Biol. 1984;56:413-425.

[25] Neote K, Mak JY, Kolakowski LF, Schall TJ. Functional and biochemical analysis of the cloned Duffy antigen: identity with the red blood cell chemokine receptor. Blood. 1994;84:44-52. doi:10.1016/S0887-7963(05)80035-5.

[26] Carvalho GB de, Carvalho GB de. Duffy blood group system and the malaria adaptation process in humans. Rev Bras Hematol Hemoter. 2011;33:55-64. doi:10.5581/1516-8484.20110016.

[27] Reid ME, Lomas-Francis C. The blood group antigen Factbook. Elsevier Academic Press; 2004. doi:10.1007/s13398-014-0173-7.2.

[28] Tournamille C, Colin Y, Cartron JP, Kim CL Van. Disruption of a GATA motif in the Duffy gene promoter abolishes erythroid gene expression in Duffy-negative individuals. Nat Genet. 1995;10:196-201.

[29] Welch SG, McGregor IA, Williams K. The duffy blood group and malaria prevalence in Gambian west africans. Trans R Soc Trop Med Hyg. 1977;71:295-296.

[30] Isaac IZ, John RT, Udomah FP, Imoru M, Erhabor O, Femi A. Duffy Blood Group Distribution among Patients in a Malaria Endemic Region. Int J Trop Dis Heal. 2016;19:1-5.

[31] Erhabor O, Shehu CE, Alhaji YB, Yakubu A. Duffy Red Cell Phenotypes among Pregnant Women in Sokoto, North Western Nigeria. J Blood Disord Transfus. 2014;5:7-11.

[32] Howes RE, Patil AP, Piel FB, Nyangiri OA, Kabaria CW, Gething PW, et al. The global distribution of the Duffy blood group. Nat Commun. 2011;2:226-225.

[33] King CL, Adams JH, Xianli J, Grimberg BT, McHenry AM, Greenberg LJ, et al. Fya/Fyb antigen polymorphism in human erythrocyte Duffy antigen affects susceptibility to Plasmodium vivax malaria. Proc Natl Acad Sci. 2011;108:20113-20118. doi:10.1073/pnas.1109621108.

[34] Niang M, Thiam LG, Sow A, Loucoubar C, Bob NS, Diop F, et al. A molecular survey of acute febrile illnesses reveals Plasmodium vivax infections in Kedougou, southeastern Senegal. Malar J. 2015;14:281.

[35] Mendes C, Dias F, Figueiredo J, Mora VG, Cano J, de Sousa B, et al. Duffy negative antigen is no longer a barrier to Plasmodium vivax - molecular evidences from the African West Coast (Angola and Equatorial Guinea). PLoS Negl Trop Dis. 2011;5:e1192.

[36] Poirier P, Doderer-Lang C, Atchade PS, Lemoine J-P, de l'Isle M-LC, Abou-bacar A, et al. The hide and seek of Plasmodium vivax in West Africa: report from a large-scale study in Beninese asymptomatic subjects. Malar J. 2016;15:570. doi:10.1186/s12936-016-1620-z.

[37] Mbenda HGN, Das A. Molecular evidence of plasmodium vivax mono and mixed malaria parasite infections in duffy-negative native cameroonians. PLoS One. 2014;9:e103262.

[38] Michon P, Stevens JR, Kaneko O, Adams JH. Evolutionary relationships of conserved cysteine-rich motifs in adhesive molecules of malaria parasites. Mol Biol Evol. 2002;19:1128-1142.

[39] Feng X, Carlton JM, Joy DA, Mu J, Furuya T, Suh BB, et al. Single-nucleotide polymorphisms and genome diversity in Plasmodium vivax. Proc Natl Acad Sci. 2003;100:8502-8507. doi:10.1073/pnas.1232502100.

[40] Imwong M, Sudimack D, Pukrittayakamee S, Osorio L, Carlton JM, Day NPJ, et al. Microsatellite variation, repeat array length, and population history of Plasmodium vivax. Mol Biol Evol. 2006;23:1016-1018.

[41] Gruszczyk J, Kanjee U, Chan LJ, Menant S, Malleret B, Lim NTY, et al. Transferrin receptor 1 is a reticulocyte-specific receptor for *Plasmodium vivax*. Science (80-). 2018;359:48-55.

[42] Abdelraheem MH, Albsheer MMA, Mohamed HS, Amin M, Hamid MMA. Transmission of Plasmodium vivax in Duffy-negative individuals in central Sudan. Trans R Soc Trop Med Hyg. 2016;110:258-260.

[43] Dalgleish T, Williams JMG., Golden A-MJ, Perkins N, Barrett LF, Barnard PJ, et al. Dsitribution of blood groups in the east African Somali Population. J Exp Psychol Gen. 2007;136:23-42.

[44] Mathews HM, Armstrong JC. Duffy blood types and vivax malaria in Ethiopia. Am J Trop Med Hyg. 1981;30:299-303.

[45] Erhabor O, Babatunde S, Uko KE. Some haematological parameters in plasmodial parasitized HIV-infected Nigerians. Niger J Med. 2006;15:52-55.

[46] Babamale O, Ugbomoiko U. Status of malaria infection in peri-urban community of north central region of Nigeria. J Bacteriol Parasitol. 2016;07:1-6. doi:10.4172/2155-9597.1000256.

[47] Mbenda HGN, Gouado I, Das A. An additional observation of Plasmodium vivax malaria infection in Duffy-negative individuals from Cameroon. J Infect Dev Ctries. 2016;10:682-686.

[48] Ménard D, Barnadas C, Bouchier C, Henry-halldin C, Gray LR. Plasmodium vivax clinical malaria is commonly observed in Duffy-negative Malagasy people. Proc Natl Acad Sci. 2010;107:5967-5971.

[49] Rubio JM, Benito A, Roche J, Berzosa PJ, García ML, Micó M, et al. Semi-nested, multiplex polymerase chain reaction for detection of human malaria parasites and evidence of Plasmodium vivax infection in Equatorial Guinea. Am J Trop Med Hyg.

1999;60:183-187. http://www.ncbi.nlm.nih.gov/pubmed/10072133.

[50] Russo G, Faggioni G, Paganotti GM, Djeunang Dongho GB, Pomponi A, De Santis R, et al. Molecular evidence of Plasmodium vivax infection in Duffy negative symptomatic individuals from Dschang, West Cameroon. Malar J. 2017;16:74.

[51] Poirier P, Lang CD, Atchade PS, Lemoine JP, Louise M, De C, et al. The hide and seek of Plasmodium vivax in West Africa : report from a large - scale study in Beninese asymptomatic subjects. Malar J. 2016;15:570.

[52] Ryan JR, Stoute JA, Amon J, Dunton RF, Mtalib R, Koros J, et al. Evidence for transmission of Plasmodium vivax among a Duffy antigen negative population in Western Kenya. Am J Trop Med Hyg. 2006;75:575-581.

[53] Graffeo R, Masucci L, Bugli F, Damiano F, Pinnetti C, Federico G, et al. Multiple malaria infection in a pregnant woman from Nigeria: Detection by multiplex PCR. New Microbiol. 2008;31:565-567.

[54] Gunalan K, Lo E, Hostetler JB, Yewhalaw D, Mu J, Neafsey DE, et al. Role of Plasmodium vivax Duffy-binding protein 1 in invasion of Duffy-null Africans. Proc Natl Acad Sci. 2016;113:6271-6276.

[55] Auburn S, Getachew S, Pearson RD, Amato R, Miotto O, Trimarsanto H, et al. Genomic Analysis of *Plasmodium vivax* in Southern Ethiopia Reveals Selective Pressures in Multiple Parasite Mechanisms. J Infect Dis. 2019; Xx Xxxx.

[56] Menard D, Chan ER, Benedet C, Ratsimbasoa A, Kim S, Chim P, et al. Whole Genome Sequencing of Field Isolates Reveals a Common Duplication of the Duffy Binding Protein Gene in Malagasy Plasmodium vivax Strains. PLoS Negl Trop Dis. 2013;7:e2489.

[57] Chan ER, Menard D, David PH, Ratsimbasoa A, Kim S, Chim P, et al. Whole Genome Sequencing of Field Isolates Provides Robust Characterization of Genetic Diversity in Plasmodium vivax. PLoS Negl Trop Dis. 2012;6:e1811.

[58] Neafsey DE, Kevin Galinsky, Jiang RHY, Young L, Sykes SM, Saif S, et al. The malaria parasite Plasmodium vivax exhibits greater genetic diversity than Plasmodium falciparum. Nat Genet. 2012;44:1046-1050.

[59] World Health Organisation. Basic malaria microscopy. (2010).

[60] Lin, E. *et al.* Differential Patterns of Infection and Disease with P. falciparum and P. vivax in Young Papua New Guinean Children. PLoS ONE **5**, e9047 (2010).

[61] Pattanasin, S. *et al.* Evaluation of a new Plasmodium lactate dehydrogenase assay (OptiMAL-IT) for the detection of malaria. Trans. R. Soc. Trop. Med. Hyg. **97**, 672-674 (2003).

[62] Tjitra, E., Suprianto, S., Dyer, M., Currie, B. J. & Anstey, N. M. Field evaluation of the ICT malaria P.f/P.v immunochromatographic test for detection of *Plasmodium falciparum* and *Plasmodium vivax* in patients with a presumptive clinical diagnosis of malaria in eastern Indonesia. *J. Clin. Microbiol.* **37**, 2412-2417 (1999).

[63] Fransisca, L. *et al.* Comparison of rapid diagnostic test Plasmotec Malaria-3, microscopy, and quantitative real-time PCR for diagnoses of Plasmodium falciparum and Plasmodium vivax infections in Mimika Regency, Papua, Indonesia. *Malar. J.* **14**, 103 (2015).

[64] Abba, K. *et al.* Rapid diagnostic tests for diagnosing uncomplicated

non-falciparum or *Plasmodium vivax* malaria in endemic countries. Cochrane Database Syst. Rev. (2014) doi:10.1002/14651858.CD011431.

[65] Gruenberg, M. *et al.* Plasmodium vivax molecular diagnostics in community surveys: pitfalls and solutions. Malar. J. **17**, 55 (2018).

[66] Li, J. *et al.* Regulation and trafficking of three distinct 18 S ribosomal RNAs during development of the malaria parasite. J. Mol. Biol. **269**, 203-213 (1997).

[67] Wampfler, R. *et al.* Strategies for Detection of Plasmodium species Gametocytes. PLoS ONE **8**, e76316 (2013).

[68] Pinzon, C. *et al.* Real-Time Quantitative Reverse Transcription PCR for Monitoring of Blood-Stage Plasmodium falciparum Infections in Malaria Human Challenge Trials. Am. J. Trop. Med. Hyg. **86**, 383-394 (2012).

[69] Demas, A. *et al.* Applied genomics: data mining reveals species-specific malaria diagnostic targets more sensitive than 18S rRNA. J. Clin. Microbiol. **49**, 2411-2418 (2011).

[70] Hester, J. *et al.* De Novo Assembly of a Field Isolate Genome Reveals Novel Plasmodium vivax Erythrocyte Invasion Genes. PLoS Negl. Trop. Dis. **7**, e2569 (2013).

[71] Chen, S.-B. *et al.* Whole-genome sequencing of a Plasmodium vivax clinical isolate exhibits geographical characteristics and high genetic variation in China-Myanmar border area. BMC Genomics **18**, 131 (2017).

[72] Cunha, M. G. *et al.* Development of a Polymerase Chain Reaction (PCR) method based on amplification of mitochondrial DNA to detect Plasmodium falciparum and Plasmodium vivax. Acta Trop. **111**, 35-38 (2009).

[73] Batista-dos-Santos, S., Raiol, M., Santos, S., Cunha, M. G. & Ribeiro-dos-Santos, Â. Real-time PCR diagnosis of Plasmodium vivax among blood donors. Malar. J. **11**, 345 (2012).

[74] Souza, C. R. T. *et al.* Prevalence of Plasmodium falciparum and P. vivax in an area of transmission located in Pará State, Brazil, determined by amplification of mtDNA using a real-time PCR assay. *Genet. Mol. Res.* GMR **11**, 3409-3413 (2012).

[75] Haanshuus, C. G. *et al.* A novel, single-amplification PCR targeting mitochondrial genome highly sensitive and specific in diagnosing malaria among returned travellers in Bergen, Norway. *Malar. J.* **12**, 26 (2013).

[76] Katrak, S. *et al.* Performance of Loop-Mediated Isothermal Amplification for the Identification of Submicroscopic Plasmodium falciparum Infection in Uganda. Am. J. Trop. Med. Hyg. **97**, 1777-1781 (2017).

[77] Lau, Y.-L., Lai, M.-Y., Fong, M.-Y., Jelip, J. & Mahmud, R. Loop-Mediated Isothermal Amplification Assay for Identification of Five Human Plasmodium Species in Malaysia. Am. J. Trop. Med. Hyg. **94**, 336-339 (2016).

[78] Rosenberg, R. Plasmodium vivax in Africa: hidden in plain sight? Trends Parasitol. **23**, 193-196 (2007).

[79] Howes, R. E. *et al.* The global distribution of the Duffy blood group. Nat. Commun. **2**, 266 (2011).

[80] Guerra, C. A. *et al.* The international limits and population at risk of *Plasmodium vivax* transmission in 2009. *PLoS Negl.* Trop. Dis. **4**, e774 (2010).

[81] Price, R. N. *et al.* Vivax malaria: neglected and not benign. Am. J. Trop. Med. Hyg. 77, 79-87 (2007).

[82] Mendis, K., Sina, B. J., Marchesini, P. & Carter, R. The neglected burden of Plasmodium vivax malaria. Am. J. Trop. Med. Hyg. **64**, 97-106 (2001).

[83] McKenzie, F. E. & Mason, D. P. Blood-stage dynamics and clinical implications of mixed Plasmodium vivax-Plasmodium falciparum infections. Am. J. Trop. Med. Hyg. **61**, 367-374 (1999).

[84] Bruce, M. C. *et al.* Effect of Transmission Setting and Mixed Species Infections on Clinical Measures of Malaria in Malawi. PLoS ONE **3**, e2775 (2008).

[85] Kotepui, M., Kotepui, K. U., De Jesus Milanez, G. & Masangkay, F. R. Plasmodium spp. mixed infection leading to severe malaria: a systematic review and meta-analysis. *Sci. Rep.* **10**, 11068 (2020).

[86] Mbakilwa, H. *et al.* Quality of malaria microscopy in 12 district hospital laboratories in Tanzania. Pathog. Glob. Health **106**, 330-334 (2012).

[87] Frean, J. *et al.* External quality assessment of national public health laboratories in Africa, 2002-2009. Bull. World Health Organ. **90**, 191-199 (2012).

Chapter 7

Plasmodium falciparum: Experimental and Theoretical Approaches in Last 20 Years

Abhichandan Das, Upasana Pathak, Sanchaita Rajkhowa and Anupam Nath Jha

Abstract

Malaria, the severe vector-borne disease has embedded serious consequences on mankind since ages, causing deterioration of health, leading to deaths. The causative parasite has a wide distribution aligned from tropical to subtropical regions. Out of all the five species *Plasmodium vivax* and *Plasmodium falciparum* have registered about more than 600 million cases worldwide. Throughout the decades, identification of various antimalarial drugs, targets, preventive measures and advancement of vaccines were achieved. The key to executing malaria elimination is the appropriate laboratory diagnosis. Development includes positive scientific judgments for a vaccine, advanced progress of 3 non-pyrethroid insecticides, novel genetic technologies, possibilities to alter malaria parasite mediation by the mosquito, identification of drug resistance markers, initiation of *Plasmodium vivax* liver stage assessment, perspective to mathematical modeling and screening for active ingredients for drugs and insecticides. Although the last century witnessed many successful programs with scientific progress, however, this was matched with notable obstacles. The mutation in the genes has changed the overall gameplay of eradication. This chapter aims to examine the numerous experimental and theoretical works that have been established in the last two decades along with the ongoing methodologies consisting of detailed explanations necessary for the establishment of new targets and drugs.

Keywords: *Plasmodium falciparum*, vector-borne, protozoa, vaccine

1. Introduction

Malaria has been a curse to mankind since early ages. It is initiated by a protozoan parasite, infecting the human circulation system. The disease is distributed throughout the tropical and subtropical regions, with transmission caused mainly through the *Anopheles* mosquitoes [1, 2]. In 2018, there were cases of about 228 million around the world which resulted in deaths of about 405,000 people. Initially four different parasite species were reported for transmission. Recently, *Plasmodium knowlesi*, a simian parasite, has been identified as a sporadic source of certain human infections, in the areas of Southeast Asia [3, 4], thus, raising the number to five species.

The *Plasmodium falciparum* species are spread worldwide and has an ability to inhibit the host physiology during the infection, making it more fatal as compared to other species [5].

Experimental study in 1991 showed that *Plasmodium falciparum* gradually evolved from two avian parasites which later got transferred to human [6]. However, in 2011, it was found that the parasite *P. falciparum* actually arose from *P. praefalciparum* rather than directly originating from the avian parasite and eventually got segregated into human parasites. The parasite basically infects humans, gorillas and chimpanzees, and *P. falciparum* of the *Laverania* family is the only species that flourishingly got transferred from apes to humans [7].

Development of vaccines is another way to overcome the burden of malaria in lieu of drugs. Unfortunately, the complicated biology, diverse genome and the life cycle of the malarial parasite has been obstructing the vaccine development process thus; no effective vaccination (licensed) has been approved against malaria [8]. The available vaccines can be categorized into: attenuated forms of microbes, inactivated microbes or protein-based subunit [9]. Recent parasitologist had made an attempt to manufacture a vaccine that can produce entire parasites in adequate quantities to stimulate immunity [10].

1.1 Treatment regimes

A remarkable progress has been achieved in the mission of eradication of malaria from mosquito nets to artemisinin-based combination therapies (ACTs). In 1820, Quinine, the world's first anti-malarial drug was introduced. It was isolated from the cinchona's bark and was administered as tonic water. Later on, various natural as well as synthetic compounds were introduced [11]. However, the development of drug resistance for the existing drug led to a failure of the treatment. Drugs with improved efficacy and potency were introduced to deal with the resistance. Recent study on drug resistance showed that *de novo* resistances are appearing more rapidly [12, 13]. The first case of drug resistance ever reported was in 1980, it was against Quinine [14].

In order to overcome drug resistance, the antimalarial drugs were administered through a combination treatment called Artemisinin-based combination therapy (ACT). The artemisinin and its derivatives compounds are still used as antimalarial drugs during the parasite stages [15, 16]. The world health organization (WHO) still suggests the use of ACT against *falciparum* [17]. Currently, *Plasmodium falciparum* has almost developed resistance for every drug available [18]. The list of drug molecules undergoing clinical trials (last two decades) is given in **Table 1** [19]. So, there is a desperate need for new antimalarial drugs in the market.

To tackle the high morbidity and mortality caused by malarial parasites chiefly in young children, a global malaria control strategy, prompt and explicit diagnosis with treatment of malaria is indispensable to accomplish a convenient cure, along with developing numerous drugs against it. However, various surveys described and reported resistance for pretty much all available antimalarial drugs that broaden the vital requirement for the development of new antimalarial drugs against substantiated existing targets, and to initiate search for novel targets in order to eradicate the speedily mutating parasites.

In this chapter, we have discussed the recent computational as well as experimental procedures that have taken place in order to facilitate the diagnosis along with the development of new antimalarial drugs in the last two decades.

Drug Name	Year	Mechanism of Action
AQ 13	2007	Not resolved so far
OZ277+ Piperaquine	2007	check the *Pf*-encoded sarcoplasmic endoplasmic reticulum calcium ATPase
MMV048	2012	parasite enzyme phosphoinositol 4-kinase enzyme inhibition
Albitiazolium (SAR9727)	2012	Restricting choline transfer within the parasite
P218	2012	*Pf*DHFR inhibitor
KAF156 Ganaplacide/ lumefantrine	2014	Not yet resolved
SJ733	2014	The P-type Na + –ATPase transporter
Sevuparin (DF02)	2014	Anti-adhesive polysaccharide derived Blocks merozoite invasion and sequestration
M5717 (DDD498)	2015	It inhibits PfeEF2, where an attaching pocket for M5717 was not explained.
KAE609 (cipargamin)	2015	Na + -TPase 4 ion channel-inhibitor
Fosmidomycin + Piperaquine	2015	DOXP pathway
Artefenomel (oz439) + Piperaquine	2016	Synthetic endoperoxide
DSM265	2017	Suppress dihydroorotate dehydrogenase enzyme
Methylene Blue	2017	Inhibits *P. falciparum* glutathione reductase to check haem polymerization
MMV390048	2017	Phosphatidylinositol 4-kinase (PfPI4K) inhibitor

Table 1.
List of the ongoing clinical trial carried out for as drug against malaria in the last two decades (2000–2020).

2. Experimental approaches concerning detection of malaria

For the detection and diagnosis of malaria-parasite infections and to tackle it effectively, multiple experimental procedures have been established to meet the specific demands during the entire diagnosis process. In this chapter we have mentioned the recently reviewed and developed strategies of standard means which include microscopic procedures, RDT or the rapid diagnostic tests, immunochromatographic tests, and molecular level identification, signified by systems based on PCR, additionally its limitations with recent trends on several new methodologies. These analyses provide practical comparisons, clarification and the feasibility between distinct diagnostic tests.

2.1 Routine laboratory diagnosis

Instant malaria diagnosis with productive outcomes reduces the probability of infection and minimizes community spreading as well. Hence, malaria is initially identified in the laboratory, employing different techniques. These procedures possess several advantages along with some shortcomings due to which recent modifications and new laboratory methodologies are being applied for future operations.

2.1.1 Blood smear as stained films

For malaria recognition, the laboratory procedure undertaken is the preparation with microscopic analysis of Giemsa, Field's or Wright's stained films of blood. Thick and thin smear of blood are taken either by needling a finger or an earlobe. Evolved trophozoites are measured by their densities which are prominent in blood mainly in the regions where abundant capillaries are found; hence, it is the ideal specimen. Blood acquired by puncture of veins, gets accumulated in the covering of EDTA or heparin anticoagulant channel, is sustainable whenever it is utilized for the closure in the modification of the leukocytes structure along with the parasites [20, 21].

2.1.1.1 Blood film (thin)

Methanol and Giemsa or Wright's stain (diluted) is used to fix and stain respectively for the preparation of thin blood smear (film) and moderate water is employed at pH of 7.2. Since, in this technique, fixed RBC monolayer is obtained, parasite recognition by morphology is done at the stage of species and the particularity is raised in comparison to the study by the thick film. Further infections, where reactions for remedy can be examined, are done by the capability to add parasites in the sequential blood films.

2.1.1.2 Blood film (thick)

The red blood cells are centralized by the thick blood smear on the compact side and are stained as an immense composition by staining with Field, Wright or Giemsa techniques. This blood film method has very intense sensitivity as the blood elements are more concentrated. This is due to the thick smear of blood and is used for the observation of less quantity of parasitemia. It is vastly superior than the thin film with returning the passing on of parasites throughout the infectious phase restoration or degeneration [22].

2.1.1.3 Application example of microscopic inspection of blood smears

A comparative analysis was undertaken by Cortés et al., in 2018 of the technique originated and put forward by the world health organization, and employed for the pre-elimination programs and detection with cure of malaria in Colombia. The acceptable procedure was the thick film (two) composition which is stained by the improved Romanowsky stain in the same slide with its technical characteristics, of storage, low cost, usage along with a cure for the diagnosis of malaria which was from the consequences after the investigation [23].

2.1.2 Fluorescence microscopy

Substitute methodologies are established to intensify the blood film based recognition of malarial parasites. Specific dyes that are fluorescent have empathy for the genetic material present in the nucleus of the parasite that must affix in its nuclei. The nucleus becomes excessively luminant when UV light is used at a proper distance to excite it. Fluorochromes often used are acridine orange as well as benzothiocarboxypurine, both when energized gives fluorescence of yellow or apple green at 490 nm. Rhodamine-123 is beneficial in order to evaluate the parasite's feasible condition, when in consideration to the absorption that depends on the entire working parasitic membrane [24].

2.1.2.1 Acridine orange (AO)

AO is a staining technique which is directed or combined to an assembly practice like the thick smear of blood employed in numerous procedures. By employing a particular long focal length objective accompanying a fluorescence microscope, the capillary tube can be helpful for the verification of the parasites. Within the passage of the transmitted beam of light an excitation filter is organized and enrolled by the simpler Kawamoto technique as well as permitting the affected wavelength of AO which is 470 to 490 nm, to move through the film stained. Additionally, in the ocular another filter of 510 nm has been set for making comprehensible AO stained fluorescing parasites observation.

2.1.2.2 Benzothiocarboxypurine (BCP)

BCP is another methodology utilized that can be put into a dry film of blood or in a suspension of lysed blood, unfixed along with profoundly staining the nucleic acid of feasible *P. falciparum* parasites. Inversely, the nuclei of leukocytes and RBC inclusions are not stained properly. The necessity of speedy investigation to halt precipitation of the dye is controlled by this activity, which was characteristic in some fluorescence systems. This element is noticed as a delicate and quick detection medium, similar to the staining by Giemsa stain, in various reports described mainly as *P. falciparum* having 95% sensitivity along with its specificity. Further, in the thick-film composition, the non-*P. falciparum* parasites are effortlessly recognizable compared to the QBC buffy coat. Workers having practice and performing these procedures where components with fluorochromes are involved can distinguish the parasites quickly and accurately.

Nowadays, fluorescent microscopes that are transportable and apply light emitting diode mechanization, glass slides that are pre-prepared as well as parasites labelling using fluorescent indicators, are accessible commercially [25].

2.1.3 Rapid diagnostic tests (non-microscopic)

Rapid diagnostic tests or RDTs are another very effective assay for the diagnosis of malaria which are contributing as a fascinating substitute for microscopy, detecting malaria parasite antigens and enzymes and forms the foundation of diagnosis in various impoverished areas where laboratory approaches are rare. Employing an immunochromatographic method, the RDT uses monoclonal antibodies to determine the antigen of malaria in 5 to 15 μL blood which is aimed at antigens specific utilizing a test strip for its permeation. The outcomes of these assays may be acquired in between 5 to 20 minutes that are elucidated from lines which are colored, present/absent on the strip. Aldolase (*P. falciparum* histidine rich protein II) and *Plasmodium* lactate dehydrogenase are identified by these tests. Considerably, for the differentiation of non-*falciparum* in between the *falciparum* infections, results from these procedures integrate any two among all the antigens for an attempt.The results from these test mechanisms are less accurate than outcomes obtained from microscopy achieved under routine field circumstances [26, 27].

2.1.4 Immunochromatographic assays

Immunochromatographic assays also known as Immunochromatography, over the surface of nitrocellulose membrane liquid, are relocated. In opposition to a target that is an antigen of malaria in conjugation with liposome constituting mobile phase with either gold particles or selenium dye, these methods got accepted with detainment of antigen from parasite obtained in peripheral blood and monoclonal antibodies are used in the entire process. During the immobile phase, a strip of nitrocellulose is taken where monoclonal antibodies are put in, which is the second/third capture. During the mobile phase, the antigen–antibody complex is migrated alongside the strip, which permits the antigen labeled to record through the monoclonal antibody in the immobile phase constructing a colored visible line. Various physical features of the component reagents are crucial for migration and it is clear that the system is controlled for migration when a labeled goat anti mouse antibody capture is incorporated [28, 29].

2.1.5 Immunochromatographic dipstick assays

RDT dipstick format is another assay and is commercially accessible with its kits for the investigation of malarial antigens. In many laboratory investigations, comparison of immunochromatographic as well as conclusion acquired from PCR and also microscopic procedures has been examined. Even though some constructors of HRP-2 tests exist without the availability of published records, experiments for HRP-2 detection including ParaSight, ICT Pf or Pf/Pv together with PATH *falciparum* Malaria IC analysis was carried out on a large scale which are commercial dipstick trials.

For the *P. falciparum* identification in samples of blood, average sensitivity between 77% and 98% in attendance of 100 parasites/1micro liter with 0.002% parasitemia was resulted from experimental methodologies using ParaSight F immunochromatographic process of HRP-2. When compared with microscopic technique of thick blood smear, specificity between 83% and 98% for *P. falciparum* was obtained. The incapability of the viewer for the parasite exposure employing microscopic tests at densities reduced to 200 parasites/l or the failure of indistinct positive lines observation from the test strip is reflected by the insignificant level of sensitivity from multiple analysis [30, 31].

2.1.5.1 Application example of Rapid diagnostic tests

Speculative treatment with anti-malarial to all feverish patients gives rise to enormous over-treatment. Accordingly, it was directed to reduce drastically over-treatment with antimalarials on its prescription to evaluate malaria rapid diagnostic tests execution consequences at urban Tanzania, which was studied by D'Acremont *et al.*, in 2011. Clinician experts with appropriate encouragement assemble with guidance of negative result patients for not treating them. Thus, to prevent unjustifiable use of antibiotics, execution of mRDT should be unified closely besides instructions for the control of various fever origins [27].

For the extraction of overall nucleic acid from operated mRDTs, Guirou *et al.* recently investigated and constructed and considerably estimated a technique. The observation along with the measurement of *P. falciparum* from patients with asymptomatic behavior by reverse transcription quantitative PCR which is allowed by the isolation of nucleic acids from low volumes of blood retained (dried) on the RDTs. Based on the procedure of separation they assembled Extraction of Nucleic Acids with RDTs procedure, an absolute advancement of extensive molecular malarial supervision. ENAR furnishes a strong mechanism to examine RNA and DNA from numerous RDTs in a high throughput and standardized way, disclosed during a review of malaria benchmarks employing RDTs collected. Finally, they got various novel and previously existed polymorphisms spreading in the Bioko Island of Equatorial Guinea, which were of single nucleotide and non-synonymous in the propeller zone of the kelch 13 gene [32].

2.1.6 Molecular diagnostic procedures

Molecular diagnostic techniques are the inspections where genetic material or the nucleic acids are being targeted and are verified as frequent, certain and acute processes. Nucleic acid tests choose gene sequences like the *P. falciparum* STEVOR multigene family, 18 s ribosomal RNA gene sequences, telomere-associated repetitive component and mitochondrial DNA. Recent progresses in various molecular biological mechanisms including PCR and loop-mediated isothermal amplification (LAMP) have allowed considerable description of the malaria parasite which is bringing new approaches for malaria diagnosis.

2.1.6.1 PCR based methods

Recently, a number of PCR assays came into existence during malaria detection at a molecular level and among various other methods, it is manifested considerably as very sensitive and distinct techniques, particularly for low parasitemia or mixed infection examples. Beneficial knowledge is offered by multiplex and nested PCR mechanisms when demanding structural issues occur throughout the strive to recognize the species level parasites. A minimum of 1 to 5 parasites/µl blood approximated about 50 to 100 parasites/µl blood from RDT and microscopy can be recognized by PCR techniques. The species picked out is validated from the methods using reverse transcription PCR along with nested PCR. Parasites of malaria can be detected upto species level even in patients of minimum parasitemia level, and is the chief benefit of employing techniques that are PCR based. And these systems mostly investigate mutations and strain variation. Moreover, PCR can assist spot and examine parasite genes interrelated to mixed infections or drug resistance and also maximum numbers of specimens might be automated [33, 34].

2.1.6.2 LAMP technique

The Loop-mediated isothermal amplification (LAMP) technique is an additional nucleic acid method. This process has the possibilities of making adjustable strategies field based on nucleic acid, since low PCR with instrumentation is only needed and is effortless. Unlike PCR, amplification takes place at a constant temperature in LAMP and is an isothermal procedure.

In comparison to PCR, LAMP utilizes primers of three sets thus, challenging PCR in terms of quantity of DNA. The amplification can be determined in real time by checking the rise in the magnesium pyrophosphate quantity viz. turbidimetry. PCR is expensive and less sensitive than LAMP, which is also an uncomplicated approach, yet it has the downside for the necessity of a low temperature repository of reagents [35, 36].

2.1.6.3 Application example of PCR based methods

A study by Calderaro *et al.*, in 2018 analyzed the current mode of imported malaria with revised inquiry as well as described the case results with their treatment, throughout January 2013 to June 2017, in Parma, Italy, with surveying the differentiation of the three indicative methods employed detection of malaria: microscopic techniques, Real-time PCR and immunochromatographic tests identifying, *Plasmodium malariae*, *Plasmodium falciparum, Plasmodium vivax, Plasmodium knowlesi, Plasmodium ovale curtisi and Plasmodium ovale wallikeri*. In their research, within the non-endemic areas, without multiple classic symptoms in different cases, the clinicians might get encouraged from the data described to doubt as malaria and to explain by parasitologists, the outcome of microscopic methods, other recommended procedures, and methodologies of molecular level to keep away from mis-detection [37].

A research from the Reference Laboratory for final malaria interpretation resembled the identification from laboratories of peripheral Belgian by Loomans *et al.*, in 2019. The records of The Reference Laboratory for each specimen submitted in 2013–2017 were examined. As a result, very adequate malaria recognition mostly of *P. falciparum* was provided by the laboratories in a malaria non-endemic environment, with *P. falciparum* parasite density calculations and standard identification of non-*falciparum* infection [38].

2.2 Disadvantages and recent trends

The microscopic inspection in smears of blood, RDTs or rapid diagnostic tests with molecular or nucleic acid based methods consists of particular defects and restrictions in constructive utilization at environments where sufficient resources are not available. The enrichment and detachment without disrupting the parasite, which could not be acquired from these systems, might be crucial in malaria parasite study. To intensify the observation of iRBCs, further new practices were implemented by some research teams. Utilization of non-woven fabric size based filtration is one of the simple and inexpensive methodologies. Out of numerous other procedures, magnetophoretic with dielectrophoretic concepts are possessing pleasing prospects in the verification of malarial parasite recently, because of individual conversions with magnetic as well as electrical effects of hRBCs in contrast to iRBCs.

Furthermore, other procedures, in particular, deformability in addition to cell morphology, seemed acceptable for future use as biomarkers. An excessive magnetic field gradient can be generated by a Magnetic-field generating system throughout an immense region [39]. Next explanation is a mixture of more than two diagnostic assays, to raise the specificity to iRBCs, thus amplifying the capacity to detect and separate malaria and infected erythrocyte respectively.

3. Computational approaches against eradication of *P. falciparum*

Potential inhibitors against *P. falciparum* have been identified using different approaches like high-throughput screening (HTS) and drug discovery based on target approach. The HTS approach consists of identification of novel and effective inhibitors which facilitates the development of hits and validation of leads. The action mechanism of the leads, once validated, is identified. The advantage of this mechanism is that it helps to directly identify active compounds. Once the active compounds are successfully identified, the targets of only those compounds are validated. Another approach to drug discovery is target-based. This approach exploits the information of the target and thus, identifies new inhibitors using this information.

3.1 System biology approach

Establishing a target is a crucial part in drug discovery. In the past two decades few targets have been established as potential targets against antitubercular drugs. Target identification is mostly achieved by biochemical methods, genetic interaction or any other computational methods. In computational methods, target establishment involves gaining a detailed knowledge at atomic level along with study of structures of proteins, sequences of genes, pathways (metabolic) and protein–protein interactions (PPI) [40]. In a nutshell, finding a protein/receptor as a target, where a lead compound, a potent drug, may bind. Using the genetic data, various techniques have been approved for searching a potent drug target. They can be summarized into four groups: *Gene-to-Target* method, *Disease-to-Target* method, Gene network and protein–protein interaction network.

3.1.1 Gene-to-target method

Initially, the common drug target classes were selected, later, computational techniques have been used to determine a new target and predict its function. Kinases protein, G-protein coupled receptors (GPCRs), the ions channel, and nuclear receptors are successfully established target classes.

After target class identification screening of possible new gene candidates is done from the sequence database. New gene candidates not only allow us in discovering new targets but also help us in understanding the disease at molecular level.

The human genome database contains a vast number of gene coding new proteins, thus, data mining the database can reveal new essential candidates of the target class. BLAST is the most commonly used technique for finding the similar sequence from the database. Sometimes more sophisticated approach viz., PRINTS are used. However, this limitation can be controlled using various *in-silico* techniques which include features like physiochemical properties, amino acid compositions etc.

The expressed sequence tags (ESTs) allow us resources for characterization of gene, identification of new gene and expression of gene with specific tissue. The EST database (dbEST) not only helps in identifying new genes of the class target but also expression of gene Wittenberger *et al.* illustrated an EST database method to search for a new member of the superfamily, GPCR. They have found about 14 new members as new putative for GPCRs [41].

Gene function identification is one of the most essential parts for drug discovery. Function prediction is proved to be a difficult task, even species like *Escherichia coli* contain about ~30% genes whose-of gene's functions are still unknown. Similarly, in *Plasmodium falciparum* about ~60% of the genes are lacking their function [42]. The approaches for gene function prediction are still way back than lagging behind as compared to the progress that has been made in genome sequencing [43].

3.1.2 Disease-to-target method

Identifying a target requires the study of the origin of the disease and their relation with the system. This method initially focuses on one specific disease and later on various approaches like expression of gene and analysis of linkage are acquired for identifying disease related genes along with potent targets for drugs.

Hundreds of gene expressions can be generated and utilized to identify disease related genes and potent target thorough microarray. Microarray techniques, apart from identifying gene targets and pathways, also allow us to understand the biological process of the disease. Identification of the target can be done by understanding how a potent drug or compound influences a particular metabolic pathway or regulates a network in cellular metabolism.

Predicted disease models that are used during experimentation can be used for validating a target. Thus, a disease model at the molecular level predicts the compounds that are best against the disease and also to perform the binding of the ligand through *in-silico*. Pettipher *et al.* have used this approach to find out inflammatory diseases associated with GPCRs. This leads to identification of new targets associated with genetics [44].

3.1.3 Gene network method

This method deals with the modeling of signaling, endogenous metabolic and regulatory networks along with potent drugs interacting with targets. This helps in recognizing if a target is inhibited and it resulted in inhibition of other activities which are in relation with that pathway. The interactions of genes are essential for studying the structure, functions and the organism's response. There is a possibility of deducing the gene network predictive model by the over expression of the gene present in the network and calculating the overall expression result of the entire gene during a stable state in the gene network. Simulation and analysis through mathematics can make a successful prediction. Various computational approaches have been approved as equation models, Bayesian networks and Boolean networks for deducing regulatory gene networks.

3.1.4 Protein–protein interactions (PPIs) network

In the drug discovery process proteins act as the main target. The expression of protein on both the normal and the diseased one plays a crucial role in drug targets and drugs development. PPI network is one of the methods for identifying essential drug targets. The interaction map of protein shows the important pathways which can be studied for target identification. They are further validated in the biological model. Although there are hundreds of pathways associated with a disease metabolism, the main role is picking out an essential node in the complex gene or protein network which can be utilized as a potent target [45]. The graphical representation of the pathway can estimate the overall topology and target node but the behavior of cell response is quite limited. To overcome this kinetic model approach was adapted.

In the static network method the constructed network is analyzed using various topological analyses which can be related to various functions and regulation mechanisms. Further a constructed static network can be compared with a well-known network thus, revealing various unknown biological functions of the system [46]. Some examples are Cytoscape, String and Gephi.

Kinetic model is also known as the mathematical approach used to determine the dynamics of the biological system. The model can be validated under various environments. The kinetic model uses some of the reaction parameters viz. Michaelis constant (K_m), turnover number (K_{cat}) and enzyme concentration (E_0). In absence of experimentally estimated parameters, parametric estimation methods and Monte Carlo are used [47].

In this context, Bora *et al.* have selected about 39 proteins out of which 15 proteins were screened out for further studies. This protein's interaction was retrieved from the STRING database. The filtered proteins along with their interacting protein are subjected to cytoscape to create a network. Further for mutant modeling and structure analysis the Adenylosuccinate lyase (ADSL) is selected. The docking resulted in ADSL complex, docked with AMP. MD simulation is performed for stability analysis [48]. Bora *et al.* have performed a computational study on *Leishmania donovani*, integrating PPI with metabolic pathways. Purine salvage pathway was considered for the study and the overall biochemical reactions were taken from the KEGG database, then the kinetic model was subjected to simulation in "COPASI". Finally, the PPI of *L. donovani* is derived from "STRING version 10.5" which was analyzed in Cytoscape using the cytohubba plugin [49].

3.1.4.1 Application examples of target identification against P. falciparum using systems biology approach

P. falciparum PPIs were identified using high-throughput kind of yeast-two hybrid assay. LaCount *et* al. identified about 2,846 new interactions of which most of them were uncharacterized proteins. Further, the *in-silico* analysis of PPIs connectivity of the network, gene expression which are coding for interacting segments and Gene Ontology were done to identify protein interacting with mRNA, transcription, modification of chromatin and those taking part in the invasion of the host cell [50]. Proteins having topology associated with significant graphs and high degree were considered as drug targets.

Saha *et al.* have made a case study of pathogens (*P. falciparum*) with host (Human). PPIs of both interacting with each other are derived from the STRING database. The node weight and edge weight has been computed simultaneously. Protein's centrality and connectedness values play a crucial role in organization of function. The node and network centrality identifies the most important protein in the network. Around 457 new interactions were identified of which 198 bait proteins and 217 prey proteins were mapped to the STRING database. Further, PANTHER was used for the analysis of functional similarity [51].

3.2 Bioinformatics approach

Bioinformatics approach facilitates identification of targets for drugs, drug molecules and screening of compounds. In addition to this it also scrutinized the side effects along with prediction of resistance of drugs. It covers almost every aspect of mechanism drug discovery through data of high throughput [52]. Apart from this homology modeling and protein simulation covers the field for more vivid virtual screening and docking studies.

3.2.1 Protein structure prediction

Tertiary structure of protein is the most essential requirement for studying the folding, unfolding along with the function of a protein. But determining the structure is not always easy. X-ray crystallography, nuclear magnetic resonance (NMR spectroscopy) and Cryo-electron microscopy (Cryo-EM) are the major techniques used for prediction of the protein 3D structure. But each of them has its own limitation keeping aside the cost part. In the past few decades computational techniques have developed quite a lot. Predicting the 3D structure not only allows studying the folding and unfolding of the protein but also may facilitate new function in a protein. The tertiary structure of proteins is mainly achieved in three ways:

3.2.1.1 Based on empirical energy calculations

Energy minimization, also known as *ab-initio,* is a way of predicting protein structure. The structure is established by the minimum energy of a protein structure at thermodynamics equilibrium. Rather than making an account on the theory of the amino acid properties it aims in locating the protein's free energy global minima as it resembles the conformation of the naive protein. Some of the essential force fields used are CHARMM, GROMOS, AMBER, ECEPP, and ROSETTA-ab initio.

3.2.1.2 Based on experimentally determined 3D structure Knowledge approaches

Knowledge based approaches are another way of predicting the 3D structures. Currently, comparative modeling or better known as homology modeling is the most common and powerful technique utilized for predicting the tertiary structure of proteins. It compares the query sequence of protein with a similar sequence to that of a known crystal structure. Thus, a precise model can be established based on sequence similarities along with building the model and energy minimization. MODELER and Distance geometry are the most commonly used analysis tools.

Another approach is the threading which aims for selecting the most possible fold of the query sequence or recognizing the possible sequences which fold into the structure. Recognizing a fold needs the perfect alignment of query sequence to that of a folding motif's amino acids. Precise structure can be designed only if atomic level details of the folds are available [53].

3.2.1.3 Hierarchical methods

The last alternate approach for predicting protein structure is the Hierarchical approach which uses the overall hierarchy, i.e., primary to tertiary structure. Here the prediction of the secondary structure is done for understanding the association between the primary sequence and the 3D structure. Few methods based on physicochemical feature approach, statistical approach, combinatorial approach, information on evolution and artificial intelligence approach have been adopted for predicting the secondary structure. Even though, using these algorithms the accuracy rate is still at 80% [54].

Intensive study of chloroquine (CQ) drug resistance in *P. falciparum* identified transporter protein (*Pf*CRT) association with the resistance. Antony *et al.* modeled both the wild and mutant type of *Pf*CRT 3D structure in Robetta and I-TASSER using threading [53]. Similar work has been performed by Sanasam and Kumar. An essential protein of *P. falciparum* AMR1 has been identified as a potential vaccine candidate. They predicted the 3D structure of AMR1 in ROSETTA using an *ab-initio* approach. Further, they predicted the best B-cell and T-helper epitopes of the protein [55]. Borah *et al.* analyzed the sequence of HopS2 protein which revealed many essential regions of the protein secondary structure. The target is then subjected to homology modeling in Swiss model but for lack of low coverage of the sequence the target has been modeled using an *ab-initio* approach. MD simulation in 100 ns has validated the stability of the target protein [56].

3.2.2 Computer-aided drug design approaches

Experimentally screening thousands of compounds along with their targets is quite laborious as well as time consuming too. As a result, *in-silico* methods were adopted, to identify the perfect hits and also improvise the probability of finding a precise drug molecule. For initiating drug discovery and design, various techniques are available, which are mostly: ligand-based (LBDD) and structure-based (SBDD) drug designing. LBDD approach involves methods such as pharmacophore modeling and quantitative structure–activity relationships (QSAR) whereas the SBDD approach involves methods such as molecular docking and molecular dynamics simulation.

3.2.2.1 Quantitative structure–activity relationships (QSAR)

Development of a quantitative structure–activity relationship equation is entirely based on the assumption that the molecular structure can be quantitatively correlated with the molecule's physicochemical or biological activity. Thus, the working concept behind this methodology is the differences observed in the biological activity of a series of compounds which can be quantitatively correlated with the differences in their molecular structure [57]. The final outcome of a logical and mathematical procedure is known as the molecular descriptor and it should be able to transform the chemical information, encoded in a molecular symbolic representation [58].

Some of the commonly used descriptors are the **hydrophobic descriptors** which represent the whole molecule size or lipophilicity [59] using properties like the molecular weight, volume and logarithm of partition coefficient in 1-octanol and water (log P), etc. **Steric descriptors** are those which explain both the shape and size of the molecules and the substituents. Some commonly used steric descriptors are the Taft's steric constant Es, molar refractivity (MR), surface areas, molecular volume, etc. **Topological descriptors** are obtained from hydrogen-depleted molecular graphs. Wiener index, structural information content, Chi index, molecular similarity, electro-topological state atom (ETSA) indices and Kappa index, etc. are some of the commonly used Topological descriptors [60]. **Electronic descriptors** are those that can justify the electronic properties of a molecule and are represented by descriptors such as, the Hammett constant (σ, σ-, σ+), charge transfer constants, dipole moments, ionization constant pKa, ΔpKa parameters derived from molecular spectroscopy and parameters derived from quantum chemical calculation. The quantum chemical descriptors based on **density functional theory (DFT)** and semi-empirical methods have been found to play a major role in QSAR studies. Some of the commonly used DFT-based descriptors are the chemical potential (μ), global hardness (η), global softness, electrophilicity index (ω), etc. The study for artemisinin (an important class of antimalarial drugs) and its derivatives using the DFT based descriptors confirmed that one of the molecules (molecule-13) was the most reactive considering the electronic configuration [61].

3.2.2.2 Pharmacophore modeling

Pharmacophore modeling is the assembling of all the frameworks of a particular molecule which are necessary features for a molecule to inhibit a target's biological response. Over the course of time this methodology has become crucial tools in drug discovery and designing. Designing a model can be accomplished by using **ligand based** where the active molecules are superimposed and similar electronic and steric features of importance are considered and **structure based** where the interaction between the target and the ligand are explored [62]. Manhas *et al.* did a pharmacophore study where they attempted to identify novel inhibition against *P. falciparum* dihydroorotate dehydrogenase (*Pf*DHODH) and also utilized docking and MD [63].

3.2.2.3 Molecular docking

SBDD is based on the target and the ligand's 3D data whereas LBDD can be implied in absence of targets 3D structure. Here, the ligands were known which remained bound with the targets. Further, the targets were analyzed to decrypt the structural as well as chemical properties of the ligands. Molecular docking is divided into three types: flexible, semi-flexible and rigid docking. During the past decades, different types of approaches have been made like conformational sampling and induced fit models [64, 65]. Some examples are: GBVI/WSA, LUDI, Monte Carlo, GoldScore and AutoDock.

Hazarika and Jha have considered three different types of docking programs viz. Molegro Virtual Docker, Glide and GOLD, a set of ligands screened out based on the druglikeness properties are considered for docking against the target protein influenza endonuclease, RNA binding protein. The resulting target-ligand complexes lists are considered based on their scoring functions. Among the top 20 compounds, 10 compounds were common in the mentioned software. Thus, indicating some consent of the compounds [66]. Thillainayagam *et al.* carried out an *in-silico* study by screening the set of pyrazole-pyrazoline against the target Histo aspartic protease (HAP). The target is docked with the set of the ligand (Asp 215, His 32 and Ser 35) as their binding site in Auto dock version 4.2. Further, MD simulation revealed HAP-ligand as more stable than HAP [67].

3.2.2.4 Molecular dynamics

Molecular dynamics (MD) simulation technique allowed us to understand the time-dependent behavior of protein-ligand interactions. MD simulation mimics the moment of an atom; the fundamental unit of a molecule, and what it does in real life. In MD simulation, which is based on Newtonian mechanics, forces on each atom are computed provided we know the energy function and positions of the atoms in a system. Generally, 2 fs (femtosecond) is applied for simulating the atom which is integrated with the numerical movement. The common and popular engines available are: GROMACS, DESMOND, CHARMM, NAMD and AMBER. Their integration with message passing interface (MPI) has significantly reduced the overall computational time by making the engines utilize the cores simultaneously [68].

Hazarika and Jha have utilized molecular dynamics in measuring the interactivity of silver nanoparticles on human serum albumin (HSA), a transport protein. Sudden change in its structure can barricade the overall function. The HSA sequence analysis was done using BLASTP and MSA followed by the secondary structure analysis of HSA. Further, MD simulation was performed in GROMACS 2016.4 version for checking the functionality of the nanoparticles with HSA [69]. In order to effectively challenge Epstein-Bar virus, Jakhmola *et al*. have applied molecular docking and MD simulation of glycoprotein H with different phytochemicals and showed their potentials as virus specific therapeutics [70]. Saikia *et al*. performed MD along with molecular docking to check the dynamics of pyrazinamide (PZA) and PZA-functionalized graphene interaction with pncA protein. A total of five sets of systems were subjected to MD simulation. Using Gromacs package 4.5.0 along with OPLS-AA force-field MD was performed [71].

3.2.3 Application examples of drug discovery against P. falciparum using Bioinformatics Approach

P. falciparum falcipains act on hemoglobin degradation, making it a potential target for drugs. Musyoka *et al.* performed an *in-silico* study on falcipain-2, falcipain-3 and their homologs. Using MODELER 9.10 homology models were prepared and docking was done in Autodock 4.2 using the 23 natural compounds against 11 target proteins. Based on docking energies 3D similar search is performed in ZINC. Further, MD simulation confirms the interaction of the derivatives with the targets. Overall they provided a more effective derivative of the compounds, making it well tolerated among humans [72].

Phosphatidylinositol-4-OH kinase (PI(4)K) type IIIβ, a type of lipid kinase has been recognized as an essential imidazopyrazines target. Unavailability of crystal structure posed a challenge for drug development. So, Rajkhowa *et al.* performed an *in-silico* where they utilized homology modeling to model the *Pf*PI(4)KIIIβ 3D structure. And they validated the structure using MD simulations. Moreover, taking the toxicity and hERG liabilities as priorities screening was done for 178 compounds from PubChem database. The ligand and target were subjected to molecular docking in AutoDock 4.2. MD simulation was further utilized against the target-ligand complexes to check stability. The study reported a total of three inhibitors based on the analysis done [73].

4. Conclusion

Malaria, the world's most regular and dreadful tropical disease, considerable actions have been undertaken to arrest or cure malaria from several decades. Diverse *in silico* attempts including high throughput screening that has screened out a number of novel drug molecules like phytochemicals which can be a potent antimalarial drug in near future, antimalarial target determination, modeling of target proteins using homology modeling, Pharmacophore modeling of derivatives in the existing resistant drugs, Ligand and structure based drug designing strategies for the development of potent drugs, along with several experimental techniques. However, it provides sensitivity along with specificity that varies resembling recent technical advances. RDTs are convenient and currently implemented in many remote settings but could lead to overdiagnosis and overtreatment, demanding upgraded quality control. Molecular-biological methodologies put forward the best sensitivities, they can be utilized to identify the development of drug-resistance, are useful for species identification, and also for quantifying parasite density with low parasitemia. However, out of reach to most and are restricted to clinical research. There are various possibilities and a wide range of applications of CRISPR/Cas9 systems evolved in prokaryotes. Using this technique, gene drives to make mosquitoes resistant to malaria have already been planned and further study can be carried out with proper examinations. Also genetically engineered mosquitoes can be developed that produces almost entirely male offspring, consequently helping in malaria eradication. To lessen the parasite would call diagnostic tools which are non-invasive highly sensitive, vigorous and go with the environment established in particular regions.

Acknowledgements

ANJ would like to acknowledge the NECBH project through IITGhy, funded by Department of Biotechnology (DBT) (project number BT/COE/34/SP28408/2018 with Project ID: 116), Govt. of India for providing computational facilities and Tezpur University for financial support.

Author details

Abhichandan Das[1], Upasana Pathak[1], Sanchaita Rajkhowa[1] and Anupam Nath Jha[2*]

1 Centre for Biotechnology and Bioinformatics, Dibrugarh University, Dibrugarh, Assam, India

2 Department of Molecular Biology and Biotechnology, Tezpur University, Tezpur, Assam, India

*Address all correspondence to: anjha@tezu.ernet.in

References

[1] Carter R, Mendis KN. Evolutionary and historical aspects of the burden of malaria. Clin Microbiol Rev. 2002; 15(4):564-594.

[2] Taylor T, Agbenyega T. Malaria. Hunter's Trop Med Emerg Infect Dis Ninth Ed. 2012;695-717.

[3] Singh B, Sung LK, Matusop A, Radhakrishnan A, Shamsul SS, Cox-Singh J, et al. A large focus of naturally acquired *Plasmodium knowlesi* infections in human beings. Lancet. 2004;363(9414):1017-24.

[4] White NJ. *Plasmodium knowlesi*: The fifth human malaria parasite. Clin Infect Dis. 2008;46(2):172-3.

[5] Hanssen E, Goldie KN, Tilley L. Ultrastructure of the asexual blood stages of *Plasmodium falciparum*. Methods in Cell Biology. 2010;96: 93-116

[6] Waters AP, Higgins DG, McCutchan TF. *Plasmodium falciparum* appears to have arisen as a result of lateral transfer between avian and human hosts. Proc Natl Acad Sci U S A. 1991;88(8):3140-4.

[7] Otto TD, Gilabert A, Crellen T, Böhme U, Arnathau C, Sanders M, et al. Genomes of all known members of a Plasmodium subgenus reveal paths to virulent human malaria. Nat Microbiol. 2018;3(6):687-97.

[8] Mahmoudi S, Keshavarz H. Malaria vaccine development: The need for novel approaches: A review article. Iran J Parasitol. 2018;13(1):1-10.

[9] Hill AVS. Vaccines against malaria. Philos Trans R Soc B Biol Sci. 2011;366(1579):2806-14.

[10] Hoffman SL, Billingsley PF, James E, Richman A, Loyevsky M, Li T, et al. Development of a metabolically active, non-replicating sporozoite vaccine to prevent *Plasmodium falciparum* malaria. Hum Vaccin. 2010;6(1):37-41.

[11] Butler AR, Khan S, Ferguson E. A brief history of malaria chemotherapy. J R Coll Physicians Edinb. 2010;40(2):172-7.

[12] Edwards RL, Odom John AR. Muddled mechanisms: Recent progress towards antimalarial target identification. F1000Research. 2016;5(0):1-10.

[13] Corey VC, Lukens AK, Istvan ES, Lee MCS, Franco V, Magistrado P, et al. A broad analysis of resistance development in the malaria parasite. Nat Commun. 2016;7(1):1-9.

[14] Bunnag D, Karbwang J, Na-Bangchang K, Thanavibul A, Chittamas S, Harinasuta T. Quinine-tetracycline for multidrug resistant *falciparum* malaria. Southeast Asian J Trop Med Public Health. 1996;27(1):15-8.

[15] Paloque L, Ramadani AP, Mercereau-Puijalon O, Augereau JM, Benoit-Vical F. *Plasmodium falciparum*: multifaceted resistance to artemisinins. Malaria Journal. 2016;15:149.

[16] Cui L, Su XZ. Discovery, mechanisms of action and combination therapy of artemisinin. Expert Review of Anti-Infective Therapy. 2009;7:999-1013.

[17] Cui L, Mharakurwa S, Ndiaye D, Rathod PK, Rosenthal PJ. Antimalarial drug resistance: Literature review and activities and findings of the ICEMR network. American Journal of Tropical Medicine and Hygiene. 2015;93:57-68.

[18] Ridley RG. Medical need, scientific opportunity and the drive

for antimalarial drugs. Nature. 2002;415:686-93.

[19] Belete TM. Recent progress in the development of new antimalarial drugs with novel targets. Drug Des Devel Ther. 2020;14:3875-89.

[20] Tangpukdee N, Duangdee C, Wilairatana P, Krudsood S. Malaria diagnosis: A brief review. Korean J Parasitol. 2009;47(2):93-102.

[21] Phillips A, Bassett P, Zeki S, Newman S, Pasvol G. Risk factors for severe disease in adults with *falciparum* malaria. Clin Infect Dis. 2009;48(7):871-8.

[22] Bailey JW, Williams J, Bain BJ, Parker-Williams J, Chiodini PL. Guideline: The laboratory diagnosis of malaria. Br J Haematol. 2013;163(5):573-80.

[23] Cortés LJ, Muñoz L, Ayala MS. Comparison of methodologies for microscopic malaria diagnosis. Biomedica. 2018;38(2):244-52.

[24] Ohrt C, Tang D. Impact of microscopy error on protective efficacy estimates in malaria prevention trials. Clin Pharmacol Ther. 1999;65(2):134.

[25] Adeoye GO, Nga IC. Comparison of Quantitative Buffy Coat technique (QBC) with Giemsa-stained thick film (GTF) for diagnosis of malaria. Parasitol Int. 2007;56(4):308-12.

[26] Basu S, Sahi PK. Malaria: An Update. Indian J Pediatr. 2017;84(7):521-8.

[27] D'Acremont V, Kahama-Maro J, Swai N, Mtasiwa D, Genton B, Lengeler C. Reduction of anti-malarial consumption after rapid diagnostic tests implementation in Dar es Salaam: A before-after and cluster randomized controlled study. Malar J. 2011;10(1):107.

[28] Sondo P, Derra K, Lefevre T, Diallo-Nakanabo S, Tarnagda Z, Zampa O, et al. Genetically diverse *Plasmodium falciparum* infections, within-host competition and symptomatic malaria in humans. Sci Rep. 2019;9(1):1-9.

[29] Yamamoto T, Hashimoto M, Nagatomi K, Nogami T, Sofue Y, Hayashi T, et al. Development of a quantitative, portable, and automated fluorescent blue-ray device-based malaria diagnostic equipment with an on-disc SiO2 nanofiber filter. Sci Rep. 2020;10(1):1-12.

[30] Garrido-Cardenas JA, Cebrián-Carmona J, González-Cerón L, Manzano-Agugliaro F, Mesa-Valle C. Analysis of global research on malaria and *Plasmodium vivax*. Int J Environ Res Public Health. 2019;16(11).

[31] Jin X, Luong TL, Reese N, Gaona H, Collazo-Velez V, Vuong C, et al. Comparison of MDCK-MDR1 and Caco-2 cell based permeability assays for anti-malarial drug screening and drug investigations. J Pharmacol Toxicol Methods. 2014;70(2):188-94.

[32] Guirou EA, Schindler T, Hosch S, Donfack OT, Yoboue CA, Krähenbühl S, et al. Molecular malaria surveillance using a novel protocol for extraction and analysis of nucleic acids retained on used rapid diagnostic tests. Sci Rep. 2020;10(1):1-14.

[33] Lucchi NW, Narayanan J, Karell MA, Xayavong M, Kariuki S, DaSilva AJ, et al. Molecular Diagnosis of Malaria by Photo-Induced Electron Transfer Fluorogenic Primers: PET-PCR. PLoS One. 2013;8(2):1-7.

[34] Talundzic E, Maganga M, Masanja IM, Peterson DS, Udhayakumar V, Lucchi NW. Field evaluation of the photo-induced electron transfer fluorogenic primers (PET) real-time PCR for the detection

of *Plasmodium falciparum* in Tanzania. Malar J. 2014;13(1):1-6.

[35] Bhatt S, Weiss DJ, Cameron E, Bisanzio D, Mappin B, Dalrymple U, et al. The effect of malaria control on *Plasmodium falciparum* in Africa between 2000 and 2015. Nature. 2015;526(7572):207-11.

[36] Gordon EB, Hart GT, Tran TM, Waisberg M, Akkaya M, Skinner J, et al. Inhibiting the mammalian target of rapamycin blocks the development of experimental cerebral malaria. MBio. 2015;6(3):1-17.

[37] Calderaro A, Piccolo G, Montecchini S, Buttrini M, Rossi S, Dell'Anna ML, et al. High prevalence of malaria in a non-endemic setting: Comparison of diagnostic tools and patient outcome during a four-year survey (2013-2017). Malar J. 2018;17(1):1-9.

[38] Loomans L, Conesa Botella A, D'Hondt A, Verschueren J, Van Den Bossche D, Van Esbroeck M, et al. Accuracy of malaria diagnosis by clinical laboratories in Belgium. Malar J. 2019;18(1):1-7.

[39] Kasetsirikul S, Buranapong J, Srituravanich W, Kaewthamasorn M, Pimpin A. The development of malaria diagnostic techniques: A review of the approaches with focus on dielectrophoretic and magnetophoretic methods. Malar J. 2016;15(1).

[40] Schenone M, Dančík V, Wagner BK, Clemons PA. Target identification and mechanism of action in chemical biology and drug discovery. Nature Chemical Biology. 2013;9:232-40.

[41] Wittenberger T, Schaller HC, Hellebrand S. An expressed sequence tag (EST) data mining strategy succeeding in the discovery of new G-protein coupled receptors. J Mol Biol. 2001;307(3):799-813.

[42] Aggarwal K, Lee KH. Functional genomics and proteomics as a foundation for systems biology. Briefings Funct Genomics Proteomics. 2003;2(3):175-84.

[43] Jiang Z, Zhou Y. Using bioinformatics for drug target identification from the genome. Am J PharmacoGenomics. 2005;5(6):387-96.

[44] Pettipher R, Mangion J, Hunter MG, Mackay I. Identification of G-protein-coupled receptors involved in inflammatory disease by genetic association studies. Curr Opin Pharmacol. 2005;5(4 SPEC. ISS.):412-7.

[45] Rain JC, Selig L, De Reuse H, Battaglia V, Reverdy C, Simon S, et al. The protein-protein interaction map of Helicobacter pylori. Nature. 2001;409(6817):211-5.

[46] Sharan R, Ideker T. Modeling cellular machinery through biological network comparison. Nat Biotechnol. 2006;24(4):427-33.

[47] Miskovic L, Tokic M, Fengos G, Hatzimanikatis V. Rites of passage: Requirements and standards for building kinetic models of metabolic phenotypes. Curr Opin Biotechnol. 2015;36:146-53.

[48] Bora N, Nath Jha A. An integrative approach using systems biology, mutational analysis with molecular dynamics simulation to challenge the functionality of a target protein. Chem Biol Drug Des. 2019;93(6):1050-60.

[49] Bora N, Jha AN. In silico Metabolic Pathway Analysis Identifying Target Against Leishmaniasis – A Kinetic Modeling Approach. Front Genet. 2020;11:1-11.

[50] LaCount DJ, Vignali M, Chettier R, Phansalkar A, Bell R, Hesselberth JR, et al. A protein interaction network of the malaria parasite

Plasmodium falciparum. Nature. 2005;438(7064):103-7.

[51] Saha S, Sengupta K, Chatterjee P, Basu S, Nasipuri M. Analysis of protein targets in pathogen-host interaction in infectious diseases: a case study on *Plasmodium falciparum* and *Homo sapiens* interaction network. Briefings in functional genomics. 2018;17:441-50.

[52] Xia X. Bioinformatics and Drug Discovery. Curr Top Med Chem. 2017;17(15):1709-26.

[53] Antony HA, Topno NS, Gummadi SN, Siva Sankar D, Krishna R, Parija SC. In silico modeling of *Plasmodium falciparum* chloroquine resistance transporter protein and biochemical studies suggest its key contribution to chloroquine resistance. Acta Trop. 2019;189:84-93.

[54] Kaur H, Raghava GPS. Prediction of α-Turns in Proteins Using PSI-BLAST Profiles and Secondary Structure Information. Proteins Struct Funct Genet. 2004;55(1):83-90.

[55] Sanasam BD, Kumar S. In-silico structural modeling and epitope prediction of highly conserved *Plasmodium falciparum* protein AMR1. Mol Immunol. 2019;116:131-9.

[56] Borah SM, Jha AN. Identification and analysis of structurally critical fragments in HopS2. BMC Bioinformatics. 2019;19(Suppl 13).

[57] Rosenberg B, VanCamp L, Trosko JE, Mansour VH. Platinum compounds: A new class of potent antitumour agents. Nature. 1969;222:385-6.

[58] Todeschini R, Consonni V. Handbook of molecular descriptors. Methods and principles in medicinal chemistry. Eur J Med Chem. 2001;36(11-12):966.

[59] Buchwald P, Bodor N. Octanol-water partition: searching for predictive models. Curr Med Chem. 1998;5(5).

[60] Devillers J, Balaban AT. Novel Strategies in the Search of Topological Indices. In: Topological Indices and Related Descriptors in QSAR and QSPAR. 2020:413-64.

[61] Rajkhowa S, Hussain I, Hazarika K, Sarmah P, Deka R. Quantitative Structure-Activity Relationships of the Antimalarial Agent Artemisinin and Some of its Derivatives – A DFT Approach. Comb Chem High Throughput Screen. 2013;16(8):590-602.

[62] Yang SY. Pharmacophore modeling and applications in drug discovery: Challenges and recent advances. Drug Discov Today. 2010;15(11-12):444-50.

[63] Manhas A, Lone MY, Jha PC. Multicomplex-based pharmacophore modeling in conjunction with multi-target docking and molecular dynamics simulations for the identification of *Pf*DHFR inhibitors. J Biomol Struct Dyn. 2019;37(16):4181-99.

[64] Hazarika Z, Rajkhowa S, Nath Jha A. Role of Force Fields in Protein Function Prediction. In: Homology Molecular Modeling - Perspectives and Applications. 2020:20.

[65] Rajkhowa S, Deka RC. Protein-ligand docking methodologies and its application in drug discovery. In: Oncology: Breakthroughs in Research and Practice. 2016:891-914.

[66] Hazarika Z, Jha AN. A Comparative Evaluation of Docking Programs using Influenza Endonuclease as Target Protein. 2020 Int Conf Comput Perform Eval ComPE 2020. 2020:321-6.

[67] Thillainayagam M, Ramaiah S, Anbarasu A. Molecular docking and dynamics studies on novel benzene

sulfonamide substituted pyrazole-pyrazoline analogues as potent inhibitors of *Plasmodium falciparum* Histo aspartic protease. J Biomol Struct Dyn. 2020;38(11):3235-45.

[68] Rajkhowa S, Jha AN. Molecular Dynamics Simulations: A Tool to Investigate the Interactions between Biomolecules and Nanoparticles. Nov Sci Publ Inc. 2019;65-108.

[69] Hazarika Z, Jha AN. Computational Analysis of the Silver Nanoparticle-Human Serum Albumin Complex. ACS Omega. 2020;5(1):170-8.

[70] Jakhmola S, Hazarika Z, Jha AN, Jha HC. *In silico* analysis of antiviral phytochemicals efficacy against Epstein-Barr virus glycoprotein H. J Biomol Struct Dyn. 2021, DOI: 10.1080/07391102.2020.1871074

[71] Saikia N, Jha AN, Deka RC. Molecular dynamics study on graphene-mediated pyrazinamide drug delivery onto the pncA protein. RSC Adv. 2014;4(47):24944-54.

[72] Musyoka TM, Kanzi AM, Lobb KA, Tastan Bishop Ö. Structure Based Docking and Molecular Dynamic Studies of Plasmodial Cysteine Proteases against a South African Natural Compound and its Analogs. Sci Rep. 2016;6:1-12.

[73] Rajkhowa S, Borah SM, Jha AN, Deka RC. Design of *Plasmodium falciparum* PI(4)KIIIβ Inhibitor using Molecular Dynamics and Molecular Docking Methods. ChemistrySelect. 2017;2(5):1783-92.

Chapter 8

Malaria Lethality in Children under 5 Years of Age and Study of Risk Factors in MbujiMayi Paediatric Environment, a Neglected Deadly Epidemic in the Democratic of Republic of Congo

Félicien Ilunga-Ilunga, Alain Levêque, Vévé Mbuyi Kanyinda, Jean Paul Mbikayi Muya and Michèle Dramaix

Abstract

The objective of this study was to determine the risk factors for malaria lethality in the MbujiMayi paediatric environment, a follow-up study of hospitalised cases over 5 years was conducted between January 2016 and December 2020 in the four hospitals. The case rate was 6.9% for the total (139 cases of death for 2017 cases of severe malaria for 5 years,) and varied from year to year (10.7% in 2016 to 4.6% in 2020). Cox Proportional Risk Model results including significant covariates in multivariate analysis [HR (IC95%)]. In multivariate analysis, two models were considered. The case-fatality rate was independently associated with late arrival after 48 hours [3.1 (1.9–5.1); p < 0.001], types of pre-hospital recourse such as recourse to the church [1.4 (1.1–2.1),; p = 0.042) and tradipractor [3.2 (1.8–6.1); p < 0.001] for severe malaria, children under 12 months of age [1.8 (1.2–2.8); p < 0.001], those with circulatory collapse [2.6 (1.1–6.1); p < 0.001] and those in deep coma [1.9 (1.1–3.4); p = 0.016]. The second model with the number of associated syndromes, showed that the risk was 1.7 plus for children with a complex clinical picture, made up of the combination of several signs [1.7 (1.1–2.6); p < 0.001]. These results highlight the need for more information campaigns to encourage people to seek institutional care for malaria. Our results also suggest that prophylactic treatment may be advisable for children under 5 years of age.

Keywords: Severe malaria, lethality, child, Risk factors, MbujiMayi, RDC

1. Introduction

Malaria is the first global endemic parasitic disease and its transmission has been reported in about a hundred countries worldwide [1]. Africa is, by far, the most affected continent, twenty-nine countries accounted for 95% of malaria cases globally. Nigeria (27%), the Democratic Republic of the Congo (12%), Uganda (5%),

Mozambique (4%) and Niger (3%) accounted for about 51% of all cases globally Millions of people around the world still do not have access to malaria prevention and treatment, while most cases and deaths are neither reported nor recorded [1, 2]. In the Democratic Republic of Congo, malaria remains the leading cause of consultations, hospitalisations, and deaths. The 2019 National Malaria Control Programme report shows more than twenty-one million cases of malaria, including nineteen million cases of simple malaria and two million cases of severe malaria, as well as thirteen thousand seventy-two malaria-related deaths, including nine thousand eight hundred and fifty-five children under the age of five, i.e., 75% [3]. However, some progress has been noted over the last decade. Proportional morbidity in children under five years of age has decreased from 41% in 2010 to 37% in 2014. Infant mortality fell from 92‰ in 2010 to 58‰ in 2014. Despite this progress, the disease remains endemic in all twenty-six provinces of the country [4].

Many provinces are affected Thus, the proportion of positive children is highest in the Kasai (29% in Kasai Oriental, 32% in Kasai Occidental), Katanga (32%), Maniema (34%) and especially in Province Orientale (38%) [5, 6].

Malaria constitutes a heavy socio-economic burden, especially in MbujiMayi (Kasai-Oriental), where a large part of the population has been destitute since the fall of the Bakwanga mining company (Miba). In this context, access to health care is a problem for the population, which is why many Congolese people in MbujiMayi have been resorting to self-medication and others to traditional medicine to date [6].

The DRC is still paying a heavy price due to malaria. Every hour, somewhere in DRC, "at least 3 families are bereaved because of malaria and more than two children lose their lives due to malaria" [6]. In addition to the coronavirus pandemic that the DRC has been facing since 10 March 2020, the burden of severe malaria in terms of death, especially in the under-five age group, remains considerable. The country is facing an increase in the epidemiological trend of malaria and malaria deaths despite efforts to step up interventions. The development of factors associated with high malaria lethality in children would help to better guide rapid and effective management.

2. Objectives

The objectives were fixed:

- Estimate the breakdown of survival time for children under 5 years of age with severe malaria over the past 5 years,
- determine the risk factors associated with lethality explained by severe malaria in hospitalised children over the past 5 years.

3. Methods

3.1 Context of the study

The town of MbujiMayi is the provincial capital of Kasai-Oriental, which is one of the 26 provinces that make up the Democratic Republic of Congo (DRC). After the new division, this town has 10 health zones considering their demographic density, each of which has a general referral hospital. It comprises 167 health areas (AS), 166 of which are covered by functional health centres. This city covers an area of 168,126 Km2. This city is in the North and is naturally bordered by the Bipemba River, from its source to its confluence with the Muya River and from the latter downstream to its mouth in the Mbuji-Mayi River, thus forming the border with the Territory of Lupatapata. South bounded by the Kanshi River upstream to its point of intersection with the Bena Mbaya Road, a locality located in the Lupatapata Territory.

To the East by the Mbuji-Mayi River upstream to its confluence with the Kanshi River bordering the Katanda et Tshilenge Territory. To the West by the Bena Mbaya road up to the limit of the Makala village. From there to its easternmost point and from this point, straight ahead to the source of the Bipemba River bordering the Lupatapata Territory. Four hospitals were selected and are represented by black dots in **Figure 1**.

3.2 Study environment

The study was performed in four reference hospitals in MbujiMayi. we chose 3 referral hospitals and a provincial hospital: The general referral hospital Saint Jean Baptiste in the Bonzola health zone, Dipumba which is a provincial hospital, the general referral hospital Présbytérien in the Dibindi health zone and the general referral hospital Christ-Roi in the Bipemba health zone. The choice was guided by their high attendance of children aged 0–59 months suffering from severe malaria.

3.3 Target population

This study considered statistical units, all children aged 0–59 months having been admitted to the paediatric ward of three general referral hospitals and a provincial hospital for severe *Plasmodium falciparum* malaria confirmed in the period of our research. The diagnoses were confirmed by identification of the hematozoan parasite via thick smears or blood smears and diagnostic immunological tests with

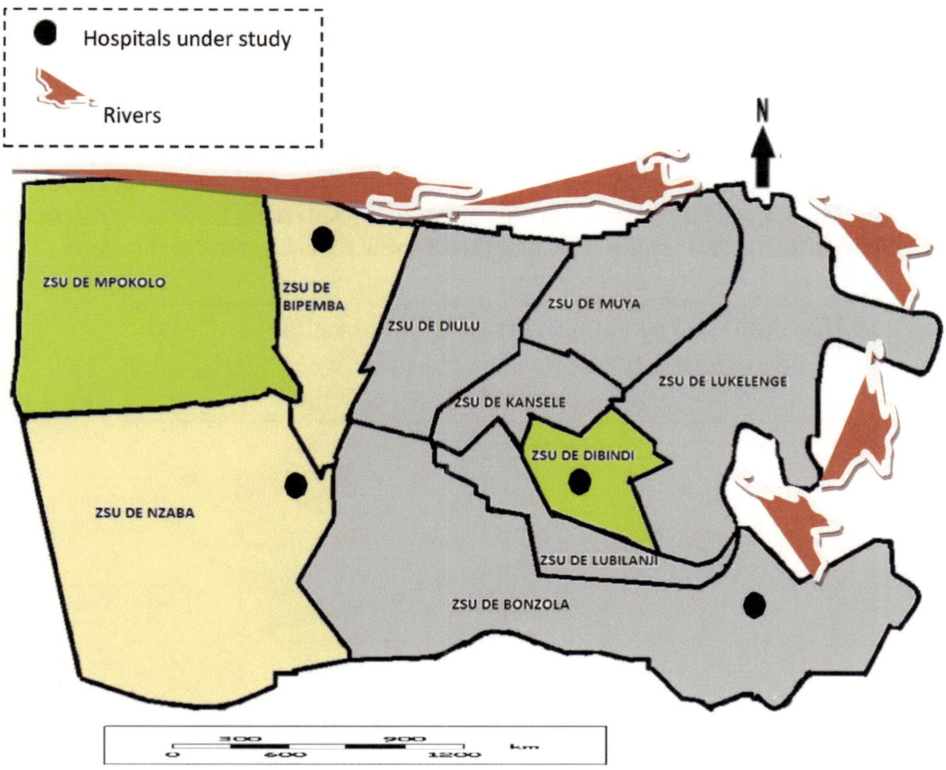

Figure 1.
Health mapping of MbujiMayi town (RDC) showing the location of the hospitals under study.

antigenic strips (i.e., immunochromatographic assay tests) that were performed on whole blood and the associated severities of clinical and biological signs (according to the WHO 2000) [7, 8].

3.4 Inclusion and exclusion criteria

This was an exhaustive sample: all children aged 0 to 59 months, 2017 children hospitalised in MbujiMayi's general reference hospitals for severe malaria from 2016 to 2020, i.e. from 1 January 2016 to 31 December 2020 were enlisted.

3.5 Statistical analyses

Quantitative data are presented as a mean ± standard deviation (SD) for monitoring data, and qualitative data as percentages. Lethality prognostic factors were analysed in uni-variate and multi-variate (Cox model). Survival analysis was carried out according to the Kaplan–Meier method. The logrank test was used to compare survival curves. The Cox model was used to express the instantaneous risk of death as a function of presumed risk factors, considering the time to death. The raw and adjusted risk ratios (HR) and their 95% confidence intervals were derived from the Cox model and the proportionality of the risks was checked by the parallelism of the curves. The statistical significance level used was 5% ($P < 0.05$). All calculations were performed with the STATATH 16 statistical software.

4. Results

The results in this study show that the average age of children with severe malaria was 31 months, statistically comparable by gender (31.3 ± 17.5 months for boys vs. 30.5 ± 17.4 months for girls, student test, $p = 0.334$). Of the 2017 children hospitalised for severe malaria, 1,150 were male or 54.8%. 59.3% lived in the peri-urban area. Nearly all had insecticide-treated mosquito net. And most of the parents were self-employed, without a permanent job, representing 18.9%, proxi of very low socio-economic level.

Evolution of case-fatality rates in children under 5 suffering from severe malaria from 2016 to 2020. The results of this **Figure 2** show that the case-fatality rate

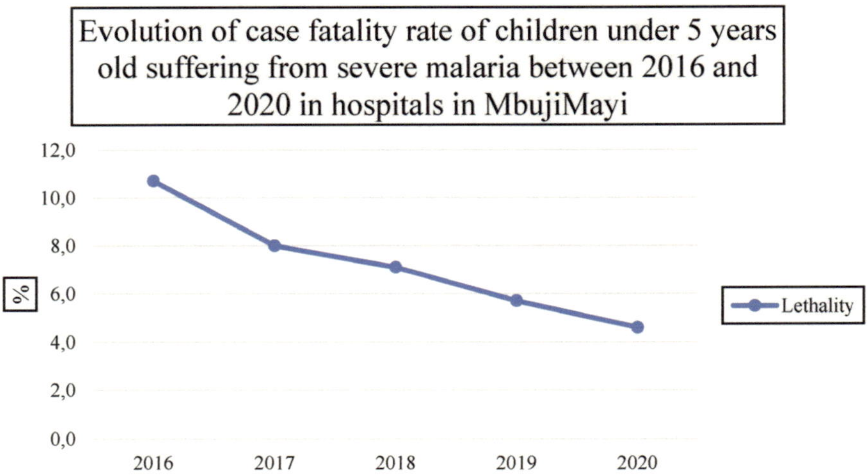

Figure 2.
Trends in case fatality rates among children under 5 years of age with severe malaria from 2016 to 2020).

was more than 6% overall (139 cases of death for 2017 cases of severe malaria for 5 years, or 6.9%) and varied from year to year. The rate decreased gradually from year to year, with a higher rate in 2016 (10.7%) and less than 6% in 2020 (4.6%).

Prognostic factors for lethality in children with severe malaria according to the Cox proportional risk model in uni-variate analysis. Severity factors associated with malaria lethality in uni-variate analysis were demonstrated: the risk of death was twice as high for children with generalised convulsions [2.6(1.8–3.8); $p < 0.001$], three times as high for those in deep coma [3.7(2.6–5.5); $p < 0.001$] and respiratory distress [3.8(2.1–7.1); $p < 0.001$]. All else being equal, the risk of death was more than 10 times higher for children with circulatory collapse (Shock) [10.8(5.1–23.3); $p < 0.001$]. late arrival after 48 hours [5.7(3.7–8.6); $p < 0.001$], and the age of the children, especially those under 12 months of age [27(18–3.9); $p < 0.001$], were also the risk factors highlighted in this study. On the other hand, possession of an insecticide-treated nets proved to be a protective factor [0.1(0.2–0.3); $p < 0.001$], so the risk of dying was less than 1. Statistically, the differences were significant. Cox Proportional Risk Model results including significant covariates in multivariate analysis.

In multivariate analysis, two models were considered. The first model with severity signs taken separately. After adjustment, the case-fatality rate was independently associated with late arrival after 48 hours, types of pre-hospital recourse such as recourse to the church and tradipractor for severe malaria, children under 12 months of age, those with circulatory collapse and those in deep coma. The second model with the number of associated syndromes, adjusted for age, sex, type of

parameters	Hazard Adjusted Ratio (IC95%)	P
Model 1		
Late arrival ≥48 h	3,1(1,9-5,1)	<0,001
Pre-hospital appeal		
Self-medication	1	
churches	1,4(1,1-2,1)	0,042
Tradipraticiens	3,2(1,8-6,1)	<0,001
Age (months)		
<12	1,8(1,2-2,8)	<0,001
≥12	1	
Circulatory Collapse		
Yes	2,6(1,1-6,1)	<0,001
Not	1	
Deep Coma		
Yes	1,9(1,1-3,4)	0,016
Not	1	
Model 2		
Number of associated syndromes		
<2	1	
≥2	1,7(1,1-2,6)	0,016

Table 1.
Cox proportional risk model results including significant covariates in multivariate analysis.

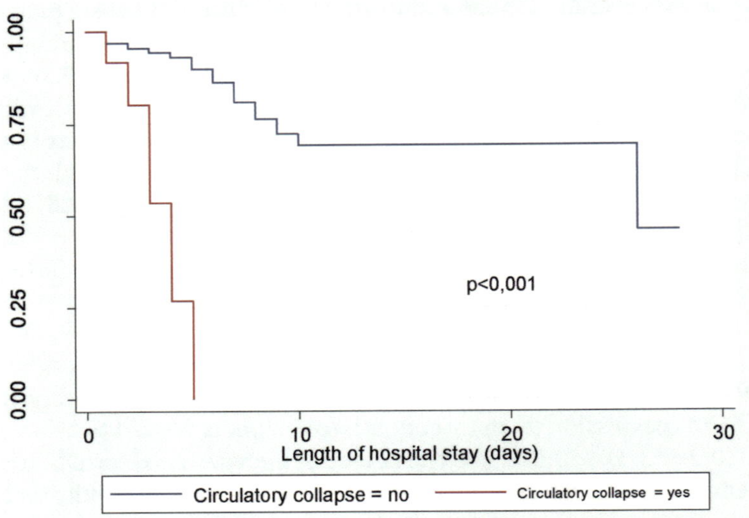

Figure 3.
Kaplan–Meier curve of the duration of follow-up without death observed in 2017 children between 2016 and 2020 depending on the presence or no circulatory collapse as a sign of severity).

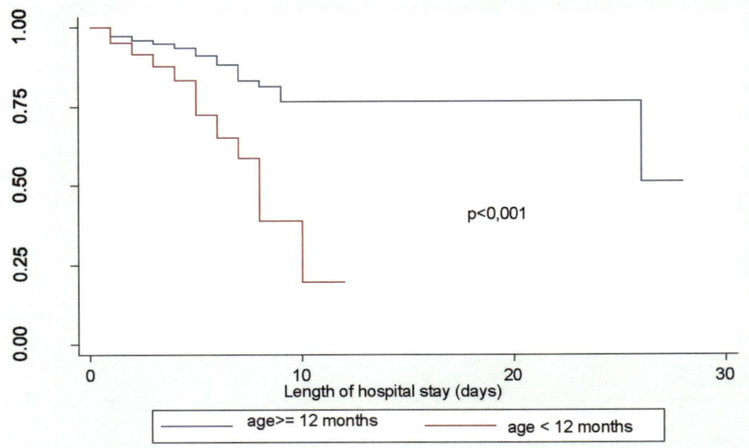

Figure 4.
Kaplan–Meier curve of follow-up without death observed in 2017 children under 12 months and 12 months and more between 2016 and 2020).

recourse and late management showed that the risk was 1.7 plus for children with a complex clinical picture, made up of the combination of several signs [1.7 (1.1–2.6); $p < 0.001$] (**Table 1**).

The different survival curves as a function of the gravity factors associated with malarial lethality in multi-variate analysis.

Figure 3 shows an early shift in the survival curve of children with circulatory collapse compared to children without circulatory collapse. Statistically, the difference was significant (log-rank test, $p < 0.001$).

Figure 4 shows an early shift in the survival curve for children under 12 months of age compared with that of children aged 12 months and over. Statistically, the difference was significant (log-rank test, $p < 0.001$).

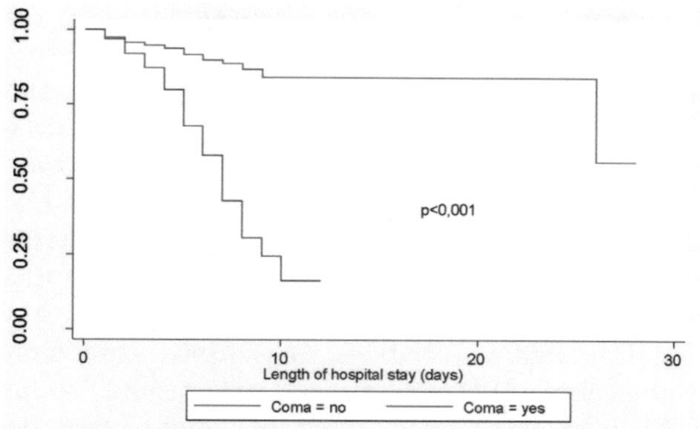

Figure 5.
Kaplan–Meier curve of the duration of follow-up without death observed in 2017 children between 2016 and 2020 with coma or not as a sign of severity.

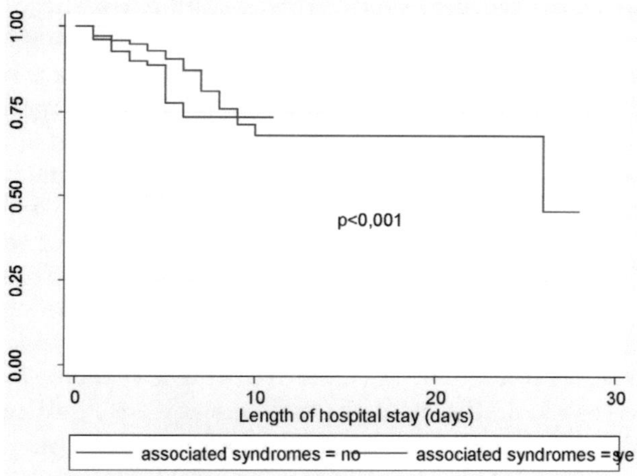

Figure 6.
Kaplan–Meier curve of follow-up duration without death observed in 2017 children between 2016 and 2020 with associated syndrome or without associated syndrome.

Figure 5 shows an early shift in the survival curve of children with coma compared to children without coma. Statistically, the difference was significant (log-rank test, $p < 0.001$).

Figure 6 shows an early shift in the survival curve of children with associated syndromes compared to children without associated syndromes. Statistically, the difference was significant (log-rank test, $p < 0.001$).

5. Discussion

In the present study, the case fatality rate was significantly related to the number of associated clinical syndromes and in many studies conducted elsewhere [9, 10], clinical polymorphism has been shown to be a poor prognostic factor. A complex clinical picture, consisting of a combination of two or more syndromes, has a poor prognosis, especially if management is delayed. The case fatality rate due to severe malaria in children aged 0–59 months in Mbujimayi and its evolution was observed on a sample of 2017 cases hospitalised for severe malaria from 2016 to 2020. During this period, 139 cases of death, i.e. a case-fatality rate of 6.9%, were recorded. As for the evolution over the last 5 years, our results show that the case-fatality rate was more than 6% overall and varied according to the year. The rate decreased progressively from year to year, higher in 2016, less than 6% in 2020. However, this does not mean that the case-fatality rate has decreased over the years. Many cases die without the possibility to be consulted due to lack of financial means [9]. Families are forced to bleed themselves dry to meet the exorbitant cost of treatment, which is a factor in the lack of recourse to modern facilities.

Malaria case fatality remains variable across countries and circumstances. In their studies Ilunga and al [8] found a case-fatality rate of about 5.3% in the city-province of Kinshasa. Considering the importance of signs of severity and the syndrome associated with malaria lethality, our study reveals that the lethality rate was independently associated with late arrival after 48 hours and that the types of pre-hospital recourse such as recourse to church and traditional healers for severe malaria, children under 12 months of age, those with circulatory collapse and those in deep coma. In addition to this, the number of associated syndromes, adjusted for age, sex, type of referral and late management, showed that the risk was 1.7 more for children who presented with a complex clinical picture, consisting of a combination of several signs. All of these were also the risk factors identified in this study for children who were managed. The duration of hospitalisation (delay) is the time elapsed between the onset of the disease and the hospitalisation of the patient. Our results show that this time varies between 2 and 3 days, which confirms the hypothesis that the delay in the management of severe malaria is an important factor in the positive evolution of severe malaria cases in the DRC (malaria becomes very lethal). The results of studies in other African countries also note the same types of risks linked to the lethality of severe malaria. According to the results obtained in our study, the possession of insecticide-treated nets was found to be an effective protective factor in that the risk of dying was less than 1. Statistically, the differences were significant. However, the misuse of this important input by the population for such purposes as football post nets, fishing nets, curtains, poultry rearing, and many other uses should be noted with regret.

Lengeler and al [10] notes that the use of LLIN reduces overall mortality by about 6 lives of children aged 0–59 months that are saved annually. LLIN also reduces clinical episodes of uncomplicated malaria due to *Plasmodium falciparum* and *Plasmodium vivax* by 50%. The effectiveness of LLIN has been widely demonstrated through several other studies whose consistent results have led WHO to recommend it to the various countries affected by this malaria scourge [11].

This lethality observed in the reference hospitals of MbujiMayi is similar to that found in Kinshasa [8] and in other African countries, notably Uganda [12] and Benin [13], but remains lower than that found by several authors in the DRC and in other contexts [11, 14–17]. The study of severity factors associated with malaria lethality in multivariate analysis leads to results like those of univariate analyses. In our study, as in those of other authors [8, 14, 15], prognosis also depends on late hospital admission.

Late hospitalisation of patients contributed to a significant increase in case fatality in our study. Raobijaona et al. [18] showed that the mortality rate was 45% if the delay in care was more than 3 days compared to 8.5% if the child was hospitalised within 24 hours [8, 19]. Our results confirm the frequency and prognostic value of the neurological form. The relevance of this factor in children has been highlighted in other African countries with higher endemicity, such as the DRC [13, 20, 21].

6. Conclusion

The morbid and deadly burden of severe malaria is enormous. As for the evolution of case-fatality rates among children under 5 years old suffering from severe malaria from 2016 to 2020, our results show that the case-fatality rate was over 6% overall and varied from year to year. The rate decreased progressively from year to year, with a higher rate in 2016, less than 6% in 2020.

Compared to the prognostic factors of lethality in children with severe malaria according to the Cox proportional risk model in Uni-variate analysis, we found the results that the severity factors associated with malaria lethality show that the risk of death was 2 times higher for children with generalised convulsions, 3 times higher risk of death for those in deep coma and respiratory distress. All other things being equal, the risk of death was more than 10 times higher for children with circulatory collapse. Late care, the types of pre-hospital care, the age of the children, especially those under 12 months of age, were also the risk factors highlighted in this study.

Rapid and effective management seems necessary if the burden of severe malaria is to be drastically reduced. This epidemic is becoming increasingly neglected with the advent of Codiv 19 and the situation is likely to be out of control with the negative repercussions in the fight against malaria.

Acknowledgements

Our thanks to the first-degree students of Istm Kinshasa and to the authorities of the hospital institutions of the city of MbujiMayi for having facilitated the task of data collection.

Conflict of interest

"The authors declare no conflict of interest."

Author details

Félicien Ilunga-Ilunga[1,2*], Alain Levêque[2], Vévé Mbuyi Kanyinda[3], Jean Paul Mbikayi Muya[3] and Michèle Dramaix[2]

1 Institut Supérieur des Techniques Médicales de Kinshasa, DR Congo

2 School of Public Health, Research Centre in Epidemiology, Biostatistics and Clinical Research, Université Libre de Bruxelles, Brussels, Belgium

3 Institut Supérieur des Techniques Médicales de MbujiMayi, DR Congo

*Address all correspondence to: feilunga@yahoo.fr

References

[1] World.Health.Organization.World. malaria.report.2020.(Available: https:// www.who.int/publications/i/item/ 9789240015791/. Accessed 20 december August 2020).

[2] Rowe AK, Rowe SY, Snow RW, Korenromp EL, Schellenberg JR, Stein C, Nahlen BL, Bryce J, Black RE, Steketee RW. The burden of malaria mortality among African children in the year 2000. Int J Epidemiol, 2006. 35(3): 691-704.

[3] Ministère de la santé publique de la RDC. Plan Stratégique National de Communication 2017-2020, (Available : http://acpcongo.com/acp/plan-strategique-national-de-communication-2017-2020-antipaludique-rdc/ Accessed 20 december August 2020). [In French]

[4] Ministère du Plan et Suivi de la Mise en œuvre de la Révolution de la Modernité (MPSMRM), Ministère de la Santé Publique (MSP) et ICF International, 2014. Enquête Démographique et de Santé en République Démocratique du Congo 2013-2014. Rockville, Maryland, USA : MPSMRM, MSP et ICF International. (Available: https://www. unicef.org/drcongo/media/1046/file/ EDS-RDC%20II%202013-2014.pdf) (Accessed 21 december 2020).[in french]

[5] République Démocratique du Congo, Programme National de Lutte contre le Paludisme (P.N.L.P.). (2016). Rapport annuel des activités de lutte contre le Paludisme 2015. Kinshasa : PNLP.41 [in french]

[6] Programme National de Lutte contre le Paludisme (PNLP). (2010). Plan stratégique national de lutte contre le paludisme 2011-2015. Kinshasa: PNLP.

[7] World Health Organisation. Severe falciparum malaria. Royal Soc of Trop Med and Hyg 2000; 94:90

[8] Ilunga-Ilunga F, Levêque A, Donnen P, Dramaix M. [Children hospitalized with severe malaria in Kinshasa (Democratic Republic of the Congo): Household characteristics and factors associated with mortality] Med Sante Trop Jan-Mar 2015;25(1):75-81. doi: 10.1684/mst.2014.0416.

[9] Ilunga-Ilunga F, Levêque A, Okenge Ngongo L, Tshimungu Kandolo F, Dramaix M. Costs of treatment of children affected by severe malaria in reference hospitals of Kinshasa, Democratic Republic of Congo. J Infect Dev Ctries. 2014 Dec 15;8(12):1574-1583. doi: 10.3855/ jidc.4622.

[10] Lengeler, C, Snow, R.W., 1996, « From efficacy to effectiveness: thé case of insecticide-treated bed nets in Africa », *Bulletin de l'Organisation mondiale de la santé,* vol. 74, n° 3.

[11] Müller O, Traoré C, Kouyaté B, Yazoumé Y, Frey C, Coulibaly B, Becher H. Effets de l'utilisation de moustiquaires de lit imprégnées d'insecticide au cours des premiers mois de la vie dans une zone à transmission palustre intense en Afrique : essai contrôlé randomisé. Bulletin de l'OMS : 202, 5(99) :321-404

[12] Idro R, Aloyo J, Mayende L, Bitarakwate E, John C, Kivumbi G. Severe malaria in children in areas with low, moderate, and high transmission intensity in Uganda, Trop Med Int Health 2006;11:115-124.

[13] Ayivi B, Toljkoljrolj F, Gansey R. Le paludisme grave chez l'enfant au CNHU de Cotonou, Bénin Médical 2000, 14 : 146-152.

[14] Lyke C, Diallo D, Licko A, et al. Association of intaleukocytic Plasmoduim falciparum malaria pigment with disease severity, clinical

manifestations, and prognosis in severe malaria. Am. J. Trop. Med. Hyg 2003 ; 69 :253-59.

[15] Kouéta F, Lassina D, Diarra Y, et al. Facteurs de risque de décès au cours du paludisme grave chez l'enfant au Centre hospitalier universitaire pédiatrique Charles de Gaulle de Ouagadougou (Burkina Faso), Cahiers Santé 2007 ; 17 : 195-199.

[16] Haque U, Magalhães R, Dipak M, et al. The role of age, ethnicity and environmental factors in modulating malaria risk in Rajasthali, Bangladesh. Malar J 2011, 10:367.

[17] Msangeni H, Kamugisha M, Sembuche S, et al. Prospective study on severe malaria among in-patients at Bombo regional hospital, Tanga, north-eastern Tanzania. BMC Infectious Diseases 2011; 11:256.

[18] Raobjaona H, Randrianotahina C, Razanamparany M. Le paludisme de l'enfant au service de pédiatrie du Centre Hospitalier de Befelatanana à Antananarivo (Madagascar) en 1996-1998. Arch Inst Pasteur 2000 ; 66 :23-25.

[19] Mehta U, Durrheim D, Blumberg L, et al. Malaria deaths as sentinel events to monitor healthcare delivery and antimalarial drug safety. Trop Med Int Health 2007;12: 617-628.

[20] Mulumba MP, Muhindo MH, Mandoko AS. Estimation du taux de létalité imputable au paludisme chez les enfants âgés de moins de cinq ans dans les hôpitaux de référence de Kinshasa. Ann Afr Med 2009 ; 2 :143-154.

[21] Camara B, Gueye A, Faye P, et al. Critères de gravité et facteurs pronostiques du paludisme chez l'enfant à Dakar, Médecine et maladies infectieuses 2011 ; 41 :63-67.

Section 3

Policy and Prevention

Chapter 9

New Challenges in Malaria Elimination

Susanta Kumar Ghosh and Chaitali Ghosh

Abstract

In recent years, efforts to eliminate malaria has gained a tremendous momentum, and many countries have achieved this goal — but it has faced many challenges. Recent COVID-19 pandemic has compounded the challenges due to cessation of many on-field operations. Accordingly, the World Health Organization (WHO) has advocated to all malaria-endemic countries to continue the malaria elimination operations following the renewed protocols. The recent reports of artemisinin resistance in *Plasmodium falciparum* followed by indication of chloroquine resistance in *P. vivax*, and reduced susceptibility of synthetic pyrethroids used in long lasting insecticide nets are some issues hindering the elimination efforts. Moreover, long distance night migration of vector mosquitoes in sub-Saharan Africa and invasion of Asian vector *Anopheles stephensi* in many countries including Africa and Southeast Asia have added to the problems. In addition, deletion of histidine rich protein 2 and 3 (*Pfhrp2/3*) genes in *P. falciparum* in many countries has opened new vistas to be addressed for point-of-care diagnosis of this parasite. It is needed to revisit the strategies adopted by those countries have made malaria elimination possible even in difficult situations. Strengthening surveillance and larval source management are the main strategies for successful elimination of malaria. New technologies like Aptamar, and artificial intelligence and machine learning would prove very useful in addressing many ongoing issues related to malaria elimination.

Keywords: Malaria, *Plasmodium vivax*, *P. falciparum*, drug resistance, vector invasion, night migration, insecticide resistance, gene deletions, surveillance, larval source management, elimination, Aptamar, Artificial intelligence, machine learning, COVID-19

1. Introduction

In the past two decades, tremendous progress has been made in the fight against malaria. A great deal of new knowledge on malaria parasite [1], insights in vector biology and control have helped target interventions resulting in substantial transmission reduction globally [2–4]. In 2019, World Health Organization (WHO) estimated 229 million malaria cases and 409,000 deaths in 87 malaria-endemic countries with large concentration of the total malaria burden (94%) in Africa [5]. Global malaria cases declined by 27% between 2000 and 2015, and only 2% between 2015 and 2019 indicating the slow progress rate in this period (**Figure 1**) [5]. Of the 29 countries that contributed 95% of the global malaria cases, Nigeria alone accounted for the highest at 27% followed by Democratic Republic of the Congo (12%), Uganda (5%), Mozambique (4%) and Niger (3%). A compiled data of global malaria cases

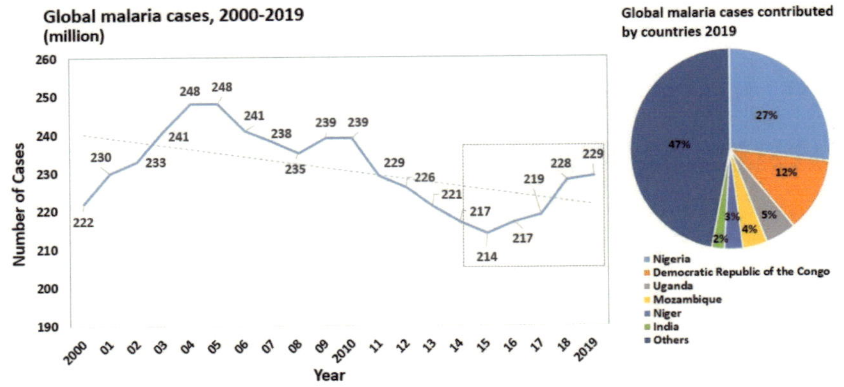

Figure 1.
Trends of global malaria 2000 to 2019. Nigeria alone continue to contribute majority of the cases; in 2019 contributed 27% of total global malaria cases. Compiled from WHO data.

from 2000 to 2019 showed a declining trend (**Figure 1**). But the trend between 2015 and 2019 is not a good indication of malaria elimination goal from 2016 to 2030, as envisaged by the Global Technical Strategy (GTS) of WHO. The population at risk living in the WHO African Region increased from about 665 million in 2000 to 1.1 billion in 2019. The WHO South-East Asia Region (SEAR) accounted for about 3% of the burden of malaria cases globally. India is the major contributor in this region sharing 2% of the total global malaria cases. On the other hand, seven countries namely Algeria, Kyrgyzstan, Uzbekistan, Argentina, Paraguay, Maldives and Sri Lanka have been certified malaria free by WHO from 2015 to 2019 [6]. Among the E-2020 countries: China, Iran, Timor-Leste, Malaysia and El-Salvador reported zero malaria in 2018 setting a precedent that malaria elimination is possible by strengthening surveillance system (**Figure 2**) [7]. In 2020, the whole world experienced an unprecedented situation of COVID-19 pandemic threatening malaria elimination efforts. Most of the public health services were diverted towards managing and containing this severe form of infection caused by SARS-COV-2 virus. Aims and aspirations are high for living in the malaria-free world, yet there are multiple challenges for realizing the goal of malaria elimination by 2030. Enumerated below are some of

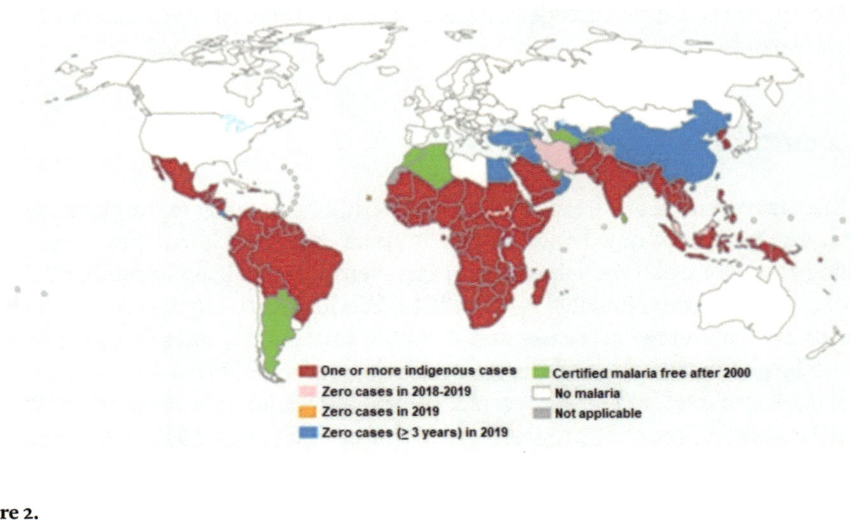

Figure 2.
Global malaria burden. Countries with indigenous cases in 2000 and their status by 2019. Source WHO [5].

issues which should be addressed to strengthen the health systems for the achieving coveted goal of malaria elimination in due time.

2. Search methods

Searched MEDLINE (PubMed); CABS Abstracts; checked the reference lists of all studies identified by the search. Also performed Google Search on specific topics. Examined references listed in review articles and previously compiled bibliographies.

3. The challenges

Besides the current impending threat of COVID-19, many more challenges are being faced in defeating malaria. Some of these are: (a) deletions of *PfHPR2/3* genes in *Plasmodium falciparum* at the point-of-care diagnosis, (b) drug resistance to parasites, (c) migration of parasite strains to newer areas, (d) migration of drug-resistant parasites in low-transmission settings, (e) multi-insecticide resistance in vector mosquitoes, (f) poor disease surveillance, (g) invasion of *Anopheles stephensi* in Africa and elsewhere, (h) long-distance migration of vector mosquitoes in sub-Saharan Africa, and (i) unmet funding drift.

3.1 Gene deletions compromising performance of Rapid Diagnostic Test (RDT) Kits

Rapid diagnostic tests (RDTs) detect species-specific antigens of *P. falciparum* and *P. vivax* parasites present in the blood of infected patients. Histidine rich protein 2 and 3 (*Pfhrp2*, *Pfhrp3*) are widely used in RDTs for point-of-care diagnosis of *P. falciparum*. Naturally occurring deletions of these genes are emerging threat to malaria detection and treatment, management and elimination. *Pfhrp2/3* deletions are increasingly reported from all malaria-endemic regions. Deletion of *Pfhrp2/3* genes in *P. falciparum* is one of the major issues for diagnosis of this dominant species globally. A recent detailed global review by WHO clearly showed a huge problem exists in Amazon basin and Eritrea [8, 9].

In India, two major studies reported the problem is limited to 0 to 23% [10, 11]. The global distribution and prevalence of these deficient genes is presented in **Figures 3** and **4**. In the Peruvian Amazon, there was emergence of a drug-resistance profile BV1 clonal lineage that was distinctly different from the previous genotype found in the region [12]. The BV1 lineage profile posed a significant problem because the strain is multidrug-resistant and escapes detection by *Pfhrp2*-based RDTs secondary to *Pfhrp2/3* deletions. The hypothesis was that the BV1 strain had emerged as a successful parasite lineage for transmission by different vectors and had contributed to the increased malaria burden recently observed in some Amazonian regions [13].

As per the report of WHO, of the 39 reports published in 39 countries, 32 (82%) reported *Pfhrp2* deletions. However, deletions are still unclear when variable methods in sample selection and laboratory analysis are performed. From the 16 published documents in 15 countries between 2019 and September 2020, *Pfhrp2/3* deletions were confirmed in 11 countries from 12 reports. These countries are China, Equatorial Guinea, Ethiopia, Ghana, Myanmar, Nigeria, Sudan, Uganda, United Kingdom (imported malaria cases from various malaria endemic countries), the United Republic of Tanzania and Zambia. However, no deletions were detected in France (among returning travelers), Haiti, Kenya and Mozambique [5].

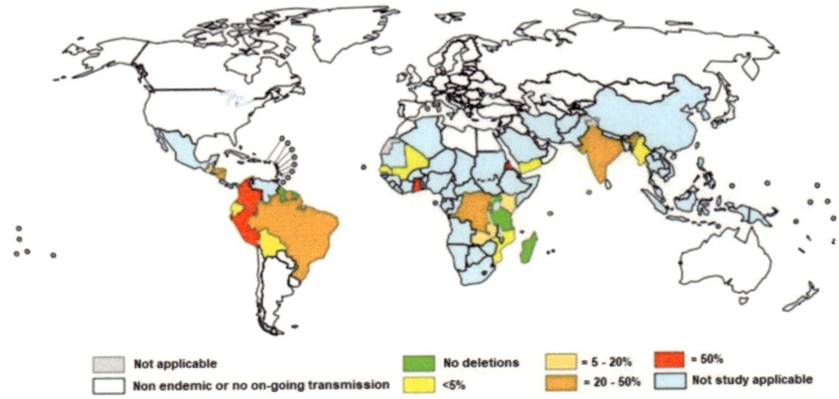

Figure 3.
Highest percentage of Pfhrp2 deletions in P. falciparum cases tested. Source: WHO [8] and Thompson et al. [9].

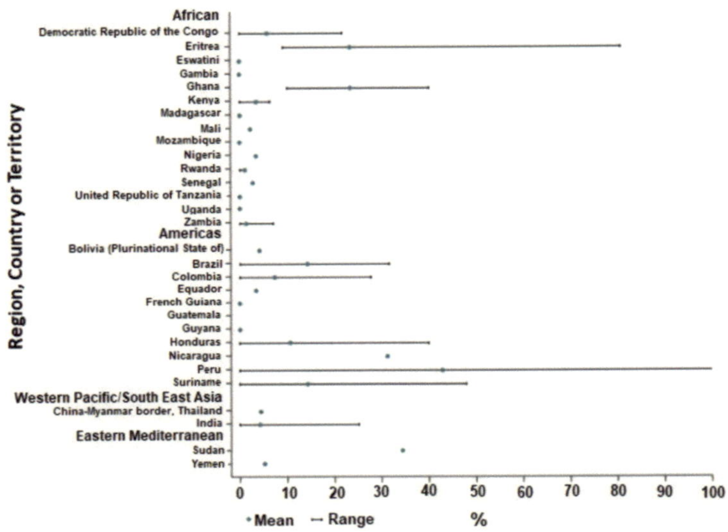

Figure 4.
Weighted average estimates for Pfhrp2 deletions in P. falciparum patients tested by country. Source: WHO [8] and Thompson et al. [9].

3.2 Drug resistance

The WHO recognises that drug resistance is one of the main concerns which requires periodic monitoring and appropriate drug policy in place to stay a step ahead arresting development and spread of drug-resistant malaria. In recent years, molecular monitoring and surveillance of mutant markers has gained pace to help the programme significantly providing an early indication of possible drug failure helping institutes alternated therapeutic regimen for radical cure [14]. *P. falciparum* and *P. vivax* are the two common human malaria parasite species, of which the former is widespread and continually evolving to be drug-resistant (**Figure 5**).

3.2.1 Plasmodium falciparum

Among all human malaria parasite species, *P. falciparum* is the most dominant species especially in sub-Saharan Africa. Recent first high-resolution global map of

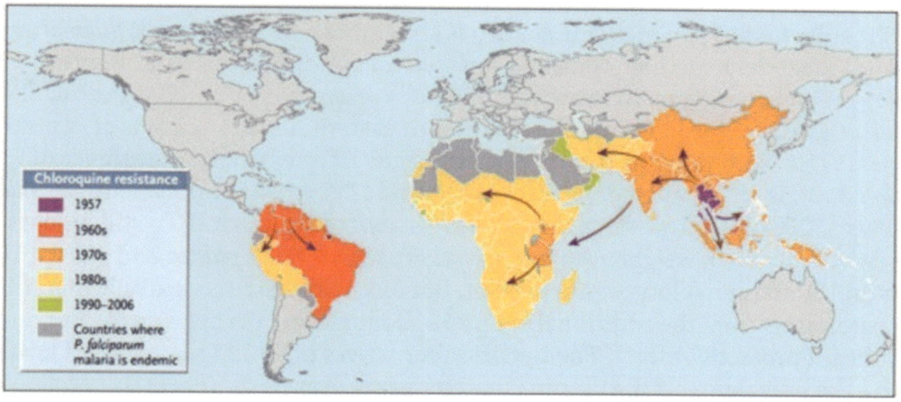

Figure 5.
History of Chloroquine-resistant P. falciparum malaria. Origin of resistance in 1957 from South East Asia and global spread in subsequent years. Source: Packard [16].

falciparum mortality, prevalence and incidence illustrated a rapid decline in burden between 2005 and 2017. However, 90.1% of people continue to reside within sub-Saharan Africa which accounted for 79.4% of cases and 87.6% of deaths in 2017 [15].

Besides *in-vivo* follow-up studies for monitoring therapeutic efficacy, the Technical Consultation Committee of WHO recommended the use of malaria molecular surveillance (MMS) for implementation in malaria elimination and control. Monitoring of molecular marker and therapeutic efficacy studies help to identify and track the prevalence of molecular mutations associated with drug resistance.

3.2.1.1 Chloroquine resistance markers

Once Chloroquine was a first-line drug for malaria treatment but has become obsolete for treatment of *P. falciparum*. Chloroquine-resistant falciparum malaria first reported in Thailand in 1957 (**Figure 5**). Subsequently, it spread through South and Southeast Asia and by the 1970s in sub-Saharan Africa and South America [16]. In India, predominant SVMNT haplotype of *PfCRT* K76Tmutation was first reported in 2004 [17]. Presence of SVMNT haplotype rather than CVIET specific of the African/Southeast Asian haplotype in India was suggestive of prevalence of chloroquine resistance in Indian strains of *P. falciparum* [17]. This helped replacing chloroquine as first-line drug for *P. falciparum* malaria to artemisinin-based combination therapy (ACT). But a study in 2020 in Mizoram (bordering Myanmar), reported prevalence of CVIET haplotype indicating its presence in this region of India [18]. Molecular surveillance of markers has helped trace the route of migration of drug-resistant malaria in the world (**Figure 5**).

3.2.1.2 Sulfadoxine-Pyrimethamine (SP) resistance markers

Dihydropteroate synthase (*dhps*) inhibitors, such as sulfadoxine, and dihydrofolate reductase (*dhfr*) inhibitors, such as pyrimethamine, disrupt parasite's folate synthesis. Antifolate resistance has been associated with point mutations in the *pfdhps* and *pfdhfr* genes. Point mutations at codons 16, 51, 59, 108 and 164 of *pfdhfr* inhibit its activity, and the parasite becomes resistant to pyrimethamine. Two mutations C59R and S108N in *pfdhfr* were recorded to be prevalent in India. While mutations at 436, 437, 540, 580 and 613 of *pfdhps* reduce the substrate binding capacity and confer resistance to sulfadoxine. Three mutations S436A, A437G and K540E were found associated with *pfdhps* [19].

Intermittent preventive treatment in pregnant women (IPTp) and in infants (IPTi) sulfadoxine-pyrimethamine (SP) is recommended to prevent *P. falciparum* malaria in moderate to high transmission areas of sub-Saharan Africa. But the major problem lies on resistance of SP to *P. falciparum*. As per WHO protocol, SP is no more effective for IPTp and IPTi in most of eastern Africa and parts of central Africa. WHO recommends countries to withdraw IPTp when the prevalence of *pfdhps* 540E is >95% and *pfdhps* 581G >10%, and ITPi when the prevalence of *pfdhps* 540E is >50% [20]. However, a recent meta-analysis found that IPTp still reduces the risk of low birth weight even in areas where high level of *pfdhps* and *pfdhfr* quintuple mutant haplotypes are present. But in areas where the sextuple mutant parasite harbouring the additional *pfdhps* 581G mutation ITPi appears to have no significant protective effect. Therapeutic alternatives to SP-IPTp are needed in areas where the prevalence of the sextuple mutant parasite exceeds 37% [21].

3.2.1.3 Artemisinin resistance marker

Artemisinin-based combination therapy (ACT) is presently the drug of choice for treatment of resistant *P. falciparum* malaria. Mutation at *Pfkelch13* propeller gene (*K13*) responsible for its role in Artemisinin resistance supposedly originated in Southeast Asia [22]. WHO has prepared a list of validated *PfKelch13* mutations of partial resistance to artemisinin. These are F446I, N458Y, M476I, Y493H, R539T, I543T, P553L, R561H, P574L and C580Y, and also the candidate markers P441L, G449A, C469F/Y, A481V, R515K, P527H, N537I/D, G538V, V568G, R622I and A675V [5]. A recent review in the *NEJM,* a worldwide map of *K13*-propeller polymorphism found no evidence of Artemisinin resistance outside Southeast Asia and China, where resistance-associated *Pfkelch13* mutations were confined [23]. Later, after comparing the *Pfkelch13* R561H genome sequence to other samples taken from all over Africa, and sequences taken from South America and Bangladesh, it was observed that the artemisinin-resistant strain of the parasite is tightly clustered with Rwandan parasites indicating artemisinin resistance in Africa [24].

In 2019, a report from eastern India indicated the presence of two mutations G625R and R539T in 5/72 *P. falciparum* cases treated with artemisinin that linked to its presence of resistance [25]. But C580Y in *kelch13* in Southeast Asia and Mekong Delta areas were predominant [26]. Following high rates of Artesunate (AS) + Sulfadoxine-Pyremethamine (SP) treatment failure in the north-eastern provinces in 2013, India changed its treatment policy in those provinces to Artesunate-Lumefantrine (AL); while AS+SP remains effective elsewhere in the country [5]. Moreover, a specific lineage of plasmepsin amplification (*PLA1*) has been detected that caused dihydroartesunate-piperquine (DHA-PPQ) treatment failure in western Cambodia due to its use as mass drug administration campaign [5]. Both the lineages of k13 (*KEL1*) and *PLA1* have compounded the problem of DHA-PPQ resistance in this region [13]. In Guyana, between 2010 and 2017, the C580Y mutation also emerged independently. However, recent studies indicated 100% of samples were found to be wild type, indicating that the mutation may be disappearing in Guyana. There is no indication of lumefantrine failure in Africa [5].

3.2.2 Plasmodium vivax

P. vivax was believed to be a benign malaria, but this phenomenon has changed in recent years for its appreciable causes of morbidity and mortality [27]. In recent years, this species has amounted to cause a significant public health burden [28, 29]. Even though there has been a considerable decrease on the burden, still over four billion people are living at risk of this infection. In 2017, vivax transmission was reported from 49 countries across Central and South America, the Horn of Africa, Asia, and the Pacific islands. *P. vivax* is the predominant species in almost two-thirds of co-endemic countries. Recent estimates, incorporating national surveillance data, prevalence surveys, and geospatial mapping, have revised the global burden to between 13.7 and 15 million cases in 2017 [30, 31]. It is assumed that ACT is widely used across Africa to combat falciparum malaria that may be favouring adaptive selection for *P. vivax* for its failure. Additionally, a better understanding is needed on the mechanism of erythrocytes invasion in Duffy-negative individuals who were previously thought to be protected against *P. vivax* malaria [32]. An estimated 82% (11.7 million cases) of the global vivax burden comes from four high-burden countries, i.e. India, Pakistan, Ethiopia, and Sudan [33].

In most countries, chloroquine is still being used for the treatment of blood stages of *P. vivax* malaria. However, chloroquine-resistant (CQR) *P. vivax* has emerged in many areas with variable degree of clinical efficacy [34]. High-grade chloroquine resistance is reported from the intense transmission area of the island of Papua (Indonesia and Papua New Guinea), and Sabah (Malaysia) where malaria elimination is well within reach [33]. To combat the declining susceptibility of *P. vivax* to chloroquine, five countries that include Indonesia, Papua New Guinea, Solomon Islands, Vanuatu and Cambodia have adopted a policy of universal ACT for both *P. falciparum* and *P. vivax* [33]. In other areas where CQR is low-grade and transient, chloroquine remains the main drug of choice for treatment of *P. vivax* malaria including four high-burden countries [33, 34].

Molecular monitoring of chloroquine resistance in *P. vivax* is an integral part of national malaria control programme. The *P. vivax* ortholog of *pfcrt*, referred as *pvcrt-o*, was characterized nearly two decades ago [35]. A lysine (AAG) insertion at amino acid 765 position 10 (K10) was discovered in Southeast Asian strains and suggested to be associated with chloroquine resistance where high dose of chloroquine is recommended [36].

In India, chloroquine is still effective for treating *P. vivax* malaria. Almost half of the malaria cases are due to *P. vivax* mostly present in low transmission settings [28]. A study in 2013 in Kolkata by Ganguly et al. observed non-synonymous polymorphism in *pvcrt-o* and *pvmdr1* and concluded no indication of chloroquine resistance in *in vivo* study [37]. But the report in 2018 from Mangalore indicated the presence of chloroquine resistance involving two genes in K10 insertion in *pvcrt-o* and F1076L mutations in *pvmdr1* [38]. Subsequently, such mutants were also detected in Puducherry, Mangaluru (Mangalore), Cuttack and Jodhpur [39]. A study in Chandigarh, North India reported double mutations in K10 insertions at 17.5% and 9.5%, in complicated and uncomplicated *P vivax* groups, respectively. *Pvmdr-1* gene analysis revealed 100% double mutants (T958M/F1076L) in the complicated, and 98.7% in the uncomplicated group, respectively. Presence of a single triple mutant T958M, F1076L and Y1028C was observed in the uncomplicated group [40]. More number of such cases were reported from Peru in amino acid changes at positions 976F and 1076 L for pvmdr1 [41], Afghanistan [42], Malaysia [43], Australia (among travellers) [44] and Brazilian Amazon [45].

Tackling *P. vivax* malaria is a herculean task due to its complex biology of hypnozoites that cause relapse. Primaquine – an 8 aminoquinoline is widely used for radical cure of malaria. But its use has been restricted in infants, pregnant women and also in G6PD-deficient individuals. WHO recommends to administer primaquine for radical cure of vivax relapse. More than 180 different G6PD deficiency alleles reported [5]. Cytochrome P450 2D6 is an enzyme that in humans is encoded by the CYP2D6 gene. CYP2D6 is primarily expressed in the liver, and is associated with primaquine tolerance [46]. So, both G6PD deficiency and CYP2D6 are contraindications to primaquine administration. In certain situations, high-dose primaquine regiments are currently recommended for radical cure of vivax malaria in Southeast Asia and Oceania [47].

Mutations at the *pvdhps* and *pvdhfr* loci leading to antifolate resistance are commonly found in *P. vivax* isolates from *P. vivax*-infested areas. DHFR mutations in *Plasmodium vivax* in Indonesia failed to therapeutic response to SP [48]. Triple mutations in *pvdhfr* was reported in Mangalore, India [49]. Thus, antifolates are not currently recommended as a first-line treatment of vivax malaria [50].

4. Invasiveness of *Anopheles stephensi*

Anopheles stephensi was originally described by Liston in 1901 from a village Ellichpur (now Achalpur) in Amravati district, Maharashtra state of India. This species is a principal malaria vector in urban India, and is considered imminent threat to malaria elimination efforts [51]. This species has three variants i.e. type, intermediate and *mysorensis* based on its egg morphometric analysis. Both type and intermediate forms are efficient vectors in rural and urban settings, but type form is the main and very efficient vector in urban settings, whereas variety *mysorensis* is considered as a rural vector with limited role. Laboratory studies have shown that all the three variants are capable of harbouring rodent malaria *P. berghei* [52] and *P. yoelii nigeriensis* [53] parasites respectively. *An. stephensi* is an efficient vector for transmitting *P. falciparum* and *P. vivax* malaria equally in the field [54].

Recent reports indicate that *An. stephensi* is expanding its geographical range crossing from the Arabian Gulf into the Horn of Africa where it has been reported in Djibouti City in 2012 [55], in Ethiopia in 2016 [56] and the Republic of Sudan [57]. In 2016, type form of this species was found for the first time in Sri Lanka [58]. Emergence of *An. stephensi* has been associated epidemiologically with an unusual resurgence in local malaria cases in Djibouti city [55]. This species is basically a container breeder and sympatric co-share breeding with *Aedes aegypti* [59]. In Sri Lanka, *An. stephensi* has been found to breed in salt water [58]; while it breeds in clear water in central regions of urban setting of Africa, but with all probability it

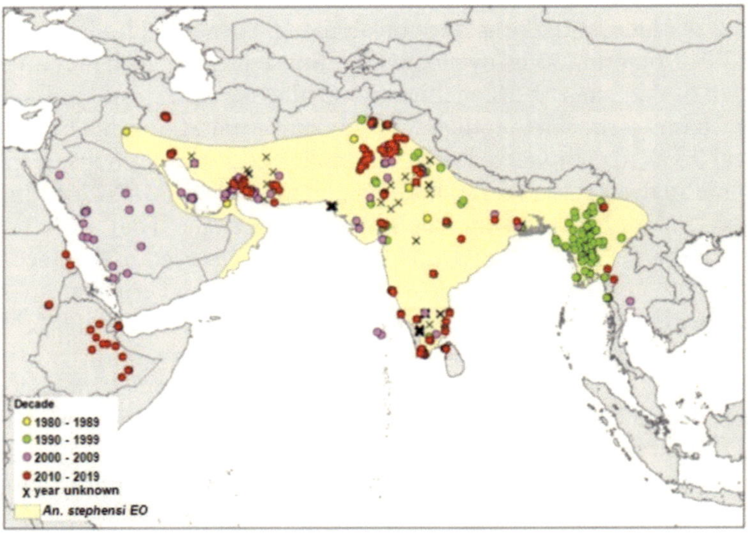

Figure 6.
The new "out of range" occurrence of An. stephensi in the Arabian Peninsula and Horn of Africa showing the 358 An. stephensi site locations used in final species distribution models (SDMs) colour coded by the decade in which they were sampled. Source: Sinka et al. [61] with permission.

may even breed in polluted water in Africa where most malaria vectors breed in such waters [60]. Sinka et al. prepared evidence-based maps predicting the possible locations of *An. stephensi* across Africa where it could establish if its spread is unchecked. The high probability maps predict the presence of *An. stephensi* in many urban cities across Africa where an estimated over 126 million people live (**Figure 6**) [61].

5. Long-distance travel of mosquitoes

Transportation of mosquitoes from one place to other through surface transportation or air route is well known. The accidental invasion of *An. gambiae* in 1930 in Natal, Northeast Brazil from Dakar, Senegal most likely adult mosquitoes that travelled in planes or ships, as no larvae were found is one such example [62]. Generally, mosquitoes can fly within a few kilometers from their breeding habitats. But long-distance migration across hundreds of kilometers during night hours is very revealing, and have implications in malaria eradication efforts. Recent study in Sahel desert of Mali in Africa, Huestis et al. reported that mosquitoes could possibly migrate up to 300 kilometers for 9-hour flight duration. Sticky nets tethered to helium-filled balloons fixed in the study villages suspended at set altitudes ranging from 40 to 290 metres above mean sea level were launched at about 10 consecutive nights each month over a span of 22–32 months. Ten species, including the primary malaria vector *An. coluzzii*, were identified among 235 Anopheline mosquitoes that were captured during 617 nocturnal aerial collections. Annually, the estimated number of mosquitoes that possibly could have migrated at altitude that cross a 100-km line perpendicular to the prevailing wind direction included 81,000 *Anopheles gambiae ss*, 6 million *An. coluzzii* and 44 million *An. squamosus*. Females accounted for more than 80% of all of the mosquitoes, and 90% of them had taken a blood meal before their migration, and studies suggest mosquito infection rates in the region are between 0.1% and 5% [63, 64]. Annually, the estimated numbers of mosquitoes at altitude that cross a 100-km line perpendicular to the prevailing wind direction. The authors concluded that millions of malaria vectors that have previously fed on blood may migrate frequently over hundreds of kilometers, and spread malaria [64]. Thus the successful elimination of malaria depends on how the sources of migrant vectors can be identified and controlled.

6. Insecticide resistance

Resistance to insecticides in vector mosquitoes is an organic *de novo* biological process. This has caused a major setback in achieving malaria elimination. Recently an update at global scale on insecticide resistance in malaria vectors has been enumerated [65]. WHO documented a cumulative total of 82 countries reported data on insecticide resistance from 2010 through 2019. Resistance of malaria vectors to insecticides threatens malaria control and elimination efforts. Commonly used insecticides are synthetic pyrethroids, organophosphates, carbamates and the rarely used organochlorine dichlorodiphenyltrichloroethane (DDT) [5].

Sources of insecticides in the environment include the application of insecticide-based vector control interventions for public health such as Indoor Residual Spray (IRS) and the application of agricultural insecticides, which include the same class of insecticide as those used in vector control programme [66]. Also pesticide contamination in water bodies is also a cause of selection pressure for resistance in mosquito larvae [67]. In response to the Roll back malaria (RBM) initiative, long lasting insecticide nets (LLIN) coverage increased markedly across Africa from 2005 [68], while

IRS usage has been restricted in smaller areas [69]. Either permethrin or deltamethrin was used initially in insecticide-treated nets (ITNs), and now α-cypermethrin is most commonly used in LLINs. Deltamethrin, λ-cyhalothrin, and DDT have been used for IRS for over 20 years. In 2003, first α-cypermethrin was used in mass campaigns. Deltamethrin has been the sole pyrethroid along with DDT and other non-pyrethroid insecticides are used in IRS from 2015 [69]. There are conflicting reports on the cause of insecticide resistance in field mosquitoes following the introduction of LLINs, IRS or both. Some studies documented an increase in resistance [70]; whereas others observed no such evidence after implementation of these intervention strategies [71].

Anopheles culicifacies is the main vector out of six primary malaria vectors and responsible for 2/3 malaria cases distributed across rural India. An tempo-spatial analysis of insecticide susceptibility status between 1991 and 2016 from 145 districts in 21 states indicated resistance to at least one insecticide in 70% (101/145) of the districts – mostly to DDT and malathion whereas, its resistant status against deltamethrin varied across the districts [72]. Similar trend was also reported in Odisha – a highly malaria-endemic state in India [73].

In India, National Vector Borne Disease Control Programme (NVBDCP) has distributed about 50 million LLINs to malaria-endemic communities for intervention during 2016–2018, and to 126 million population at risk [74]. The lower efficacy of synthetic pyrethroids to vector mosquitoes is a matter of concern. Certain major drawbacks of LLINs include feelings of suffocation in humid tropical climate, and some traditional practices compelling the users to wash the nets more frequently than prescribed protocol. Another risk of using LLINs is host switching and possible horizontal transmission potential in the endemic areas [73].

Resistance of malaria vectors to pyrethroids may pose a serious problem in achieving the malaria elimination goal. The six countries Cambodia, China (Yunnan Province), the Lao People's Democratic Republic (PDR), Myanmar, Thailand and Viet Nam of the Greater Mekong Subregion (GMS) have made significant gains in their battle to eliminate malaria by 2030. In recent years, there has been a remarkable progress towards elimination of the disease. Between 2012 and 2018, the reported number of malaria cases fell by 74%; malaria deaths fell by 95% over the same period. However, Cambodia contributes almost half of malaria in this zone of which 85% are *P. vivax*. This may be due to high degree resistance of pyrethroids [75] (**Figure 7**).

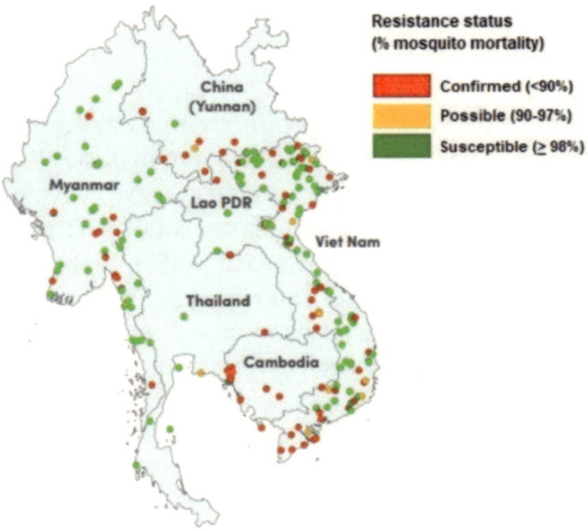

Figure 7.
Resistance of malaria vectors to pyrethroids in the Greater Mekong Subregion, 2010–2019. Source: WHO [75].

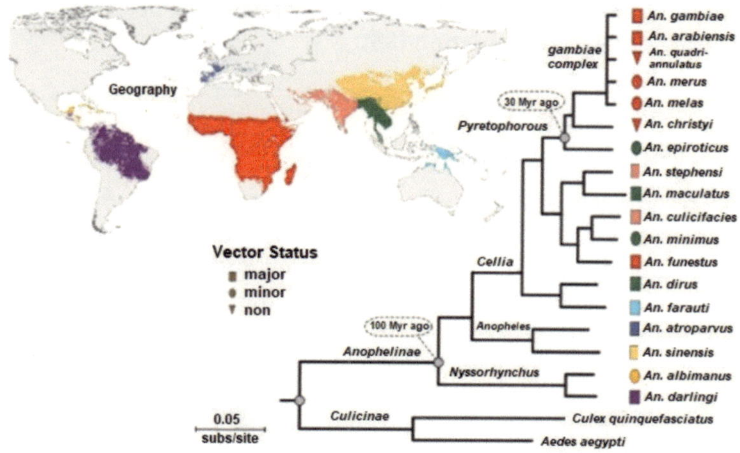

Figure 8.
Comparative genomics of vector mosquitoes to understand difference in vectorial capacity. Source WHO [13].

Another important aspect is to understand and track gene flow in Anopheline mosquitoes. This is complex given the amount of genetic diversity that exists within mosquito populations. **Figure 8** depicts a clear picture how comparative genomics can be applied to understand differences in vectorial capacity and their impact on malaria transmission [13].

7. Poor disease surveillance

Disease surveillance is the key intervention strategy to support malaria elimination. A new guideline promulgated by WHO in 2018 reinforced the GTS and framework for elimination principle that identified surveillance as the main elimination strategy. But poor surveillance continues to derail the elimination efforts. Strengthening surveillance system in many countries eliminated malaria successfully. Aiming malaria elimination, a standardized surveillance system landscaping compared with ideal system were conducted in 16 countries aiming malaria elimination. Assessment was done in 2015 and 2016 across the Greater Mekong Subregion (Cambodia, Laos, Myanmar, and Vietnam), Southern Africa (Botswana, Mozambique, Namibia, South Africa, Swaziland, and Zimbabwe), Hispaniola (Dominican Republic and Haiti), and Central America (Costa Rica, Guatemala, Honduras, and Panama). This landscaping analysis provided a clear framework that identified multiple gaps in current malaria surveillance systems. It is important to close these gaps identified which will allow countries to deploy resources more efficiently, track progress, and accelerate towards malaria elimination [75]. Rapid reporting and information on geolocation have been the strength of malaria control system in Zanzibar for over a decade resulting in low transmission of malarial cases [76]. However, falciparum malaria remains a problem in Zanzibar and Swaziland [77–79]. China adopted and continues the `1-3-7' surveillance strategy, whereby case notification occurs within one day, case investigation within three days and foci investigation and targeted action within seven days. To avoid transmission and re-establishment, monthly bulletins are issued on reported and detected cases. Training, technical support and supervision are provided regularly to sustain capacity [80]. In Mangalore, India a `1-3-7-14' strategy is under operation using digital TAB-based smart surveillance which focuses on real time micromanagement of each malaria positive case and vector control operation [81, 82]. Digital surveillance and bridging the surveillance gaps are two major issues have been advocated to accelerate towards malaria elimination [83].

8. Discussion

In the last five years the GTS milestone has drawn a detailed road-map to eliminate malaria from 2016 to 2030. It can be seen from the **Table 1** that all the 58 countries in the Europe and Central Asia territories, and in other territories around 50% achieved malaria elimination except Sub-Saharan Africa. This means the real problem still exists in this territories [83]. This also reflects in the world malaria report. In November 2018, WHO together with RBM Partnership to End Malaria has launched the 'high burden to high impact' (HBHI) approach – a targeted malaria response in all 11 high malaria burden countries, and India is one such country outside Africa. **Figure 9** shows how HBHI countries have initiated high-level political engagement and support [5]. In a recent virtual meeting of MPAC of WHO commended the efforts made so far in the COVID-19 pandemic. Training should aim to increase the sub-national capacity for evidence-driven decision-making and translating those decisions into actions [13].

Over 100 countries have successfully eliminated malaria in the last century. In the past two decades a lot of initiatives have been launched to contain and eliminate malaria, viz., Roll Back Malaria (RBM), President's Malaria Initiative (PMI), Asia Pacific Malaria Elimination Network (APMEN), E-2020, Malaria Elimination Research Alliance (MERA) - India [84, 85]. Many countries have developed national elimination goals. Regional networks have been formed to facilitate collaboration [86]. Leaders from the Asia Pacific Leaders Malaria Alliance (APLMA) in November 2014 and the African Leaders Malaria Alliance in January 2015 endorsed regional goals for malaria elimination by 2030 [87, 88]. In 2009, the APMEN was established initially in 10 countries (Bhutan, China, Democratic People's Republic of Korea (DPR Korea), Indonesia, Malaysia, the Philippines, Republic of Korea, Solomon Islands, Sri Lanka, and Vanuatu), and now have expanded to 18 countries adding Bangladesh, Cambodia, Lao People's Democratic Republic (Lao PDR), India,

Indicator	Americas and Caribbean	South Asia and East Africa and Pacific	Europe and Central Asia	Middle East and North Africa	Sub-Saharan Africa	Total
Total number of Countries	46	38	58	23	45	211
1900	2	13	3	1	1	20
1900–1949	0	0	9	0	0	9
1950–1978	23	5	35	4	1	68
1979–1990	0	1	2	2	1	6
1991–2019	4	2	9	7	0	22
Total number of malaria-free countries	29	21	58	14	3	125

Table 1.
Number of countries and territories that eliminated malaria by region, 1900–2019. Compiled from Shretta et al. [84] and WHO [8].

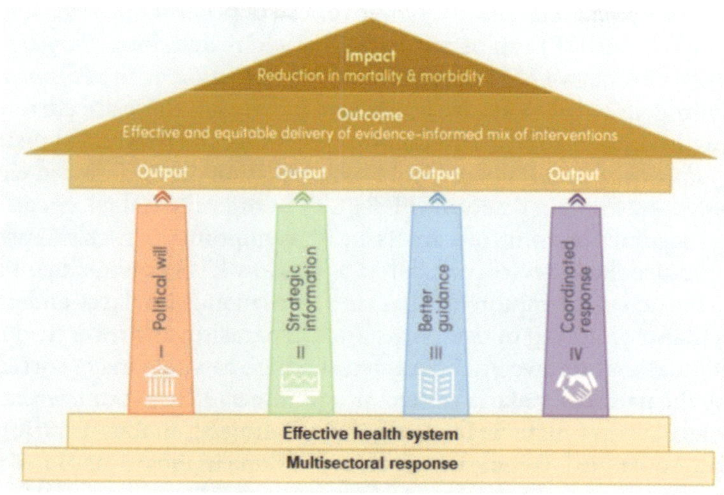

Figure 9.
Schematic presentation how 'High burden to high impact' countries get back on track to achieve the GTS 2015 milestone. Source WHO. [5].

Nepal, Papua New Guinea, Thailand, and Vietnam. Among these, India contributes maximum malaria cases explaining the importance of malaria elimination in this country [89]. But China (Yunnan), Cambodia, Thailand, Myanmar, Lao PDR and Viet Nam in Greater Mekong Subregion greatly reduced falciparum malaria [85] and now the Mekong Malaria Elimination Programme is ready for the last mile of malaria elimination [90].

The real malaria burden lies in the sub-Saharan Africa region. There were significant impact of malaria control from 2000 to 2015, but the situation has plateaued between 2015 and 2019 largely attributed to emerging synthetic pyrethroid (PY) resistance in the principal malaria vector *An. gambiae*. Adding piperonyl butoxide (PBO) enhances the efficacy of PY, but the requirement is huge, and costs have risen substantially amidst financial gap. In high insecticide resistance areas, pyrethroid-PBO nets increase mosquito mortality and reduce blood feeding rates that leads to lower malaria prevalence. But the impact of pyrethroid-PBO LLINs on mosquito mortality was not sustained over 20 washes. There is a little evidence to support higher entomological efficacy of pyrethroid-PBO nets in areas where the mosquitoes show lower levels of resistance to pyrethroids [91]. This warrants routine monitoring of insecticide resistance to take appropriate decisions by the national programme managers.

In India the total global burden has reduced from 4% in 2018 to 2% in 2019 of total malaria cases. But it still falls under the `high burden to high impact' countries outside Africa. India contributed 87.9% of total malaria cases and 86% of malaria deaths in the South East Asia region of WHO [5]. This requires a special attention for the high burden states with high *P. falciparum* cases. For example, malaria cases in Karnataka state, India fell 98.95% in 2019 compared with 1995 data, but 70 to 80% of reported cases from Mangalore city alone requires concerted efforts. Now, a special action plan with digital surveillance has been initiated for the last five years, which is showing some results. Hopefully, Karnataka can declare malaria elimination by 2025 ahead of India's deadline of 2027 [81, 82]. Such strong surveillance system can be implemented to find a solution to get freedom from malaria.

In recent years many innovative intervention strategies have been shown to be promising. Finding the reasons for *Pfhrp2/3* deletions and drug resistance in *P. falciparum* is an important step to address this major issue. BV1 lineage is associated with these two important issues [8]. Moreover use of other more advanced RDT like malaria-RDT (mRDT) can be an alternative where deletions *Pfhrp2/3* are low [92]. However, alternative RDT options based on detection of the *Plasmodium* lactate dehydrogenase [pLDH]) are limited; in particular, there are currently no WHO-prequalified non-*Pfhrp2* combination tests that can detect and distinguish between *P. falciparum* and *P. vivax* [5]. In such situation photo-induced electron transfer- polymerase chain reaction (PET-PCT) or microPCR devices can be applied with highest accuracy at point-of-care. Issue of asymptomatic malaria cases can addressed because these devices can detect a very low level of parasitaemia [93, 94].

Besides, burden of asymptomatic parasite cases in most malaria-endemic countries, molecular monitoring of drug resistance in parasites and insecticide resistance in vector populations are two vital parameters which can help make correct policy decisions by the national malaria control programmes. Many countries have initiated for molecular surveillance; for example in Haiti [93], in Asia-Pacific countries [95] and Cambodia [96]. Genome analysis is not done in most situations due to its prohibitive cost. Now very sensitive and low-cost oxford nanopore platform is very useful and many researchers are using this to find out the gene flow and genetic diversity in parasites and vectors [97]. SNP barcode is used instead of microsatellite technology using this platform [98]. Scientists in Africa have been working on these issues on Pathogens Genomic Diversity Network Africa [99]. Such platforms must work on other regions also to provide guidance to the national malaria programme from time to time for taking corrective measures to change the policy decisions. Similarly, vector resistance to insecticide pattern can also established to take correct selection of effective insecticide [100].

Monitoring of insecticide resistance allows targeting of specific interventions with pyrethroid-PBO nets, and resistance mechanisms finding mixed-function oxidase (MFO) resistance mechanisms over time. Such monitoring also enables programmes to assess the value of different insecticide resistance management strategies like IRS rotation, new types of ITNs and LLINs or other effective tools. Using genotyping to detect insecticide resistance is quicker to implement than phenotypic assays that require rearing of larvae, even wild type adults can be used when available in sufficient numbers. It is possible that resistance could be underestimated due to unknown age of the mosquito. With this approach, shifts in allele frequencies may be easier to detect than shifts in phenotype over short time periods [13].

Finding origin of the parasites and gene flow in the elimination era is a challenging task. Genetic relatedness studies using metrics of identity-by-state (IBS) and identical-by-descent (IBD) - alleles that are genetically the same, and alleles that come from a common ancestor, respectively can address this issue [101]. This requires a number of informative markers (molecular barcode genotyping) that vary depending on the level of transmission in the geographic area under examination. A barcode is considered informative for relatedness by IBS at >0.95 relatedness. When using this measure in a low transmission setting, relatedness can serve as a key indicator for distinguishing imported and local transmission and understanding the persistence of transmission in the area [13].

In high falciparum areas an alternative approach to understanding receptivity risk for imported and onward indigenous transmission of malaria is to investigate parasite markers in parasite-vector interactions that determine whether the parasite can successfully infect the mosquito. Pfs47 is a target of interest allows the ookinete to evade the immune response of the mosquito midgut and successfully develop into an oocyst. The allele is polymorphic with signatures of natural selection relevant to the geographic origin of the parasite. *P. falciparum* isolates are more compatible with *Anopheles* species from their region of origin. Pfs47 single nucleotide polymorphisms (SNPs) can therefore be used to predict the transmission risk of imported *P. falciparum* and help establish its geographic origin. Specific SNPs for vivax malaria is warranted [13].

Now time has come act judiciously to eliminate malaria at subnational to achieve elimination target at national level. Again surveillance that can capture and report individual cases in time to investigate and take action [81, 82]. The Chinese national malaria elimination programme, now approaching WHO certification used effectively in subnational initiatives to interrupt malaria transmission followed by validations of elimination [102] Similarly, Kenya has established a national strategic action plan 2019–2023 to achieve malaria elimination in targeted countries by 2030 [103]. Malaysia has successfully launched malaria elimination partnering between the public and commercial sectors in Sabah [104], but the rising threat of zoonotic *P. knowlesi* is a matter of concern [105].

Time has come to look back the success stories of malaria elimination efforts. In October 1998, the Director-General of WHO launched the RBM initiative. It was established through a partnership between WHO, the World Bank, the United Nations Children's Fund (UNICEF) and the United Nations Development Programme (UNDP) [106]. The purpose of launching RBM initiative was in this direction. In Karnataka, India we successfully implemented larvivorous fish-based malaria elimination campaign [107, 108]. We need to repurpose the larval source management strategy. The best historical example is the successful eradication of accidentally introduced African vector *Anopheles gambiae* in 54000 km^2 of largely ideal habitat in Northeast Brazil (Natal) from Dakar, Senegal in the 1930s and early 1940s. This outstanding success was achieved through an integrated programme but relied overwhelmingly upon larval control. The success of Frederick Lowe Soper and Rockeller Foundation's International Health Division campaigned with anti-larval chemical Paris Green and eliminated *An. gambiae* before the scheduled timeline [62]. It was a significant watershed in the history of malaria control, and revived the faith in vector control strategies that paved the way for the application of eradication methods in the fight against malaria following World War II. This experience was soon repeated in Egypt and another larval control programme successfully suppressed malaria for over 20 years around a Zambian copper mine [109]. It is important to revisit all such success stories implemented earlier. Today, with the development of advanced technology, we have more options like application of a new anti-larval product Aquatain AMF™ for use in LSM. It is a silicon-based liquid formulation that forms a very thin film on stagnant water. The mosquito larvae are killed due to physical and mechanical action. Drone technology are now used for anti-larval applications [110]. Rhamnolipids – a class of glycolipid may be applied as anti-larval agent especially against *Ae. aegypti* and may be against *A. stephensi* [111].

Efforts are also being made to develop technology for diagnosis of malaria parasites and identification of vector mosquitoes using artificial intelligence and machine learning. [112, 113]. Aptamer technology can be applied which has the potential to revolutionize biological diagnostics and therapeutics. This technology can be used for malaria diagnosis in place of HRP2 which is facing certain problems [114, 115]. This also be used in malaria as adjunct therapy [116]. Other most prospective gene editing technology in vector mosquitoes especially in *An. gambiae* in Africa where most malaria exists, and also in *An. stephensi* – the most invasive malaria vector. [61, 110, 117]. It is important to find new drug molecules to counter drug resistance challenge in parasites. Medicines for Malaria Venture (MMV) has been working for more than two decades in this front. *P. vivax* liver stage assays platform was initiated by MMV to discover new molecules for anti-relapse drugs to work against hypnozoites. India was one of the partners under this initiative [118]. A new vaccine candidate R21 with adjuvant Matrix-M™ developed by Novamax has shown a new hope for an effective vaccine that could be used in malaria elimination. A Phase 2B trial on 450 children aged 5-17 months in Burkina Faso, West Africa showed 77% efficacy [119].

Now, all resources have been diverted to COVID-19 even WHO alerted in the beginning of the pandemic. In a recent article published in *Nature* emphasized the need to create a general attention like COVID-19 to all tropical diseases including malaria. The author has expressed concerns about the reversing the impact on malaria elimination achieved so far especially in Sub-Saharan Africa [120]. It may be mentioned that in March 2020, as the COVID-19 pandemic spread rapidly around the globe, WHO convened a cross-partner effort to mitigate the negative impact of the corona virus in malaria-affected countries and contribute to the COVID-19 response otherwise, much of the progress against malaria was under enormous risk, with the potential to wipe out 20 years of malaria gains [120].

Funding in malaria elimination efforts is an important component. Sufficient and timely release of allocated funds would ease out many constraints for which strict financial management is utmost necessary. The total annual financial resources needed were estimated at US$ 4.1 billion in 2016, rising to US$ 6.8 billion in 2020 to achieve the GTS milestone. An additional funding of US$ 0.72 billion is estimated to be required annually for global malaria research and development (R&D). In 2019, the total funding for malaria control and elimination in was estimated at US$ 3.0 billion, compared with US$ 2.7 billion in 2018 and US$ 3.2 billion in 2017. The amount invested in 2019 falls short of the US$ 5.6 billion estimated to be required globally. In recent years, the funding gap between the amount invested and the resources needed has widen dramatically, increasing from US$ 1.3 billion in 2017 to US$ 2.3 billion in 2018, and to US$ 2.6 billion in 2019 [5].

9. Conclusion

In the renewed efforts to eliminate malaria more needs to be done following the strategies and technologies adopted by those countries successfully eliminate malaria. High burden to high impact countries need special attentions. If these countries in Africa and India are free from malaria over 80% of malaria burden can be curtailed. There are several roadblocks namely gene deletions in *Pfhrp2/3*, insecticide resistance, drug resistance in *P. falciparum* and also in *P. vivax* need to be addressed following new technologies like gene editing and Aptamar technologies. There are many gaps in surveillance for which smart digital surveillance is an important strategy that need to be implemented on priority. Artificial intelligence and machine learning should find proper place to solve many ongoing problems of diagnosis and effective implementation, monitoring of the elimination programme. Routine malaria molecular surveillance of parasites and vectors at subnational and regional levels must be carried out to take correct and appropriate measures policy decision makers. As long distance night travel and invasiveness of vector mosquitoes have been established or otherwise, LSM must find priority. Like COVID-19, other tropical diseases like malaria must be given priority with proper funding provisions.

Acknowledgements

The authors are grateful to Dr. Vas Dev, Former Senior Scientist, ICMR-National Institute of Malaria Research, New Delhi, India for suggestions and interest in this article.

DOI: http://dx.doi.org/10.5772/intechopen.96532

Conflict of interest

The authors declare no conflict of interest.

Author details

Susanta Kumar Ghosh[1*] and Chaitali Ghosh[2]

1 ICMR-National Institute of Malaria Research, Bengaluru, India

2 Tata Institute for Genetics and Society, Bengaluru, India

*Address all correspondence to: ghoshnimr@gmail.com

References

[1] Malaria – Biology in the Era of Eradication. A subject collection from Cold Spring Harbor Perspectives in Medicine (Wirth DF, Alonso PL, Eds.), Cold Spring Harbor Laboratory Press, New York, USA. 2017; pp. 1-315

[2] Anopheles mosquitoes – New Insights into Malaria Vectors. Manguin S (Ed.). Available from: InTech Open Access (www.intechopen.com, http://dx.doi.org/10.5772/3392), Croatia. 2013; p. 813

[3] Towards Malaria Elimination - A Leap Forward (Manguin S and Dev V, Eds.). Available from: InTech Open Access (https://www.intechopen.com/books/towards-malaria-elimination-a-leap-forward), London. 2018; p. 429.

[4] Vector Biology and Control. An Update for Malaria Elimination Initiative in India, New Delhi, Dev V (Ed.), The National Academy of Sciences, India. 2020; p. 272

[5] WHO. World Malaria Report 2020. 2020. Available from: https://www.who.int/docs/default-source/malaria/world-malaria-reports/9789240015791-double-page-view.pdf?sfvrsn=2c24349d_5.

[6] WHO. Countries and territories certified malaria-free by WHO. Certification of malaria elimination, 1955-2019. 2019. Available from: https://www.who.int/teams/global-malaria-programme/elimination/countries-and-territories-certified-malaria-free-by-who.

[7] WHO. E-2020. Eliminating malaria: 21 countries, a common goal. 2020. Available from: https://www.who.int/teams/global-malaria-programme/elimination/e-2020-initiative-of-malaria-eliminating-countries

[8] WHO. Response plan to *Pfhrp2* gene deletions. 2019. https://www.who.int/malaria/publications/atoz/response-plan-pfhrp2-gene-deletions/en/

[9] Thomson R, Parr JB, Cheng Q, Chenet S, Perkins M, Cunningham J. Prevalence of *Plasmodium falciparum* lacking histidine-rich proteins 2 and 3: a systematic review. Bulletin of the World Health Organization. 2020; **98(8)**:558-568

[10] Kumar N, Pande V, Bhatt RM, Shah NK, Mishra N, Srivastava B, Valecha N, Anvikar AR. Genetic deletion of HRP2 and HRP3 in Indian *Plasmodium falciparum* population and false negative malaria rapid diagnostic test. Acta Tropica. 2013; **125(1)**:119-121.

[11] Bharti PK, Chandel HS, Ahmad A, Krishna S, Udhayakumar V, Singh N. Prevalence of pfhrp2 and/or pfhrp3 gene deletion in *Plasmodium falciparum* population in eight highly endemic states in India. PLoS One. 2016; **11(8)**:e0157949.

[12] Okoth SA, Chenet SM, Arrospide N, Gutierrez S, Cabezas C, Matta JA, Udhayakumar V. Molecular investigation into a malaria outbreak in Cusco, Peru: *Plasmodium falciparum* BV1 lineage is linked to a second outbreak in recent times. American Journal of Tropical Medicine and Hygiene. 2016; **94(1)**: 128-131.

[13] WHO. Technical consultation on the role of parasite and Anopheline genetics in malaria surveillance. Malaria Policy Advisory Committee Meeting 2-4 October 2019, Geneva, Switzerland Background document for Session 7. 2019. Available from: https://www.who.int/malaria/mpac/mpac-october2019-session7-report-consultation-on-genomics.pdf

[14] Ghosh SK. Molecular monitoring of antimalarial drug resistance in India. Indian Journal of Medical Microbiology. 2017; **35(2)**:155-156.

[15] Weiss DJ, Lucas TCD, Nguyen K Nandi AK, Donal Bisanzio D, et al. Mapping the global prevalence, incidence, and mortality of *Plasmodium*

falciparum, 2000-17: a spatial and temporal modelling study. Lancet. 2019; **394**: 322-331.

[16] Packard RM. The origins of antimalarial-drug resistance. New England Journal of Medicine. 2014; **371**: 397-399.

[17] Vathsala PG, Pramanik A, Dhanasekaran S, Usha Devi C, Pillai CR, Subbarao SK, Ghosh SK, Tiwari SN, Sathyanarayan TS, Deshpande PR, Ranjit MR, Dash AP, Rangarajan PN, Padmanavan G. Chloroquine resistant PfCRT haplotype (SVMNT) is wide-spread in *Plasmodium falciparum* malaria in India. American Journal of Tropical Medicine and Hygiene. 2004; **70**:256-259.

[18] Zomuanpuii R, Hmar CL, Lallawmzuala K et al. Epidemiology of malaria and chloroquine resistance in Mizoram, northeastern India, a malaria-endemic region bordering Myanmar. Malaria Journal. 2020; **19:** 95.

[19] Patel P, Bharti PK, Bansal D, Ali NA, Raman RK, Mohapatra PK, Sehgal R, Mahanta J, Sultan AA, Singh N. Prevalence of mutations linked to antimalarial resistance in *Plasmodium falciparum* from Chhattisgarh, Central India: A malaria elimination point of view. Scientific Reports. 2017; **30;7(1): 16690**. doi: 10.1038/s41598-017-16866-5.

[20] Amimo F, Lambert B, Magit A, et al. *Plasmodium falciparum* resistance to sulfadoxine-pyrimethamine in Africa: a systematic analysis of national trends. BMJ Global Health. 2020; **5:e003217**. doi:10.1136/ bmjgh-2020-003217.

[21] van Eijk AM, Larsen DA, Kayentao K, Koshy G, Slaughter DEC, et al. Effect of *Plasmodium falciparum* sulfadoxine-pyrimethamine resistance on the effectiveness of intermittent preventive therapy for malaria in pregnancy in Africa: a systematic review and meta-analysis. Lancet Infectious Diseses. 2019; **19(5)**:546-556.

[22] Ashley EA, Dhorda M, Fairhurst RM, Amaratunga C, Lim P, et al. Spread of artemisinin resistance in *Plasmodium falciparum* malaria. New England Journal of Medicine. 2014;**371(5)**:411-423.

[23] Ménard D, Khim N, Beghain J, Adegnika AA, Shafiul-Alam M, et al. A worldwide map of *Plasmodium falciparum* K13-Propeller polymorphisms. New England Journal of Medicine. 2016; **374(25)**: 2453-2464.

[24] Uwimana A, Legrand E, Stokes BH, Ndikumana JM, Warsame M, et al. Emergence and clonal expansion of in vitro artemisinin-resistant *Plasmodium falciparum* kelch13 R561H mutant parasites in Rwanda. Nature Medicine. 2020; **26**:1602-1608.

[25] Das S, Saha B, Hati AK, Roy S. Evidence of artemisinin-resistant *Plasmodium falciparum* malaria in Eastern India. New England Journal of Medicine. 2018;**379(20)**:1962-1964.

[26] Imai K, Tarumoto N, Runtuwene LR, et al. An innovative diagnostic technology for the codon mutation C580Y in kelch13 of *Plasmodium falciparum* with MinION nanopore sequencer. Malaria Journal. 2018; **17**:217.

[27] Baird JK. Evidence and implications of mortality associated with acute *Plasmodium vivax* malaria. Clinical Microbiology Reviews. 2013;26: 36-57.

[28] Sharma VP, Dev V, Phookan S. Neglected *Plasmodium vivax* malaria in northeastern States of India. Indian Journal of Medical Research. 2015;**141**: 546-55

[29] Anvikar AR, Shah N, Dhariwal AC, Sonal GS, Pradhan MM, Ghosh SK, Valecha N. Epidemiology of *Plasmodium*

vivax Malaria in India. American Journal of Tropical Medicine and Hygiene. 2016; **95 (Suppl.)**, 108-120.

[30] Battle,KE, Lucas TCD, Nguyen M, Howes RE, Nandi AK, et al. 2019. Mapping the global endemicity and clinical burden of *Plasmodium vivax*, 2000-17: a spatial and temporal modelling study. Lancet. 2019; **394**:332-343.

[31] Twohig KA, Pfeffer DA, Baird JK, Price RN, Zimmerman PA, Hay SI, et al. Growing evidence of *Plasmodium vivax* across malaria-endemic Africa. PLoS Negl Trop Diseses. 2019; **13(1)**: e0007140.

[32] Oboha MA, Oyebola KM, Idowub TE, Badianea AS, Otubanjo OA, Ndiayea D. Rising report of *Plasmodium vivax* in sub-Saharan Africa: Implications for malaria elimination agenda. Scientific African. 2020; **10**: e00596.

[33] Price RN, Commons RJ, Battle KE, Thriemer K, Mendis K. *Plasmodium vivax* in the era of the shrinking *P. falciparum* map. Trends in Parasitology. 2020; **36(6)**: 560-570.

[34] Price RN, Douglas NM, Anstey NM. New developments in *Plasmodium vivax* malaria: severe disease and the rise of chloroquine resistance. Current Opinion in Infectious Diseases. 2009; **22(5)**: 430-435.

[35] Nomura T, Carlton JM, Baird JK, del Portillo HA, Fryauff DJ, et al. Evidence for different mechanisms of chloroquine resistance in 2 *Plasmodium* species that cause human malaria. The Journal of Infectious Diseases. 2001; **183**; 1653-1661.

[36] Lu F, Wang B, Cao J, Sattabongkot J, Zhou H, Zhu G, Kim K, Gao Q, Han ET. Prevalence of drug resistance-associated gene mutations in *Plasmodium vivax* in Central China. Korean Journal of Parasitology. 2012; **50**: 379-384.

[37] Ganguly S, Saha P, Guha SK, Das S, Bera DK, et al. *In vivo* therapeutic efficacy of chloroquine alone or in combination with primaquine against vivax malaria in Kolkata, West Bengal, India, and polymorphism in *pvmdr1* and *pvcrt-o* genes. Antimicrobial Agents and Chemotherapy. 2013; **57:** 1246-51.

[38] Joy S, Mukhi B, Ghosh SK, Achur RN, Gowda DC, Surolia N. Drug resistance genes: *pvcrt-o* and *pvmdr-1*polymorphism in patients from malaria endemic South Western Coastal Region of India. Malaria Journal. 2018; **17**:40.

[39] Anantabotla VM, Antony HA, Parija SC, Rajkumari N, Kini JR, Manipura R, Nag VL, Gadepalli R, Chayani N, Patro S. Polymorphisms in genes associated with drug resistance of *Plasmodium vivax* in India. Parasitology International. 2019; **70**: 92-97.

[40] Kaur H, Sehgal R, Kumar A, et al. Distribution pattern of amino acid mutations in chloroquine and antifolate drug resistance associated genes in complicated and uncomplicated *Plasmodium vivax* isolates from Chandigarh, North India. BMC Infectious Diseases. 2020; **20**: 671.

[41] Villena FE, Maguiña JL, Santolalla ML, et al. Molecular surveillance of the *Plasmodium vivax* multidrug resistance 1 gene in Peru between 2006 and 2015. Malaria Journal. 2020; **19:** 450.

[42] Mosawi SH, Dalimi A, Safi N, Fotouhi-Ardakani R, Ghaffarifar F, Sadraei J. An unlabelled probe-based real time PCR and modified semi-nested PCR as molecular tools for analysis of chloroquine resistant *Plasmodium vivax* isolates from Afghanistan. Malaria Journal. 2020; **19**:253.

[43] Grigg MJ, William T, Menon J, Barber BE. Efficacy of Artesunate-mefloquine for chloroquine resistant *Plasmodium vivax* malaria in Malaysia: an open-label, randomized, controlled trial. Clinical Infectious Diseases. 2016; **62(11)**:1403-1411.

[44] Noisang C, Meyer W, Sawangjaroen N, Ellis J, Lee R. Molecular detection of antimalarial drug resistance in *Plasmodium vivax* from returned travellers to NSW, Australia during 2008-2018. Pathogens. 2020; **5;9(2)**:101. doi: 10.3390/pathogens9020101.

[45] Silva SR, Almeida ACG, da Silva GAV, et al. Chloroquine resistance is associated to multi-copy *pvcrt-o* gene in *Plasmodium vivax* malaria in the Brazilian Amazon. Malaria Journal. 2018; **17:** 267.

[46] Bennett JW, Pybus BS, Yadava A, Tosh D, Sousa JC, McCarthy WF, et al. Primaquine failure and cytochrome P-450 2D6 in *Plasmodium vivax* malaria. New England Journal of Medicine. 2013 **369**: 1381-1382.

[47] Chu C, White NJ. Management of relapsing *Plasmodium vivax* malaria. Expert Review of Anti-infective Therapy. 2016;**14**: 885-900.

[48] Hastings MD, Porter KM, Maguire JD, Susanti I, Kania W, et al. Dihydrofolate reductase mutations in *Plasmodium vivax* from Indonesia and therapeutic response to sulfadoxine plus pyrimethamine. The Journal of Infectious Diseases. 2004; **189**: 744-750.

[49] Joy S, Ghosh SK, Achur RN, Gowda DC, Surolia N. Presence of novel triple mutations in the *pvdhfr* from *Plasmodium vivax* in Mangaluru city area in the southwestern coastal region of India. Malaria Journal. 2018; **17**:167.

[50] WHO. Guidelines for the Treatment of Malaria. 3rd edition. Geneva: 2015. Available from: https://www.who.int/publications/i/item/ 9789241549127.

[51] Ghosh SK. *Anopheles* (*Cellia*) *stephensi* Liston 1901: the vector of urban malaria – an imminent threat to malaria elimination in India. In: Vector Biology and Control-An Update for Malaria Elimination Initiative in India, New Delhi (Dev V, Ed.), The National Academy of Sciences, India. 2020. pp. 69-82.

[52] Basseri HR, Mohamadzadeh Hajipirloo H, Mohammadi Bavani M, Whitten MM. Comparative Susceptibility of Different Biological Forms of *Anopheles stephensi* to Plasmodium berghei ANKA Strain. PLoS ONE. 2013 **8(9)**: e75413

[53] Ghosh C. Studies on the genetic basis of Fenitrothion resistance and comparative susceptibility of *anopheles stephensi*, Liston to rodent malaria parasite. Phd Thesis, Bangalore University, December 2002, Bangalore, India.

[54] Thomas S, Ravishankaran S, Justin NJ, Asokan A, Mathai MT, Valecha N, et al. Resting and feeding preferences of *Anopheles stephensi* in an urban setting, perennial for malaria. Malaria Journal. 2017; **16**:111.

[55] Faulde MK, Rueda LM, Khaireh BA. First record of the Asian malaria vector *Anopheles stephensi* and its possible role in the resurgence of malaria in Djibouti, Horn of Africa. Acta Tropica. 2014; **139**: 39-43.

[56] Carter TE, Yared S, Gebresilassie A, et al. First detection of *Anopheles stephensi* Liston, 1901 (Diptera: culicidae) in Ethiopia using molecular and morphological approaches. Acta Tropica. 2018; **188**: 180-186.

[57] WHO. Vector alert: *Anopheles stephensi* invasion and spread. 2019. Available from: https://www.who.int/publications-detail/vector-alert-anopheles-stephensi-invasion-and-spread

[58] Surendran S, Sivabalakrishnan K, Sivasingham A, et al. Anthropogenic factors driving recent range expansion of the malaria vector *Anopheles stephensi*. Frontier in Public Health. 2019; **7**: 53.

[59] Seyfarth M, Khaireh BA, Abdi AA, Bouh SM, Faulde MK. Five years following first detection of Anopheles stephensi (Diptera: Culicidae) in Djibouti, Horn of Africa: populations established—malaria emerging. Parasitology Research. 2019; **118(3)**: 725-732.

[60] Sinka ME, Bangs MJ, Manguin S, et al. The dominant Anopheles vectors of human malaria in the Asia-Pacific region: occurrence data, distribution maps and bionomic précis. Parasites & Vectors. 2011; **4**: 89.

[61] Sinka ME, Pironon S, Massey NC, Longbottom J, Hemingway J, Moyes CL, Willis KJ. A new malaria vector in Africa: predicting the expansion range of *Anopheles stephensi* and identifying the urban populations at risk. Proceedings of the National Academy of Science, U S A. 2020 117(**40**):24900-24908. doi: 10.1073/pnas.2003976117.

[62] Packard RM, Gadelha P. A land filled with mosquitoes: Fred L Soper, The Rockefeller Foundation and the *Anopheles gambiae* invasion of Brazil. Medical Anthropology. **17**: 215-238.

[63] Huestis DL, Dao A, Diallo M, Sanogo ZL, Samake D, et al. Windborne long-distance migration of malaria mosquitoes in the Sahel. Nature. 2019; **574(7778)**:404-408.

[64] Wadman M. Windborne mosquitoes may carry malaria hundreds of kilometres. 2019. doi:10.1126/science.aaz7159.

[65] Riveron JM, Tchouakui M, Mugenzi L, Menze BD, Chiang MC, Wondji CS. Insecticide resistance in malaria vectors: an update at a global scale. In: Towards Malaria Elimination - A Leap Forward (Manguin S and Dev V, Eds.), InTech Open, London, 2018. pp. 149-175.

[66] Chouaibou M, Etang J, Brevault T, Nwane P, Hinzoumbe CK, Mimpfoundi R, et al. Dynamics of insecticide resistance in the malaria vector *Anopheles gambiae s.l.* from an area of extensive cotton cultivation in Northern Cameroon. Tropical Medicine and International Health. 2008; **13(4)**: 476-486.

[67] Hien AS, Soma DD, Hema O, Bayili B, Namountougou M, Gnankine O, et al. Evidence that agricultural use of pesticides selects pyrethroid resistance within *Anopheles gambiae s.l.* populations from cotton growing areas in Burkina Faso, West Africa. PLoS ONE. 2017; **12(3)**. https://doi.org/10.1371/journal. pone.0173098.

[68] Bhatt S, Weiss DJ, Mappin B, Dalrymple U, Cameron E, Bisanzio D, et al. Coverage and system efficiencies of insecticide-treated nets in Africa from 2000 to 2017. eLife. 2015; **4**. https://doi.org/10.7554/ eLife.09672.

[69] Tangena J-A, Hendricks CJM, Devine M, Tammaro M, Trett AE, de Pina A, et al. Indoor residual spraying for malaria control in Sub-Saharan Africa 1997 to 2017: an adjusted retrospective analysis. Malaria Journal. 2020; **19**:150.

[70] Mandeng SE, Awono-Ambene HP, Bigoga JD, Ekoko WE, Binyang J, Piameu M, et al. Spatial and temporal development of deltamethrin resistance in malaria vectors of the *Anopheles gambiae* complex from North Cameroon. PLoS ONE. 2019; 14(2). https://doi.org/10.1371/journal.pone.0212024 20, 24-26.

[71] Cook J, Tomlinson S, Kleinschmidt I, Donnelly MJ, Akogbeto M, Adechoubou A, et al. Implications of insecticide resistance for malaria vector control with long-lasting insecticidal nets: trends in pyrethroid resistance during a WHO-coordinated multi-country prospective study. Parasites and Vectors. 2018; **11**. https://doi.org/10.1186/s13071-018-3101-4.

[72] Raghavendra K, Velamuri PS, Verma V, Elamathi N, Barik TK, Bhatt RM, Dash AP. Temporo-spatial distribution of insecticide-resistance in Indian malaria vectors in the last quarter-century: Need for regular resistance monitoring and management. Journal of Vector Borne Diseases. 2017; **54(2)**: 111-130.

[73] Sahu SS, Thankachy S, Dash S, Swaminathan S, Kasinathan G, Purushothaman J. Multiple insecticide resistance in *Anopheles culicifacies* s.l. (Diptera: Culicidae) in east-central India. Pathogens and Global Health. 2019; **113(8)**:352-358.

[74] National Vector Borne Disease Control Programme (NVBDCP). Malaria. Available from: https://nvbdcp.gov.in/index1.php?lang=1&level=1&sublinkid=5784&lid= 3689.

[75] WHO. Countries of the Greater Mekong zero in on falciparum malaria. Bulletin 8 of the Mekong Malaria Elimination programme18 December 2019. Available from: https://www.who.int/publications/i/item/WHO-HTM-GMP-MME-2019.04.

[76] Lourenço C, Tatem AJ, Atkinson PM, Cohen JM, Pindolia D, Bhavnani D, and Menach AL. Strengthening surveillance systems for malaria elimination: a global landscaping of system performance, 2015-2017. Malaria Journal. 2019; **18**:315.

[77] Björkman A, Shakely D, Ali AS *et al.* From high to low malaria transmission in Zanzibar—challenges and opportunities to achieve elimination. BMC Medicine. 2019; **17:** 14

[78] Morgan AP, Brazeau NF, Ngasala B, et al. Falciparum malaria from coastal Tanzania and Zanzibar remains highly connected despite effective control efforts on the archipelago. Malaria Journal. 2020; 19, 47.

[79] Cohen JM, Dlamini S, Novotny JM, Kandula D, Kunene S, Tatem AJ. Rapid case-based mapping of seasonal malaria transmission risk for strategic elimination planning in Swaziland. Malaria Journal. 2013; **12**:61.

[80] Cao J, Sturrock HJ, Cotter C, et al. Communicating and monitoring surveillance and response activities for malaria elimination: China's "1-3-7" strategy. PLoS Medicine. 2014;**11(5)**

[81] Baliga BS, Jain A, Koduvattat, N, Prakash Kumar BG, Kumar M, Kumar A, Ghosh SK. Indigenously developed digital handheld Android-based Geographic Information System (GIS)-tagged tablets TABs in malaria elimination programme in Mangaluru city, Karnataka, India. Malaria Journal. 2019;**18**: 444.

[82] Baliga BS, Jain A, Koduvattat, N, Prakash Kumar BG, Kumar M, Kumar A, Ghosh SK. Digitized smart surveillance in malaria elimination programme in Mangaluru city, Karnataka, India - a detailed account of operationalization in post-digitization years. medRxiv, 7 July 2020. https://www.medrxiv.org/content/10.1101/2020.07.06.20147405v1.

[83] Nema S, Ghanghoria P, Bharti PK. Malaria elimination in India: bridging the gap between control and elimination. Indian Pediatrics. 2020; **57**: 613-617.

[84] Shretta R, Liu J, Cotter C, Cohen J, Charlotte Dolenz JC, et al. Malaria elimination and eradication. In book chapter 12. Major Infectious Diseases – 3rd edition. (Holmes KK, Bertozzi S, Bloom BR, Jha P. Laxminarayan R, Mock CN Editors). 2017; 315-346.

[85] Ghosh SK, Rahi M. Malaria elimination in India—The way forward. Journal of Vector Borne Diseases. 2019; **56**:32-40.

[86] Newby G, Bennett A, Larson E, Cotter C, Shretta R, et al. The Path to

Eradication: A Progress Report on the Malaria-Eliminating Countries. Lancet. 2016; **387 (10029)**: 177-184.

[87] Asia Pacific Leaders Malaria Alliance (APLMA). 2015. Asia-Pacific at the Forefront of a Global Movement to Eliminate Malaria. 2015. APLMA Blog, October 7. Available from: http://aplma .org /blog/22/asia-pacific-at-the-forefront-of-a -global -movement-to-eliminate-malaria/

[88] United Nations. African Leaders Call for Elimination of Malaria by 2030. Office of the UN Secretary-General's Special Envoy for Financing the Health Millennium Development Goals and for Malaria. MDG Health EnvoyNews, 2015; February 3. Available from: http://www.mdghealthenvoy.org/african-leaders-call-for-elimination-of-malaria-by-2030/.

[89] Wangdi K and Clements ACA. Ending Malaria Transmission in the Asia Pacific Malaria Elimination Network (APMEN) Countries: Challenges and the Way Forward. In a book chapter Towards Malaria Elimination- A Leap Forward. Edited by Manguin S and Dev V. IntechOpen 2018. pp. 201-232.

[90] WHO. Countries of the Greater Mekong ready for the "last mile" of malaria elimination Bulletin 9 of the Mekong Malaria Elimination programme 21 December 2020. Available from: https://www.who.int/publications/i/item/WHO-UCN-GMP-MME-2020.05.

[91] Gleave K, Lissenden N, Richardson M, Choi L, Ranson H. Piperonyl butoxide (PBO) combined with pyrethroids in insecticidetreated nets to prevent malaria in Africa. Cochrane Database of Systematic Reviews 2018, Issue 11. Art. No.: CD012776. DOI: 10.1002/14651858.CD012776.pub2.

[92] Agaba BB, Yeka A, Nsobya S, Arinaitwe E, Nankabirwa J, Opigo J, Mbaka P, Lim CS, Kalyango JN, Karamagi C, Kamya MR. Systematic review of the status of pfhrp2 and pfhrp3 gene deletion, approaches and methods used for its estimation and reporting in *Plasmodium falciparum* populations in Africa: review of published studies 2010-2019. Malaria Journal. 2019; **18(1)**:355.

[93] Lucchi, N.W., Karell, M.A., Journel, I. *et al.* PET-PCR method for the molecular detection of malaria parasites in a national malaria surveillance study in Haiti. Malaria Journal. 2011; **13**, 462.

[94] Nair CB, Jagannath J, Pradeep AS, Prakash BN, Manoj NM, Malpani S, Pullela PK, Subbarao PV, Ramamoorthy S, Ghosh SK. Differential Diagnosis of Malaria on Truelab Uno1, a Portable, Real-Time, MicroPCR Device for Point-Of-Care Applications. PLoS One. 2016; 11(1): e014696. doi:10.1371/journal.pone.0146961.

[95] Noviyanti R, Miotto O, Barry A, et al. Implementing parasite genotyping into national surveillance frameworks: feedback from control programmes and researchers in the Asia–Pacific region. Malaria Journal. 2020; **19:** 271.

[96] Dwivedi A, Khim N, Reynes C, Ravel P, Ma L, et al. *Plasmodium falciparum* parasite population structure and gene flow associated to anti-malarial drugs resistance in Cambodia. Malaria Journal. 2016; **15**:319.

[97] Runtuwene LR, Tuda JSB, Mongan AE et al. Nanopore sequencing of drug-resistance-associated genes in malaria parasites, *Plasmodium falciparum*. Scientific Reports. 2018; **8:** 8286.

[98] Fola AA, Kattenberg E, Razook Z, et al. SNP barcodes provide higher resolution than microsatellite markers to measure *Plasmodium vivax* population genetics. Malaria Journal. 2020; **19**, 375.

[99] Amambua-Ngwa A, Amenga-Etego L, Kamau E, Amato R, Ghansah A,

et al. Major subpopulations of *Plasmodium falciparum* in sub-Saharan Africa. Science. 2019; 23; **365(6455)**: 813-816.

[100] Hancock PA, Hendriks CJM, Tangena J-A, Gibson H, Hemingway J, Coleman M, et al. (2020) Mapping trends in insecticide resistance phenotypes in African malaria vectors. PLoS Biology. 2020; 18(6): e3000633.

[101] Taylor AR, Jacob PE, Neafsey DE, Buckee CO. Estimating relatedness between malaria parasites. Genetics. 2019; **212(4)**:1337-1351.

[102] Feng J, Zhang L, Huang F, Yin JH, Tu H, Xia ZG, Zhou SS, Xiao N, Zhou XN, 2018. Ready for malaria elimination: zero indigenous case reported in the People's Republic of China. Malaria Journal 2018; **17**:315.

[103] Lindblade KA, Kachur SP. Opportunities for subnational malaria elimination in high-burden Countries. American Journal of Tropical Medicine and Hygiene. 2020; **103(6)**:2153-2154.

[104] Sanders KC, Rundi C, Jelip J, Rashman Y, Smith Gueye C, Gosling RD. Eliminating malaria in Malaysia: the role of partnerships between the public and commercial sectors in Sabah. Malaria Journal. 2014; **13**:24.

[105] Chin AZ, Maluda MCM, Jelip J, et al. Malaria elimination in Malaysia and the rising threat of *Plasmodium knowlesi*. **Journal of Physiological Anthropology**. 2020; **39**, 36.

[106] Nabarro DN, Tayler EM. The "Roll Back Malaria" campaign. Science. 1998; **280(5372)**:2067-2068.

[107] Ghosh SK, Tiwari SN, Ojha VP. A renewed way of malaria control in Karnataka, south India. Frontiers in Physiology. 2012; **3**:194.

[108] Ghosh SK. Larvivorous fish: repurposing of an old strategy for sustainable malaria vector control – a success story based in Karnataka, South India. In: Vector Biology and Control-An Update for Malaria Elimination Initiative in India, New Delhi (Dev V, Ed.), The National Academy of Sciences, India. 2020; 197-204.

[109] Killeen GF, Fillinger U, Kiche I, Gouagna LC, Knols BG. Eradication of *Anopheles gambiae* from Brazil: lessons for malaria control in Africa? Lancet Infectious Diseases. 2002; **Oct; 2(10)**:618-627.

[110] Ghosh SK, Ghosh C. New ways to tackle malaria. In a book chapter `Current Topics in the Epidemiology of Vector-Borne Diseases', 2019. IntechOpen, UK, DOI: 10.5772/intechopen.89467. Available from: https://www.intechopen.com/online-first/new-ways-to-tackle-malaria

[111] Silva V L, Lovaglio R B, Zuben C J V, Contiero J. 2015. Rhamnolipids: Solution against *Aedes aegypti*? Frontiers in Microbiology. 2015; **6:** 2-6.

[112] Das D, Vongpromek R, Assawariyathipat T, Srinamon K, Kennon K, et al. Multi-centric field evaluation of a digital malaria microscopy device based on machine-learning: EasyScan GO - a preliminary analysis. Paper presented in the 69th Annual Virtual Meeting of the American Society of Tropical Medicine and Hygiene. 2020. Abstract No. 1635. Available from: https://moticdigitalpathology.com/wp-content/uploads/2020/11/b_Multi-centric-Field-Evaluation-Of-A-Digital-Malaria-Microscopy-Device-Based-On-Machine-Learning_-EasyScan-GO-A-Preliminary-Analysis__b_.pdf.

[113] Couret J, Moreira DC, Bernier D, Loberti AM, Dotson EM, Alvarez M (2020) Delimiting cryptic morphological variation among human malaria vector species using convolutional neural networks. PLoS Neglected Tropical Diseases. 2020; **14(12)**: e0008904.

[114] Cheung YW, Dirkzwager RM, Wong WC, Cardoso J, D'Arc Neves Costa J, Tanner JA. Aptamer-mediated Plasmodium-specific diagnosis of malaria. Biochimie. 2018; **145**:131-136.

[115] Oteng EK, Gu W, McKeague M. High-efficiency enrichment enables identification of aptamers to circulating *Plasmodium falciparum*-infected erythrocytes. Scientific Reports. 2020; **10**:9706.

[116] Nik Kamarudin NAA, Mohammed NA, Mustaffa KMF. Aptamer Technology: Adjunct Therapy for Malaria. Biomedicines. 2017; **5(1)**:1.

[117] Kormos A, Lanzaro GC, Bier E, Dimopoulos G, Marshall JM, et al. Application of the relationship-based model to engagement for field trials of genetically engineered malaria vectors. American Journal of Tropical Medicine and Hygiene. 2020 Dec 21. doi: 10.4269/ajtmh.20-0868. Online ahead of print.

[118] Subramani PA, Vartak-Sharma N, Sreekumar S, et al. *Plasmodium vivax* liver stage assay platforms using Indian clinical isolates. Malaria Journal. 2020; **19:** 214.

[119] Malaria Vaccine Phase 2b Clinical Trial Results Published in Preprints with The Lancet. 23 April 2021. Available from: https://ir.novavax.com/news-releases/news-release-details/malaria-vaccine-phase-2b-clinical-trial-results-published?sf142619988=1

[120] Ntoumi F. What if tropical diseases had as much attention as COVID? Nature. 2020. **587**; 331. https://www.nature.com/articles/d41586-020-03220-5.

Chapter 10

Elimination of *Plasmodium vivax* Malaria: Problems and Solutions

Liwang Cui, Awtum Brashear, Lynette Menezes and John Adams

Abstract

Malaria is caused by multiple parasitic species of the genus *Plasmodium*. Although *P. falciparum* accounts for the highest mortality, *P. vivax* is the most geographically dispersed and the most common species outside of Africa. Several unique biological features make *P. vivax* less responsive to conventional control measures and allow it to persist even after elimination of *P. falciparum*. The ability of *P. vivax* to develop in diverse vectors at lower ambient temperatures bestows it a greater distribution range and resilience to ecological changes. Its tropism for reticulocytes often causes low-density infections below the levels detectable by routine diagnostic tests, demanding the development of more sensitive diagnostics. *P. vivax* produces gametocytes early enabling transmission before the manifestation of clinical symptoms, thus emphasizing the need for an integrated vector control strategy. More importantly, its dormant liver stage which engenders relapse is difficult to diagnose and treat. The deployment of available treatments for the liver hypnozoites, including primaquine and the recent U.S. Food and Drug Administration-approved tafenoquine, requires point-of-care diagnostics to detect glucose-6-phosphate dehydrogenase deficiency among endemic human populations. Here we review the continued challenges to effectively control *P. vivax* and explore integrated technologies and targeted strategies for the elimination of vivax malaria.

Keywords: *Plasmodium vivax*, relapse, transmission, G6PD, CYP2D6, radical cure

1. Introduction

Malaria has been an ancient scourge of humankind and efforts to mitigate the harm from malaria have been relentless. In 1955, the World Health Organization (WHO) launched the Global Malaria Eradication Program (GMEP), relying heavily on two essential tools: chloroquine (CQ), a safe and effective drug for malaria prevention and treatment, and the insecticide DDT for vector control. Despite the GMEP's enormous success in reducing malaria burden in many countries outside of sub-Saharan Africa, its failure to sustain the program resulted in malaria resurgence and discontinuation of this global campaign in 1969 [1]. The considerable gains achieved in many areas were soon lost and the world witnessed a sharp rise in malaria incidence in the following two decades. In India, for example, malaria prevalence reduced from an estimated 75 million cases to about 100,000 cases annually during the GMEP, only to rapidly expand to 6.5 million in 1976 [2, 3].

In recognition of this huge malaria burden, the Roll Back Malaria Partnership launched in 1998, marking a renewed attack on this disease resulting in a declining incidence of malaria globally. Empowered by a strong political will and enabled by financial commitment and new interventions, many national malaria control programs (NMCPs) now consider malaria elimination an attainable goal. WHO's "Global Technical Strategy for Malaria 2016-2030" provided goals for the next 15 years and specific guidelines for achieving these goals. Among them, "eliminating malaria in at least 35 countries" and "preventing the re-establishment of malaria in all countries that are malaria-free" specifically address the tasks to attain and sustain malaria elimination. Significant strides have been made toward malaria elimination in the past two decades with 19 countries attaining zero indigenous cases for 3 years or more between 2000 and 2018. These countries include Sri Lanka, Paraguay, and Uzbekistan, which were recently certified as malaria-free [4]. Despite these laudable achievements, formidable challenges still lie ahead for many endemic nations to achieve malaria elimination.

Of the six *Plasmodium* species naturally infecting humans, *P. falciparum* is usually considered the most virulent and is associated with the vast majority of deaths, while *P. vivax* is the most geographically widespread. In comparison, *P. ovale curtisi*, *P. ovale wallikeri*, and *P. malariae* are much less common, whereas the monkey malaria parasite *P. knowlesi* is primarily associated with zoonotic infections [5]. Since malaria elimination is the interruption of local malaria transmission (zero indigenous cases) in a defined geographic area, it is time to target the elimination of all malaria parasite species simultaneously to set the final stage for malaria eradication [6].

At the same time that malaria incidence is continually declining [4], malaria epidemiology is rapidly changing [7]. In countries pursuing elimination, structural changes in at-risk populations have resulted in malaria becoming geographically clustered in hard-to-reach pockets. "Border malaria" has become a shared phenomenon and malaria is increasingly an imported disease. Additionally, because of a divergent response by each species to control interventions, *P. vivax* has become the predominant parasite in malaria-endemic countries outside of Africa. Most pre-elimination countries—such as the members of the Asian Pacific Malaria Elimination Network (APMEN, www.apmen.org) — must be ready to face the ultimate challenge of eliminating vivax malaria, a potentially long and arduous process. In fact, because of the possibility of relapse, the WHO malaria-free certification requires no cases for three years [1]. Here we review the changing malaria epidemiology and discuss the challenges associated with vivax malaria elimination and solutions to address them.

2. Geographic distribution and epidemiology of vivax malaria

Outside of Africa, *P. vivax* is the most common parasite causing malaria. It accounts for 75, 50, and 29% of the malaria burden in the Americas, SE Asia, and the East Mediterranean, respectively [4]. The parasite's ability to complete its sporogonic development in mosquitoes at ambient temperatures as low as 16 °C and to lie dormant for seasonal transmission has extended its geographical range deep into the temperate zones. There is considerable spatial heterogeneity in *P. vivax* distribution at the global and local scales. SE Asia carries more than half of the global *P. vivax* burden (**Table 1**). In the Asian continent, India, Cambodia, and Myanmar have higher endogenous *P. vivax* burden, and transmission is concentrated along international borders [8]. Similarly, the southern part of South America has a relatively low burden with Paraguay and Argentina recently achieving malaria-free

	Africa	America	Eastern Mediterranean	SE Asia	Western Pacific	Total
P. vivax	704	700	1,414	3,947	690	7,500
All	213,000	929	4,900	7,900	1,980	228,000

Table 1.
Estimated cases of P. vivax *and all malaria (×1,000) by WHO region [4].*

status, whereas the northern part of the continent has a substantial *P. vivax* burden (**Figure 1**). In Africa, until recently, *P. vivax* was documented only in the Horn of Africa, and considered extremely rare or "absent" in Central and West Africa because of the dominance of the Duffy-negative blood group [10], a required receptor for erythrocyte invasion by *P. vivax* [11]. Increasing reports of *P. vivax* in Duffy-negative individuals suggests its capability to exploit Duffy-independent invasion pathways [12, 13]. In the last decade, the growing evidence of *P. vivax* transmission in all regions of Africa, including acute and asymptomatic cases, infected vectors, serological indicators, and infected international travelers, indicates more *P. vivax* transmission than previously thought [14, 15]. Although malaria control programs in Africa are justifiably focused on *P. falciparum* (given the striking morbidity and mortality associated with this species), *P. vivax* is becoming an emerging concern for malaria elimination from African nations.

Throughout history, *P. vivax* has shown extreme resilience to control measures [16], and in many areas where *P. falciparum* and *P. vivax* co-exist, *P. vivax* is becoming predominant [17, 18]. With this shift in species predominance come changes in the at-risk populations. In areas of *P. falciparum* and *P. vivax* sympatry, clinical episodes of vivax malaria rapidly decrease around 12 months of age, whereas *P. falciparum* cases continue to rise until about 3 years of age [19, 20]. Since exposure undoubtedly plays a role in the acquisition and maintenance of immunity, *P. vivax* recurrence may allow for repeated exposure from fewer infection events which may contribute to this age discrepancy. Additionally, primaquine (PQ) is not commonly given to children below 5 years, while chloroquine (CQ) underdosing is not unusual [21], resulting in repeated *P. vivax* attacks in young children. Recent studies in SE Asia showed that school-aged children had significantly increased

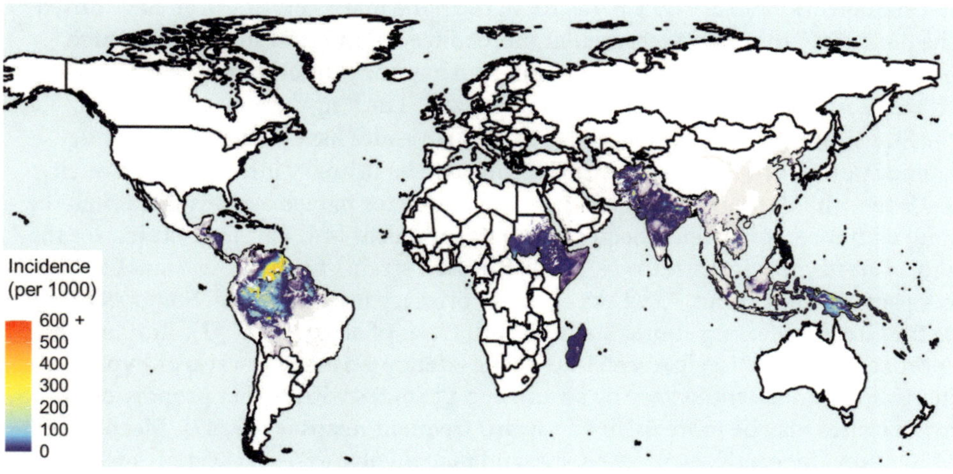

Figure 1.
Global distribution of P. vivax *malaria. Shading represents incidence in cases per 1000 people per year [8, 9]. Very low incidence areas are shaded in gray.*

odds of acquiring *P. vivax* infections [18, 22]. Because PQ is contraindicated for pregnant women, radical treatment of *P. vivax* remains difficult in this group. Consequentially, relapsing episodes of malaria during pregnancy can lead to congenital malaria [23–25]. Certain occupations such as soldiers and forest workers are also more vulnerable to malaria infections [18, 26]. A better understanding of local malaria epidemiology will be essential for implementing targeted control measures.

3. Morbidity of vivax malaria

Biologically, *P. vivax* exhibits key differences from *P. falciparum* influencing its transmission, presentation and outcome [27]. Historically, *P. vivax* malaria has been mistakenly described as "benign tertian malaria". In fact, *P. vivax* infection causes a full spectrum of disease symptoms ranging from uncomplicated febrile illness to severe and fatal malaria. Severe *P. vivax* malaria is often associated with severe anemia, a common complication, as well as thrombocytopenia, acute respiratory distress, hepatic dysfunction, renal failure, seizures or coma, and shock [28, 29]. Severe anemia is the most common complication associated with *P. vivax* malaria [30–32]. *P. vivax* has a strong preference for $CD71^{high}$ reticulocytes [33] and aggravates anemia by targeting cells immediately after replacement [34, 35]. Recurrent *P. vivax* parasitemia further elevates the risk of severe anemia [36]. Although the risk of thrombocytopenia is prevalent in all forms of malaria, evidence suggests that it is more common in *P. vivax* than *P. falciparum* patients [37, 38]. In pregnant women, *P. vivax* infection is associated with a higher risk of anemia, abortion and low birth weight [39, 40]. Furthermore, the presence of co-morbidities may exacerbate *P. vivax* infections resulting in severe and life-threatening complications.

4. Relapse

One distinctive feature of *P. vivax* that enables the parasite to evade conventional control measures designed for *P. falciparum* is the formation of a dormant liver stage, termed hypnozoite [41]. Hypnozoites persist in a non-dividing fashion within the liver where they may be awakened weeks and months later causing relapse. Recent detections of *P. vivax* parasites in the bone marrow and spleen have raised the possibility that the extravascular merozoites might be an additional source of recurrence in addition to the relapse from hypnozoite activation [42, 43]. Two latency forms of *P. vivax* strains are recognized. The long-latency strains (e.g., the St. Elizabeth strain) prevalent in temperate zones have either a ~ 9-month latency period or a 2-week incubation time for the primary infection followed by a ~ 9-month interval before the relapse, allowing for parasite survival through the long winter season when mosquito vectors are absent [44, 45]. In contrast, for the short-latency tropical strains (e.g., the Chesson strain) from SE Asia and Oceania, relapses typically occur ~3 weeks after the primary infection [46]. Some areas, such as the Greater Mekong subregion host both types of strains [46, 47]. Besides, the sporozoite inoculation load can impact the latency period. The ratio of hypnozoites to sporozoites could vary by strain, and parasites with higher proportions of hypnozoites may be more inclined toward frequent relapses [48, 49]. Mechanisms of hypnozoite reactivation are elusive and may involve external stimuli such as drugs, another malaria infection, or other infectious diseases [50]. A meta-analysis of *P. falciparum* drug efficacy trials reveals a high risk of *P. vivax* parasitemia after treatment of falciparum malaria [51].

Relapse increases the morbidity associated with *P. vivax* infections. Relapses can contribute to 50–80% of the overall vivax infections in high transmission areas [52–55]; sometimes occurring repeatedly from the same infection, such as a case from Eritrea where one patient's three episodes of vivax malaria were caused by meiotic siblings suggesting the same infection event [56]. Additionally, *P. vivax* is frequently found in highly polyclonal infections, even in areas with relatively low malaria endemicity. One study from Cambodia found that around half of polyclonal infections might have resulted from relapse [57]. Long-distance parasite migration and introduction also favor hypnozoites. When introduced by an asymptomatic human host to an area with suitable *Anopheles* vector species, relapsed parasites could spark autochthonous infections and establish new transmission foci, as observed in Greece [58].

5. Diagnosis

Accurate and timely diagnosis of malaria by species is essential for the delivery of appropriate treatments. In clinical settings, acute vivax malaria is diagnosed by microscopy or rapid diagnostic tests (RDTs). Routine microscopy has a limit of detection (LOD) of around 50 parasites/µl of blood [59, 60]. Specific training is required, as misidentification of the infecting species is fairly common [59, 61]. RDTs are a fast, affordable and efficient method for malaria diagnosis with a LOD of ~200 parasites/µl, but the sensitivity varies among brands [62]. The tropism of *P. vivax* for reticulocytes can result in parasite densities much lower than the LODs of the conventional diagnostic methods. Recently, the creation of ultra-sensitive RDTs has lowered the LOD for *P. falciparum* infection [63, 64] but one targeting *P. vivax* is still lacking.

In malaria elimination settings, malaria prevalence is often assessed through active case detection in the form of cross-sectional surveillance. Most available clinical diagnostic tools are inadequate for detecting *P. vivax* asymptomatic reservoirs with very low parasitemia. Molecular methods although sensitive to low-density infections and useful in epidemiological surveillance are not feasible in field applications [19]. The presence of microscopically subpatent infections in endemic populations may render a mass screening and treatment-based strategy ineffective if screening is based on low-sensitivity tools [65].

Hypnozoites pose a significant challenge for the elimination of vivax malaria because they defy detection by any diagnostic methods. Recently, a screen for IgG responses to a panel of 342 *P. vivax* antigens in longitudinal clinical cohorts established that antibody responses to eight proteins detected *P. vivax* infections in the previous 9 months with 80% sensitivity and specificity [66]. Modeling demonstrates that treating a serologically positive population could potentially reduce *P. vivax* prevalence by 59–69%. While this new development still awaits prospective evaluation, it offers a promising surrogate marker for hypnozoite detection and treatment.

6. Chemotherapy and drug resistance

Most antimalarial drugs in use are blood schizontocides that kill asexual blood-stage parasites, which are associated with clinical symptoms. The ability of *P. vivax* (and also *P. ovale* spp.) to form liver hypnozoites capable of causing relapses requires the addition of a hypnozoitocide to prevent relapses. For the radical cure of *P. vivax* malaria, CQ and PQ have been the companion therapies of choice for the treatment of uncomplicated vivax malaria since the 1950s. Due to the development of CQ resistance in the island of New Guinea, CQ was abandoned and replaced with an artemisinin combination therapy (ACT) there [67].

6.1 Treatment of *P. vivax* blood-stage infections

For the treatment of blood-stage uncomplicated *P. vivax* malaria, WHO recommends the use of either an ACT or CQ in areas where parasites remain CQ sensitive (CQS) or an ACT in areas where *P. vivax* is known to be CQ resistant (CQR) [68]. ACTs are contraindicated in pregnant women in their first trimester; thus for this patient population, uncomplicated vivax malaria is treated with either CQ for CQS malaria or quinine for CQR malaria. WHO recommends parenteral therapy for severe malaria with either artesunate, artemether, or quinine (listed here in the order of preference) for at least 24 h regardless of the causative *Plasmodium* species [68]. No additional drugs are needed to block transmission (as compared to the recommended low-dose PQ for blocking the transmission of *P. falciparum*) because *P. vivax* gametocytes are sensitive to most antimalarial drugs.

6.1.1 Chloroquine and unified treatment with ACTs

CQ remains the mainstay treatment for *P. vivax* malaria in most endemic countries. If low-grade or sporadic CQ resistance is identified, optimizing the treatment regimen can improve the therapeutic efficacy of CQ. A recent meta-analysis of CQ efficacy studies indicates underdosing (<25 mg of CQ/kg) among a substantial proportion (>30%) of patients [21]. Increasing the recommended dose to 30 mg/kg, especially in children under 5 years, could reduce the risk of early recurrence by more than 40% if CQ is used alone. The safety and tolerability of the increased CQ dose are substantiated by earlier studies where CQ doses of 50 mg/kg were used to treat CQR *P. falciparum* [69]. In addition to underdosing, there is accumulating evidence of emerging CQR parasites in endemic sites [70, 71]. A meta-analysis of 129 clinical trials on CQ efficacy identified CQR *P. vivax* parasites in most vivax-endemic areas, though the prevalence of resistance varied geographically [72]. The epicenter of CQR *P. vivax* is located on the island of New Guinea, where the CQR parasite was first reported in 1989 [73]. Reports of high rates of recurrent parasitemia within 28 days in subsequent years [74–76]—consistent with the WHO definition for RI resistance [77]—led to the ultimate withdrawal of CQ from treating vivax malaria in New Guinea [67]. ACTs have shown high efficacy as a treatment replacement of CQ for uncomplicated vivax malaria in many endemic sites [78–80]. Dihydroartemisinin-piperaquine treatment had a significantly lower risk of *P. vivax* recurrence at day 42 than artemether-lumefantrine [81]. These higher rates of recurrence are probably due to different pharmacokinetic profiles of the partner drugs: lumefantrine has a much shorter half-life (~4 days) than piperaquine (28–35 days) and thus offers less protection against early relapse and/or reinfection. This can be mitigated by the inclusion of PQ in the treatment [81]. In areas co-endemic for both *P. vivax* and *P. falciparum*, the deployment of a unified ACT-based strategy for both parasites provides several advantages [78]. First, the excellent clinical efficacy of ACTs against vivax malaria makes them highly suitable for areas of known or suspected CQR vivax. Second, it offers operational ease in routine practice where species misdiagnosis is a frequent issue [18]. The World Malaria Report 2020 indicated an increasing number of countries adopting ACTs as first-line therapy for *P. vivax* [82]. The reluctance to change the treatment may be due to the perceived ease of treating vivax malaria and the economic burden associated with the switch to a much more expensive drug.

6.1.2 Chloroquine resistance

To ensure the high efficacy of first-line therapy, close monitoring is essential. For *P. falciparum* malaria, this is typically done by clinical efficacy studies, *in vitro* drug assays, and molecular surveillance of resistance-conferring genetic markers. Surveillance for *P. vivax* resistance relies heavily on *in vivo* assessment of the schizontocidal therapy, conducted through follow-ups of recurrent *P. vivax* parasitemia after initial treatment for 28 days. Extending the follow-up to 42 days will allow the identification of late recrudescence [21]. After the standard treatment with CQ (3-day regimen of 25 mg/kg CQ base), the blood concentration of the active drugs (CQ and desethyl CQ) reaches the minimum inhibitory concentration (MIC, ~100 ng/ml) around 28 days, and thus recurrent parasitemia before day 28, regardless of the origin of the parasites (recrudescence, relapse or new infection), is likely due to CQR parasites [83]. Given that drug resistance is defined as the growth of the parasite in the presence of the drug above the MIC, CQ resistance must be confirmed by measurement of residual blood CQ and desethyl CQ levels on the day of recurrence.

Ex vivo measurement of drug sensitivity has been conducted in many endemic regions, but it is not ideal for routinely monitoring antimalarial drug resistance in *P. vivax* because of the difficulties in setting up the *ex vivo* assays [84, 85]. Since a long-term *in vitro* culture system is not available for *P. vivax*, *ex vivo* assays are restricted to one-time assays using fresh field isolates, making further validation of results difficult. The *P. vivax* tropism for reticulocytes means that reinvasion does not happen frequently under field conditions. As a result, *ex vivo* drug exposure is limited to one intraerythrocytic cycle. The most commonly used method to quantify parasite growth is the modified Rieckman's microtest that compares schizont maturation rates [86, 87]. Another method quantifies the production of lactate dehydrogenase by the parasites [88]. Unlike *P. falciparum* clinical samples where parasites are all at the ring stage, *P. vivax* clinical isolates contain mixed stages with various degrees of synchronicity. Since *P. vivax* trophozoites are highly tolerant to CQ [89, 90], *ex vivo* assays for CQ need to be done using isolates with no less than 80% ring stages. Despite the variability of assay results between labs, *ex vivo* assays can complement *in vivo* studies to follow temporal changes of drug sensitivities in an endemic area [91].

Molecular surveillance of putative CQR markers in *P. vivax* populations, though conducted in multiple endemic sites, is hindered by the lack of understanding of the genetic basis of resistance [71]. Initial studies focused on the orthologs of the *pfcrt* and *pfmdr1*, the main determinants of CQ resistance in *P. falciparum*. Most studies fail to show a strong correlation between *pvcrt-o* mutations and the CQR phenotype. Some studies from the Brazilian Amazon indicated an association of CQ resistance with higher expression level and gene amplification of *pvcrt-o* [92, 93], whereas such a link was not validated in Papua Indonesia with high-grade CQ resistance [94]. The relationship between the upregulation of *pvcrt-o* expression and CQ resistance was recently supported by a genetic cross of *P. vivax* strains [95]. There are also considerable controversies about the main *pfmdr1* mutations Y976F and F1076L as potentially conferring CQ resistance [96–99], suggesting that *pvmdr1* may not be a major determinant for CQ resistance in *P. vivax*. Population genomics studies of *P. vivax* populations from areas with drastically different CQ resistance have identified genomic sites under strong selection [100, 101], but their significance in mediating drug resistance remains to be determined. When using *Plasmodium knowlesi* as an *in vitro* model, some of the markers did not seem to change the drug sensitivity phenotypes in transgenic parasites [102].

6.2 Treatment of *P. vivax* liver stages

6.2.1 Primaquine and tafenoquine in anti-relapse therapy

Relapses from hypnozoite reactivation are preventable by anti-relapse therapy with 8-aminoquinoline drugs. For the prevention of relapse, WHO recommends a dose of 0.25–0.5 mg/kg body weight of PQ daily for 14 days [68]. A high dose (0.5 mg/kg/day) is needed for tropical, frequently relapsing *P. vivax* strains such as the Chesson strain that is prevalent in East Asia and Oceania, whereas a lower dose (0.25 mg/kg/day) is recommended for temperate strains. Many nations adopt low-dose PQ for fear of possible harm to unscreened patients with glucose-6-phosphate dehydrogenase (G6PD) deficiency, but suboptimal dosing may fail to prevent relapses in many endemic sites [46, 103]. Conversely, the high dose requires more detailed clinical investigations to document its efficacy [104].

The 14-day PQ treatment regimen is inevitably associated with poor adherence, which seriously compromises its public health benefit. It is estimated that the effectiveness of unsupervised PQ regimens in vivax patients from Papua, Indonesia, could be as low as 12% [105]. Unfortunately, a shortened 5-day regimen of 15 mg daily PQ did not efficaciously prevent relapse [106, 107]. However, a 7-day high PQ dose (1.0 mg/kg/day) regimen in Asia and Africa recently performed comparably to the 14-day PQ regimen (0.5 mg/kg/day), providing a possible solution to poor adherence [108, 109]. In 2018, another 8-aminoquinoline, tafenoquine (TQ), was approved by the U.S. Food and Drug Administration for radical cure of vivax malaria and malaria prophylaxis [110, 111]. TQ, administered as a single 300 mg dose, showed similar tolerability and efficacy to PQ in preventing relapse in vivax malaria [112, 113]. While TQ appears to be the best choice for travel medicine in people with normal G6PD activity, further clinical studies are needed before seeing its deployment in endemic regions.

In patients with known G6PD deficiency, PQ may be given at 0.75 mg/kg for eight weeks [68], but this should be under close medical supervision with ready access to blood transfusion services. This dosing regimen leverages the "total dose effect", discovered in the relapsing monkey malaria parasite *P. cynomolgi* [114]—it posits the same efficacious dose of PQ can be delivered in a range of schedules to achieve the same therapeutic effect. For the temperate and tropical strains, the total dose equals 210 and 420 mg PQ, respectively [115]. This regimen was tested in those carrying the G6PD A- variant experimentally infected with the Chesson strain and found to be safe and efficacious [116]. A recent trial of this regimen found that 5/18 (27.7%) G6PD deficient patients experienced >25% fractional drops in their hemoglobin concentrations, including one patient requiring transfusion [117, 118]. This study precludes the use of unsupervised weekly PQ in Cambodia (and perhaps other parts of the Greater Mekong subregion), where the regional prevalence of Viangchan (a class II G6PD variant) and other hemoglobinopathies such as hemoglobin E and β-thalassemia may predispose G6PD deficient patients to a greater risk of acute hemolytic anemia (AHA) when treated with PQ.

6.2.2 G6PD deficiency and point-of-care testing

The root problem of PQ and TQ is hemolytic toxicity in patients with G6PD deficiency [115, 119, 120]. The *G6PD* gene is extraordinarily polymorphic with at least 217 known mutations, and their effects on the stability and catalytic efficiency of the enzyme vary greatly [121–123]. The residual enzyme activity varies from 5–10% of the normal levels in the G6PD A- variant from Africa to less than 1% of the normal levels in the G6PD Mediterranean variant. As a result, the clinical spectrum of PQ toxicity can range from relatively mild and self-limiting in G6PD A- individuals to severe AHA in the G6PD Mediterranean individuals, while most variants from Southeast Asia (the Mahidol, Viangchan, and Canton variants) typically have intermediate levels of enzyme activity [124]. Evidence supporting protective advantages of the G6PD A- against *P. falciparum* [125–128] and G6PD Mahidol against *P. vivax* [129, 130] is consistent with the wide geographic distribution of G6PD deficiency and its overlap with malaria distribution [124]. G6PD deficiency affects around 8% of the global population, but its distribution is geographically heterogeneous and can range from 3 to 30% in tropical areas [131–133]. G6PD is X-linked; thus, male hemizygotes and female homozygotes have full expression of the G6PD deficiency, whereas heterozygous females display varying degrees of G6PD activity due to random X-chromosome inactivation (lyonization) resulting in red cell mosaicism. As a result, the male population displays two distinctive phenotypes, whereas the female population shows a full spectrum of G6PD activity, which has significant ramifications for the treatment with the 8-aminoquinoline drugs [134]. Because of this, cases of severe AHA have been identified in female heterozygotes receiving the high daily dose of PQ (1.0 mg/kg) even though these subjects tested as G6PD normal after screening with the qualitative fluorescent spot test (FST) [108, 109, 135]. Furthermore, even in vivax patients with a class III G6PD variant (e.g., the Mahidol variant considered mildly deficient), a low-dose PQ treatment (15 mg/kg/day) for three days could lead to AHA, requiring blood transfusions or even renal failure [117, 136, 137]. Therefore, for the goal of malaria elimination in areas with *P. vivax*, the deployment of point-of-care G6PD deficiency diagnostics is urgent [138]. Currently, FST is the most common method to screen for G6PD deficiency, which has minimum lab requirements of cold chain and electricity as well as trained personnel. The CareStart™ G6PD RDT (Access Bio) is a point-of-care screen for G6PD deficiency, but the cost (~15 USD) is prohibitive for large-scale implementation in low-resource endemic areas [139]. Of note, qualitative screening with the FST or RDT can detect G6PD deficiency below 30% of normal activity, but cannot reliably diagnose female heterozygotes with an intermediate deficiency (30–70% normal activity). Fortunately, rapidly eliminating PQ with its half-life of 6 h can be prescribed to patients with G6PD activity above 30% of normal activity [111]. However, TQ has a long half-life of 14 days, and the recommended threshold of G6PD activity is set at 70% of normal activity. Thus, for rolling out TQ in endemic areas, more stringent screening of G6PD activity with quantitative tests is needed [111, 140]. A recent cost-effectiveness analysis suggests that TQ may be deployed in endemic areas outside sub-Saharan Africa using a gender-specific strategy where G6PD-normal females can be prescribed a low-dose PQ for 14 days [141]. This approach again centers on the availability of a qualitative G6PD test.

6.2.3 Host cytochrome P450 (CYP) 2D6 activity

Another problem identified recently is that PQ efficacy depends on the host activity of the hepatic cytochrome P450 (CYP) 2D6. Failures of PQ to radically cure have been linked to reduced activity of CYP2D6 [142], which mediates activation of PQ to its active metabolite(s) [143, 144]. Follow-up studies in Indonesia have established CYP2D6-dependent metabolism of PQ as a key determinant of the efficacy against relapse [145]. Studies in Brazil similarly identified an association of the diplotype-based CYP2D6 activity score of $\leq$1.0 with increased risks of *P. vivax* recurrence within 180 days after PQ treatment [146, 147]. There are also cases of patients with impaired CYP2D6 activity suffering from multiple relapse attacks despite receiving adequate anti-relapse therapy with PQ [148, 149]. Even for the single-low-dose PQ used as a transmission-reducing strategy for *P. falciparum*, the genetic variation in CYP2D6 affects the pharmacokinetics of PQ [150], and CYP2D6 poor/intermediate metabolism is associated with prolonged gametocyte carriage [151]. Thus, it is important to determine the extent to which reduced CYP2D6 activity is responsible for PQ failures in the radical cure of vivax malaria [152].

CYP2D6 is involved in the metabolism of as many as 25% of drugs in clinical use and is also highly polymorphic [153, 154]. Over 150 CYP2D6 allelic variants have been found and grouped into four phenotypic classes of non-functional, low, normal, and increased metabolizers, with respective activity scores of 0, 0.5, 1.0, and 2.0 per allele, corresponding to diplotype activity scores of 0, 0.5, 1.0, 1.5, 2.0, and > 2.0 [155]. Individuals with diplotype activity scores of ≤1.0 are considered to be poor PQ metabolizers [156]. The proportion of poor PQ metabolizers varies geographically. In the Brazilian Amazon, ~25% of the population was found to have reduced CYP2D6 activity [146, 147]. In Cambodia, 52 and 1% of subjects were found to have intermediate and poor metabolism, respectively [157]. Most surveys are based on genotyping results, whereas direct measurement of the CYP2D6 activity using CYP2D6 substrate metabolism (dextromethorphan to dextrorphan conversion) could more accurately determine the phenotype [145]. While CYP2D6 genotypes are not routinely screened in malaria-endemic areas, knowledge of the extent of this problem will help plan for vivax elimination.

6.2.4 Primaquine resistance

PQ-resistant *P. vivax* hypnozoites have never been unequivocally demonstrated. PQ efficacy studies are complicated to conduct and possibly one reason PQ resistant parasites have not been identified. PQ alone has excellent anti-relapse activity [158], but co-administration of a schizontocide (e.g., quinine, CQ, or an ACT) has been shown to significantly potentiate PQ's anti-relapse activity [159]. This effect has been recently verified using an *in vitro P. cynomolgi* hepatic system, wherein CQ could enhance PQ's activity against schizonts and hypnozoites by ~18-fold [160]. Any therapeutic failures of PQ in *P. vivax* radical cure could plausibly result from reasons other than PQ resistance. For example, treatment may fail because of improper PQ dose, short duration of treatment, or poor adherence to the treatment regimen [80, 161, 162]. Further, with the current genotyping strategy, it is not possible to reliably determine whether a recurrent infection after day 28 is due to relapse or reinfection. In endemic areas, patients can harbor multiple genotypically different hypnozoites and a relapse infection may be from reactivation of a heterologous hypnozoite clone [163, 164]. Likewise, a genotype different from that of the primary infection may be from either relapse or reinfection. PQ efficacy studies require longer follow-up, making it difficult to exclude the possibility of reinfection in endemic areas. In studies where the possibility of reinfection can be excluded [158, 165], PQ failure requires further scrutiny, especially with the newly identified CYP2D6 effect. In 21 Indonesian patients who experienced therapeutic failure of PQ against *P. vivax* relapse, 20 were classified as CYP2D6 impaired, whereas only one with normal CYP2D6 activity and adequate PQ exposure may represent true resistance to PQ [145]. Ultimately, PQ resistance may still be rare in most endemic areas, though continued surveillance is recommended.

7. Vector control

P. vivax produces transmissible gametocytes early in infection before the development of clinical symptoms [166–168], allowing ready transmission through mosquito vectors with more efficient transmission in certain species [169, 170]. There are 71 *Anopheles* species/species complexes that are potential vectors for vivax malaria [171], and vector control is a critical component for integrated control of vivax malaria [172]. Long-lasting insecticide-treated nets (LLINs) and indoor residual spraying (IRS) are the key vector-based malaria interventions that are highly effective in sub-Saharan Africa [173, 174]. However, these measures are either under-utilized with low coverage or less effective in certain regions [82, 175]. Since many vector species exhibit early evening and outdoor biting preferences, LLINs and IRS alone are not sufficient for interrupting malaria transmission [176]. In malaria elimination settings, residual transmission often occurs in a forested habitat that lacks core mosquito control coverage [177, 178], requiring targeted vector control efforts for special populations. Further, the emergence and spread of insecticide resistance compromising the efficacy of mosquito control measures needs continual monitoring [179–181]. Successful malaria elimination programs in various regions of the world have all included vector control as one of their pillar strategies [16]. Thus, novel vector control approaches are desperately needed including larval control strategies [182, 183], incorporation of ivermectin in the mass drug administration (MDA) program to reduce the life span of mosquitoes [184, 185], topical and spatial repellents [186, 187], genetically manipulated mosquitoes for population replacement [188], and next-generation LLINs and IRS [189].

8. Technologies and strategies for supporting elimination

8.1 Experience gleaned from successful stories

Despite the unique challenges posed by *P. vivax*, elimination is achievable with integrated control measures. There are nearly 40 countries and territories that have been WHO certified as malaria-free, with 10 of those achieving certification since the turn of the century. Although they all used a combination of strategies including vector control, case management, and mass drug administration, different regions emphasized specific sets of tools at different stages of elimination. The Maldives, the first country in SE Asia to reach malaria-free status, relied heavily on vector control [190]. For Sri Lanka's battle against malaria, strong surveillance, case detection, and patient isolation with treatment were key to its highly targeted elimination strategy [191]. Sri Lanka had anti-relapse treatment as a component of its elimination plan, especially for highly mobile military members, engendering the elimination of *P. vivax* almost simultaneously with *P. falciparum* [191]. In the republics of the former Soviet Union, preventive therapy and MDA with PQ, seasonal CQ chemoprophylaxis, and IRS, were instrumental for malaria elimination [16, 192]. China eliminated indigenous malaria cases in 2017 after the declaration of the National Malaria Elimination Action Plan in 2010 [193]. In the final stage of malaria elimination, China adopted targeted MDA to eliminate vivax transmission in central provinces and developed a rigorous 1–3-7 malaria surveillance strategy [194, 195].

8.2 Strategies for vivax elimination

Management of clinical vivax malaria. Accurate diagnosis using sensitive methods is critical for proper treatment of vivax cases. More sensitive diagnostics such as the uRDTs under development may fill such a need. For the treatment of blood stages, a unified treatment with ACTs is highly recommended. The deployment of point-of-care diagnostics for G6PD deficiency will ensure the wider prescription of the anti-relapse drug PQ. For those patients with G6PD deficiency, monthly presumptive treatment or prophylaxis with a drug with a long half-life such as naphthoquine may be adopted, as it has proven to be safe and 100% effective for preventing relapse malaria parasite [196, 197].

Targeted MDA. As mass screenings and treatment-based strategies are ineffective for the final elimination phase [65], residual transmission requires targeted MDA to eliminate asymptomatic and submicroscopic parasite reservoirs. For the success of MDA, better knowledge of malaria epidemiology and strong community engagement are needed. In areas such as the Greater Mekong subregion, G6PD deficiency and CYP2D6 poor metabolizers are prevalent and may account for 30% of the population. In addition, point-of-care diagnostics for G6PD deficiency are not available, which seriously undermines the feasibility of PQ-based MDA [156]. In these regions, periodic MDA with an ACT or prophylaxis drug combination with a long eliminating half-life may be an effective alternative [196–199]. Incorporation of ivermectin in the MDA program can reduce the life span of adult mosquitoes and in turn, the transmission of the parasite [184, 185].

Vector control. Traditional control methods such as LLIN and IRS need to be implemented with high coverage. This can be supplemented with novel vector control approaches such as larval control [183]. Topical and spatial repellents [186, 187] may be used for populations at higher risk of outdoor transmission.

Surveillance system. The establishment of a stringent malaria surveillance system in the NMCPs that allows timely responses to new malaria incidence plays a crucial role in malaria elimination. This has proved highly important for many, if not all, successful malaria elimination stories. Within this system, training and capacity building are necessary to establish a malaria control network responding effectively to emerging malaria cases.

8.3 Sustaining elimination

With increased international and cross-border travel, imported malaria cases re-introduce malaria in countries where malaria has been eliminated [193, 200], potentially leading to local transmission [58]. Weakening malaria control programs have been linked to almost all resurgence events such as one that occurred in central China [201], and resource concerns are a large contributing factor [202]. Targeted elimination programs (including regular screening and extensive vector management) can be costly, and there remains a concern that countries who have achieved elimination status may be tempted to reduce their targeted vigilance in order to prioritize funding for other endeavors [203]. However, vector control programs are vital to multiple infectious disease programs, which makes them key components of an integrated response. Additionally, countries should continue to train medical workers for the diagnosis and treatment of malaria and remain vigilant to malaria re-introduction from international travelers or mobile communities. Experience from the malaria program in South Korea demonstrated the significance of good case management practice combined with stringent surveillance for reducing the resurgent malaria threat [204]. In many malaria-free nations, chemoprophylaxis is suggested for international travelers [191, 205], and introduced cases are met with an investigation to eliminate the possibility of endemic spread [206].

9. Conclusions

Several unique biological characters of the *P. vivax* parasite are responsible for its wide distribution and persistence in the face of escalating control efforts.

Problems	Solutions
Relapse from reactivation of dormant hypnozoites; long-latency strains allow for parasite survival beyond winter season	Treatment of hypnozoite stage; sustained vector control to prevent transmission
Anti-relapse treatment with PQ or TQ increases risk of acute hemolytic anemia in G6PD deficient patients with varying degrees in male vs. female	Deployment of point-of-care G6PD RDTs and gender-sensitive treatment strategies that account for differing phenotypic presentation of G6PD deficiency.
Impaired activity of CYP2D6 is associated with poor PQ efficacy	Screening for impairment in CYP2D6 activity in regions of PQ treatment failure can inform targeted treatment strategy
Lack of radical treatment for patients with G6PD deficiency, low CYP2D6 activity, and PQ contraindication	Prophylaxis with a safe drug with a long half-life (e.g., naphthoquine)
Suboptimal dosing in CQ treatment of uncomplicated malaria	Standardizing dose to 30 mg/kg, especially in children under five years can prevent early recurrence
CQ resistance in many endemic sites	Treatment with ACTs
Lack of RDTs for detecting asymptomatic reservoirs with low parasitemia	Detecting antibodies to specific *P. vivax* proteins followed by treatment may reduce *P. vivax* prevalence
Residual transmission from asymptomatic and submicroscopic parasite reservoirs	Targeted MDA following epidemiological assessment and community engagement
Vector control strategies such as LLINs and IRS have low coverage, decreased adherence and limited efficacy in some regions	Increasing coverage of LLINs and IRS. Implementing novel vector control approaches to decrease mosquito density, lifespan, and outdoor transmission
Single vertical strategy to eliminate malaria remains unsuccessful	Combined strategies of strong surveillance, early case detection, patient isolation with treatment, sustained vector control.

Table 2.
Summary of the problems and solutions in eliminating P. vivax malaria.

Table 2 summarizes the challenges in controlling and eliminating vivax malaria and potential solutions. Because of the geographical variation of the vivax malaria situation, different endemic countries are likely to emphasize one or a few control strategies. As an infectious disease involving the human-parasite-vector triad, it requires integrated approaches targeting all components of these interactions for the ultimate elimination of vivax malaria.

Acknowledgements

We thank the National Institute of Allergy and Infectious Diseases, NIH, for financial support (U19AI089672).

Author details

Liwang Cui[1,2*], Awtum Brashear[1,2], Lynette Menezes[1] and John Adams[2]

1 Department of Internal Medicine, Morsani College of Medicine, University of South Florida, Tampa, FL, USA

2 Center for Global Health and Infectious Diseases, College of Public Health, University of South Florida, Tampa, FL, USA

*Address all correspondence to: liwangcui@usf.edu

References

[1] Li XH, Kondrashin A, Greenwood B, et al. A Historical Review of WHO Certification of Malaria Elimination. Trends Parasitol. 2019;**35**:163-171.

[2] Pattanayak S, Sharma VP, Kalra NL, et al. Malaria paradigms in India and control strategies. Indian J Malariol. 1994;**31**:141-199.

[3] Baird JK. Essential guidance on malaria elimination in its history. J Vector Borne Dis. 2019;**56**:11-14.

[4] WHO. World Malaria Report 2019. https://www.who.int/publications-detail/world-malaria-report-2019. 2019.

[5] Millar SB, Cox-Singh J. Human infections with Plasmodium knowlesi--zoonotic malaria. Clin Microbiol Infect. 2015;**21**:640-648.

[6] Lover AA, Baird JK, Gosling R, et al. Malaria elimination: time to target all species. Am J Trop Med Hyg. 2018;**99**:17-23.

[7] Cotter C, Sturrock HJ, Hsiang MS, et al. The changing epidemiology of malaria elimination: new strategies for new challenges. Lancet. 2013;**382**:900-911.

[8] Battle KE, Lucas TCD, Nguyen M, et al. Mapping the global endemicity and clinical burden of *Plasmodium vivax*, 2000-17: a spatial and temporal modelling study. Lancet. 2019;**394**:332-343.

[9] Kahle D, Wickham H. ggmap: Spatial Visualization with ggplot2. The R Journal. 2013;**5**:144-161.

[10] Howes RE, Patil AP, Piel FB, et al. The global distribution of the Duffy blood group. Nat Commun. 2011;**2**:266.

[11] Miller LH, Mason SJ, Clyde DF, et al. The resistance factor to *Plasmodium vivax* in blacks. The Duffy-blood-group genotype, FyFy. N Engl J Med. 1976;**295**:302-304.

[12] Popovici J, Roesch C, Rougeron V. The enigmatic mechanisms by which *Plasmodium vivax* infects Duffy-negative individuals. PLoS Pathog. 2020;**16**:e1008258.

[13] Gunalan K, Niangaly A, Thera MA, et al. *Plasmodium vivax* infections of Duffy-negative erythrocytes: Historically undetected or a recent adaptation? Trends Parasitol. 2018;**34**:420-429.

[14] Howes RE, Reiner RC, Jr., Battle KE, et al. *Plasmodium vivax* Transmission in Africa. PLoS Negl Trop Dis. 2015;**9**:e0004222.

[15] Twohig KA, Pfeffer DA, Baird JK, et al. Growing evidence of *Plasmodium vivax* across malaria-endemic Africa. PLoS Negl Trop Dis. 2019;**13**:e0007140.

[16] Shanks GD. Control and elimination of *Plasmodium vivax*. Adv Parasitol. 2012;**80**:301-341.

[17] Cui L, Cao Y, Kaewkungwal J, et al. Malaria Elimination in the Greater Mekong Subregion: Challenges and Prospects. In: Manguin S, Dev V, editors. Towards Malaria Elimination: A Leap Forward: IntechOpen; 2018. p. 179-200.

[18] Geng J, Malla P, Zhang J, et al. Increasing trends of malaria in a border area of the Greater Mekong Subregion. Malar J. 2019;**18**:309.

[19] Lin E, Kiniboro B, Gray L, et al. Differential patterns of infection and disease with *P. falciparum* and P. vivax in young Papua New Guinean children. PLoS One. 2010;**5**:e9047.

[20] Mueller I, Galinski MR, Tsuboi T, et al. Natural acquisition of immunity

to *Plasmodium vivax*: epidemiological observations and potential targets. Adv Parasitol. 2013;**81**:77-131.

[21] Commons RJ, Simpson JA, Thriemer K, et al. The effect of chloroquine dose and primaquine on *Plasmodium vivax* recurrence: a WorldWide Antimalarial Resistance Network systematic review and individual patient pooled meta-analysis. Lancet Infect Dis. 2018;**18**:1025-1034.

[22] Li N, Parker DM, Yang Z, et al. Risk factors associated with slide positivity among febrile patients in a conflict zone of north-eastern Myanmar along the China-Myanmar border. Malar J. 2013;**12**:361.

[23] Corder RM, de Lima ACP, Khoury DS, et al. Quantifying and preventing *Plasmodium vivax* recurrences in primaquine-untreated pregnant women: An observational and modeling study in Brazil. PLOS Neglected Tropical Diseases. 2020;**14**:e0008526.

[24] Brummaier T, Gilder ME, Gornsawun G, et al. Vivax malaria in pregnancy and lactation: a long way to health equity. Malar J. 2020;**19**:40.

[25] Tao ZY, Fang Q, Liu X, et al. Congenital malaria in China. PLoS Negl Trop Dis. 2014;**8**:e2622.

[26] Sandfort M, Vantaux A, Kim S, et al. Forest malaria in Cambodia: the occupational and spatial clustering of *Plasmodium vivax* and *Plasmodium falciparum* infection risk in a cross-sectional survey in Mondulkiri province, Cambodia. Malar J. 2020;**19**:413.

[27] Adams JH, Mueller I. The Biology of *Plasmodium vivax*. Cold Spring Harb Perspect Med. 2017;**7**: a025585.

[28] Anstey NM, Douglas NM, Poespoprodjo JR, et al. *Plasmodium vivax*: clinical spectrum, risk factors and pathogenesis. Adv Parasitol. 2012;**80**:151-201.

[29] Baird JK. Evidence and implications of mortality associated with acute *Plasmodium vivax* malaria. Clin Microbiol Rev. 2013;**26**:36-57.

[30] Kotepui M, Kotepui KU, Milanez GJ, et al. Prevalence and risk factors related to poor outcome of patients with severe *Plasmodium vivax* infection: a systematic review, meta-analysis, and analysis of case reports. BMC Infect Dis. 2020;**20**:363.

[31] Tjitra E, Anstey NM, Sugiarto P, et al. Multidrug-resistant *Plasmodium vivax* associated with severe and fatal malaria: a prospective study in Papua, Indonesia. PLoS Med. 2008;**5**:e128.

[32] Rahimi BA, Thakkinstian A, White NJ, et al. Severe vivax malaria: a systematic review and meta-analysis of clinical studies since 1900. Malar J. 2014;**13**:481.

[33] Malleret B, Li A, Zhang R, et al. *Plasmodium vivax*: restricted tropism and rapid remodeling of CD71-positive reticulocytes. Blood. 2015;**125**:1314-1324.

[34] McQueen PG, McKenzie FE. Age-structured red blood cell susceptibility and the dynamics of malaria infections. Proceedings of the National Academy of Sciences of the United States of America. 2004;**101**:9161-9166.

[35] Cromer D, Stark J, Davenport MP. Low red cell production may protect against severe anemia during a malaria infection—Insights from modeling. Journal of Theoretical Biology. 2009;**257**:533-542.

[36] Douglas NM, Lampah DA, Kenangalem E, et al. Major burden of severe anemia from non-falciparum malaria species in Southern Papua: a

hospital-based surveillance study. PLoS Med. 2013;**10**:e1001575; discussion e1001575.

[37] Kochar DK, Das A, Kochar A, et al. Thrombocytopenia in *Plasmodium falciparum*, *Plasmodium vivax* and mixed infection malaria: a study from Bikaner (Northwestern India). Platelets. 2010;**21**:623-627.

[38] Tanwar GS, Khatri PC, Chahar CK, et al. Thrombocytopenia in childhood malaria with special reference to P. vivax monoinfection: A study from Bikaner (Northwestern India). Platelets. 2012;**23**:211-216.

[39] Nosten F, McGready R, Simpson JA, et al. Effects of *Plasmodium vivax* malaria in pregnancy. Lancet. 1999;**354**:546-549.

[40] Pincelli A, Neves PAR, Lourenco BH, et al. The hidden burden of *Plasmodium vivax* malaria in pregnancy in the Amazon: an observational study in northwestern Brazil. Am J Trop Med Hyg. 2018.

[41] Markus MB. Dormancy in mammalian malaria. Trends Parasitol. 2012;**28**:39-45.

[42] Obaldia N, 3rd, Meibalan E, Sa JM, et al. Bone marrow is a major parasite reservoir in *Plasmodium vivax* infection. MBio. 2018;**9**.

[43] Markus MB. Biological concepts in recurrent *Plasmodium vivax* malaria. Parasitology. 2018:1-7.

[44] Lover AA, Coker RJ. Quantifying effect of geographic location on epidemiology of *Plasmodium vivax* malaria. Emerg Infect Dis. 2013;**19**:1058-1065.

[45] Kondrashin AV, Morozova LF, Stepanova EV, et al. On the epidemiology of *Plasmodium vivax* malaria: past and present with special reference to the former USSR. Malar J. 2018;**17**:346.

[46] White NJ. Determinants of relapse periodicity in *Plasmodium vivax* malaria. Malar J. 2011;**10**:297.

[47] Yang BL, Wan WJ, Wang WR, et al. [Experimental studies on the biological characteristics of *Plasmodium vivax* in south Yunnan]. Ji Sheng Chong Xue Yu Ji Sheng Chong Bing Za Zhi. 1986;**4**:101-105.

[48] Hollingdale MR, Collins WE, Campbell CC, et al. In vitro culture of two populations (dividing and nondividing) of exoerythrocytic parasites of *Plasmodium vivax*. Am J Trop Med Hyg. 1985;**34**:216-222.

[49] Hollingdale MR, Collins WE, Campbell CC. In vitro culture of exoerythrocytic parasites of the North Korean strain of *Plasmodium vivax* in hepatoma cells. Am J Trop Med Hyg. 1986;**35**:275-276.

[50] Shanks GD, White NJ. The activation of vivax malaria hypnozoites by infectious diseases. Lancet Infect Dis. 2013;**13**:900-906.

[51] Commons RJ, Simpson JA, Thriemer K, et al. Risk of *Plasmodium vivax* parasitaemia after *Plasmodium falciparum* infection: a systematic review and meta-analysis. Lancet Infect Dis. 2019;**19**:91-101.

[52] Robinson LJ, Wampfler R, Betuela I, et al. Strategies for understanding and reducing the *Plasmodium vivax* and Plasmodium ovale hypnozoite reservoir in Papua New Guinean children: a randomised placebo-controlled trial and mathematical model. PLoS Med. 2015;**12**:e1001891.

[53] Adekunle AI, Pinkevych M, McGready R, et al. Modeling the dynamics of *Plasmodium vivax* infection and hypnozoite reactivation in vivo. PLoS Negl Trop Dis. 2015;**9**:e0003595.

[54] Betuela I, Rosanas-Urgell A, Kiniboro B, et al. Relapses contribute significantly to the risk of *Plasmodium vivax* infection and disease in Papua New Guinean children 1-5 years of age. J Infect Dis. 2012;**206**:1771-1780.

[55] Commons RJ, Simpson JA, Watson J, et al. Estimating the proportion of *Plasmodium vivax* recurrences caused by relapse: a systematic review and meta-analysis. Am J Trop Med Hyg. 2020;**103**:1094-1099.

[56] Bright AT, Manary MJ, Tewhey R, et al. A high resolution case study of a patient with recurrent *Plasmodium vivax* infections shows that relapses were caused by meiotic siblings. PLoS Negl Trop Dis. 2014;**8**:e2882.

[57] Lin JT, Hathaway NJ, Saunders DL, et al. Using Amplicon Deep Sequencing to Detect Genetic Signatures of *Plasmodium vivax* Relapse. J Infect Dis. 2015;**212**:999-1008.

[58] Spanakos G, Snounou G, Pervanidou D, et al. Genetic Spatiotemporal Anatomy of *Plasmodium vivax* Malaria Episodes in Greece, 2009-2013. Emerg Infect Dis. 2018;**24**:541-548.

[59] Mekonnen SK, Aseffa A, Medhin G, et al. Re-evaluation of microscopy confirmed *Plasmodium falciparum* and *Plasmodium vivax* malaria by nested PCR detection in southern Ethiopia. Malar J. 2014;**13**:48.

[60] WHO. Control and elimination of *Plasmodium vivax* malaria. 2015.

[61] Barber BE, William T, Grigg MJ, et al. Limitations of microscopy to differentiate Plasmodium species in a region co-endemic for *Plasmodium falciparum*, *Plasmodium vivax* and Plasmodium knowlesi. Malar J. 2013;**12**:8.

[62] Agarwal R, Choi L, Johnson S, et al. Rapid diagnostic tests for *Plasmodium vivax* malaria in endemic countries. Cochrane Database Syst Rev. 2020;**11**:CD013218.

[63] Unwin VT, Ahmed R, Noviyanti R, et al. Use of a highly-sensitive rapid diagnostic test to screen for malaria in pregnancy in Indonesia. Malar J. 2020;**19**:28.

[64] Yeung S, McGregor D, James N, et al. Performance of Ultrasensitive Rapid Diagnostic Tests for Detecting Asymptomatic *Plasmodium falciparum*. Am J Trop Med Hyg. 2020;**102**:307-309.

[65] Sutanto I, Kosasih A, Elyazar IRF, et al. Negligible Impact of Mass Screening and Treatment on Mesoendemic Malaria Transmission at West Timor in Eastern Indonesia: A Cluster-Randomized Trial. Clin Infect Dis. 2018;**67**:1364-1372.

[66] Longley RJ, White MT, Takashima E, et al. Development and validation of serological markers for detecting recent *Plasmodium vivax* infection. Nat Med. 2020;**26**:741-749.

[67] Baird JK. Resistance to chloroquine unhinges vivax malaria therapeutics. Antimicrob Agents Chemother. 2011;**55**:1827-1830.

[68] WHO. Guidelines for the treatment of malaria. Third edition. 2015:pp. 316.

[69] Ursing J, Rombo L, Bergqvist Y, et al. High-Dose Chloroquine for Treatment of Chloroquine-Resistant *Plasmodium falciparum* Malaria. J Infect Dis. 2016;**213**:1315-1321.

[70] Baird JK. Resistance to therapies for infection by *Plasmodium vivax*. Clin Microbiol Rev. 2009;**22**:508-534.

[71] Price RN, Auburn S, Marfurt J, et al. Phenotypic and genotypic characterisation of drug-resistant

Plasmodium vivax. Trends Parasitol. 2012;**28**:522-529.

[72] Price RN, von Seidlein L, Valecha N, et al. Global extent of chloroquine-resistant *Plasmodium vivax*: a systematic review and meta-analysis. Lancet Infect Dis. 2014;**14**:982-991.

[73] Rieckmann KH, Davis DR, Hutton DC. Plasmodium vivax resistance to chloroquine? Lancet. 1989;**2**:1183-1184.

[74] Sumawinata IW, Bernadeta, Leksana B, et al. Very high risk of therapeutic failure with chloroquine for uncomplicated *Plasmodium falciparum* and P. vivax malaria in Indonesian Papua. Am J Trop Med Hyg. 2003;**68**:416-420.

[75] Baird JK, Basri H, Purnomo, et al. Resistance to chloroquine by *Plasmodium vivax* in Irian Jaya, Indonesia. Am J Trop Med Hyg. 1991;**44**:547-552.

[76] Ratcliff A, Siswantoro H, Kenangalem E, et al. Therapeutic response of multidrug-resistant *Plasmodium falciparum* and P. vivax to chloroquine and sulfadoxine-pyrimethamine in southern Papua, Indonesia. Trans R Soc Trop Med Hyg. 2007;**101**:351-359.

[77] WHO. Chemotherapy of malaria: Report of the WHO Scientific Group. WHO Technical Report Series No. 375. 1967. Available from: https://apps.who.int/iris/bitstream/handle/10665/40671/WHO_TRS_375.pdf.

[78] Douglas NM, Anstey NM, Angus BJ, et al. Artemisinin combination therapy for vivax malaria. Lancet Infect Dis. 2010;**10**:405-416.

[79] Gogtay N, Kannan S, Thatte UM, et al. Artemisinin-based combination therapy for treating uncomplicated *Plasmodium vivax* malaria. Cochrane Database Syst Rev. 2013;**10**:CD008492.

[80] Baird JK, Valecha N, Duparc S, et al. Diagnosis and Treatment of *Plasmodium vivax* Malaria. Am J Trop Med Hyg. 2016;**95**:35-51.

[81] Commons RJ, Simpson JA, Thriemer K, et al. The efficacy of dihydroartemisinin-piperaquine and artemether-lumefantrine with and without primaquine on *Plasmodium vivax* recurrence: A systematic review and individual patient data meta-analysis. PLoS Med. 2019;**16**:e1002928.

[82] WHO. World Malaria Report 2020 2020. Available from: https://www.who.int/publications/i/item/9789240015791.

[83] Baird JK, Leksana B, Masbar S, et al. Diagnosis of resistance to chloroquine by *Plasmodium vivax*: timing of recurrence and whole blood chloroquine levels. Am J Trop Med Hyg. 1997;**56**:621-626.

[84] Wernsdorfer WH, Tasanor O, Wernsdorfer G. In vitro drug sensitivity testing in *Plasmodium vivax*. Wien Klin Wochenschr. 2008;**120**:30-33.

[85] Russell B, Suwanarusk R, Malleret B, et al. Human ex vivo studies on asexual *Plasmodium vivax*: the best way forward. Int J Parasitol. 2012;**42**:1063-1070.

[86] Renapurkar DM, Pradhan VR, Sutar NK, et al. Micro test for assaying sensitivity of *Plasmodium vivax* in vitro. Chemotherapy. 1989;**35**:160-163.

[87] Russell BM, Udomsangpetch R, Rieckmann KH, et al. Simple in vitro assay for determining the sensitivity of *Plasmodium vivax* isolates from fresh human blood to antimalarials in areas where P. vivax is endemic. Antimicrob Agents Chemother. 2003;**47**:170-173.

[88] Druilhe P, Brasseur P, Blanc C, et al. Improved assessment of *Plasmodium vivax* response to antimalarial drugs by a colorimetric double-site plasmodium lactate dehydrogenase antigen capture enzyme-linked immunosorbent assay. Antimicrob Agents Chemother. 2007;**51**:2112-2116.

[89] Russell B, Chalfein F, Prasetyorini B, et al. Determinants of in vitro drug susceptibility testing of *Plasmodium vivax*. Antimicrob Agents Chemother. 2008;**52**:1040-1045.

[90] Sharrock WW, Suwanarusk R, Lek-Uthai U, et al. *Plasmodium vivax* trophozoites insensitive to chloroquine. Malar J. 2008;7:94.

[91] Li J, Zhang J, Li Q, et al. Ex vivo susceptibilities of *Plasmodium vivax* isolates from the China-Myanmar border to antimalarial drugs and association with polymorphisms in Pvmdr1 and Pvcrt-o genes. PLoS Negl Trop Dis. 2020;**14**:e0008255.

[92] Melo GC, Monteiro WM, Siqueira AM, et al. Expression levels of pvcrt-o and pvmdr-1 are associated with chloroquine resistance and severe *Plasmodium vivax* malaria in patients of the Brazilian Amazon. PLoS One. 2014;**9**:e105922.

[93] Silva SR, Almeida ACG, da Silva GAV, et al. Chloroquine resistance is associated to multi-copy pvcrt-o gene in *Plasmodium vivax* malaria in the Brazilian Amazon. Malar J. 2018;**17**:267.

[94] Pava Z, Handayuni I, Wirjanata G, et al. Expression of *Plasmodium vivax* crt-o is related to parasite stage but not ex vivo chloroquine susceptibility. Antimicrob Agents Chemother. 2015;**60**:361-367.

[95] Sa JM, Kaslow SR, Moraes Barros RR, et al. *Plasmodium vivax* chloroquine resistance links to pvcrt transcription in a genetic cross. Nat Commun. 2019;**10**:4300.

[96] Suwanarusk R, Russell B, Chavchich M, et al. Chloroquine resistant *Plasmodium vivax*: in vitro characterisation and association with molecular polymorphisms. PLoS One. 2007;**2**:e1089.

[97] Orjuela-Sanchez P, de Santana Filho FS, Machado-Lima A, et al. Analysis of single-nucleotide polymorphisms in the crt-o and mdr1 genes of *Plasmodium vivax* among chloroquine-resistant isolates from the Brazilian Amazon region. Antimicrob Agents Chemother. 2009;**53**:3561-3564.

[98] Marfurt J, de Monbrison F, Brega S, et al. Molecular markers of in vivo *Plasmodium vivax* resistance to amodiaquine plus sulfadoxine-pyrimethamine: mutations in pvdhfr and pvmdr1. J Infect Dis. 2008;**198**:409-417.

[99] Shalini S, Chaudhuri S, Sutton PL, et al. Chloroquine efficacy studies confirm drug susceptibility of *Plasmodium vivax* in Chennai, India. Malar J. 2014;**13**:129.

[100] Pearson RD, Amato R, Auburn S, et al. Genomic analysis of local variation and recent evolution in *Plasmodium vivax*. Nat Genet. 2016;**48**:959-964.

[101] Brashear AM, Fan Q, Hu Y, et al. Population genomics identifies a distinct *Plasmodium vivax* population on the China-Myanmar border of Southeast Asia. PLoS Negl Trop Dis. 2020;**14**:e0008506.

[102] Verzier LH, Coyle R, Singh S, et al. Plasmodium knowlesi as a model system for characterising *Plasmodium vivax* drug resistance candidate genes. PLoS Negl Trop Dis. 2019;**13**:e0007470.

[103] John GK, Douglas NM, von Seidlein L, et al. Primaquine radical cure

of *Plasmodium vivax*: a critical review of the literature. Malar J. 2012;**11**:280.

[104] Milligan R, Daher A, Villanueva G, et al. Primaquine alternative dosing schedules for preventing malaria relapse in people with *Plasmodium vivax*. Cochrane Database Syst Rev. 2020;**8**:CD012656.

[105] Douglas NM, Poespoprodjo JR, Patriani D, et al. Unsupervised primaquine for the treatment of *Plasmodium vivax* malaria relapses in southern Papua: A hospital-based cohort study. PLoS Med. 2017;**14**:e1002379.

[106] Gogtay NJ, Desai S, Kamtekar KD, et al. Efficacies of 5- and 14-day primaquine regimens in the prevention of relapses in *Plasmodium vivax* infections. Ann Trop Med Parasitol. 1999;**93**:809-812.

[107] Yadav RS, Ghosh SK. Radical curative efficacy of five-day regimen of primaquine for treatment of *Plasmodium vivax* malaria in India. J Parasitol. 2002;**88**:1042-1044.

[108] Chu CS, Phyo AP, Turner C, et al. Chloroquine versus dihydroartemisinin-piperaquine with standard high-dose primaquine given either for 7 days or 14 days in *Plasmodium vivax* malaria. Clin Infect Dis. 2019;**68**:1311-1319.

[109] Taylor WRJ, Thriemer K, von Seidlein L, et al. Short-course primaquine for the radical cure of *Plasmodium vivax* malaria: a multicentre, randomised, placebo-controlled non-inferiority trial. Lancet. 2019.

[110] Hounkpatin AB, Kreidenweiss A, Held J. Clinical utility of tafenoquine in the prevention of relapse of *Plasmodium vivax* malaria: a review on the mode of action and emerging trial data. Infect Drug Resist. 2019;**12**:553-570.

[111] Baird JK. Tafenoquine for travelers' malaria: evidence, rationale and recommendations. J Travel Med. 2018;**25**.

[112] Lacerda MVG, Llanos-Cuentas A, Krudsood S, et al. Single-dose tafenoquine to prevent relapse of *Plasmodium vivax* malaria. N Engl J Med. 2019;**380**:215-228.

[113] Llanos-Cuentas A, Lacerda MVG, Hien TT, et al. Tafenoquine versus primaquine to prevent relapse of *Plasmodium vivax* malaria. N Engl J Med. 2019;**380**:229-241.

[114] Schmidt LH, Fradkin R, Vaughan D, et al. Radical cure of infections with *Plasmodium cynomolgi*: a function of total 8-aminoquinoline dose. Am J Trop Med Hyg. 1977;**26**:1116-1128.

[115] Baird JK. 8-Aminoquinoline therapy for latent malaria. Clin Microbiol Rev. 2019;**32**.

[116] Alving AS, Johnson CF, Tarlov AR, et al. Mitigation of the haemolytic effect of primaquine and enhancement of its action against exoerythrocytic forms of the Chesson strain of Piasmodium vivax by intermittent regimens of drug administration: a preliminary report. Bull World Health Organ. 1960;**22**:621-631.

[117] Kheng S, Muth S, Taylor WR, et al. Tolerability and safety of weekly primaquine against relapse of *Plasmodium vivax* in Cambodians with glucose-6-phosphate dehydrogenase deficiency. BMC Med. 2015;**13**:203.

[118] Taylor WRJ, Kheng S, Muth S, et al. Hemolytic dynamics of weekly primaquine antirelapse therapy among Cambodians with acute *Plasmodium vivax* malaria with or without glucose-6-phosphate dehydrogenase deficiency. J Infect Dis. 2019;**220**:1750-1760.

[119] Baird JK. Primaquine toxicity forestalls effective therapeutic management of the endemic malarias. Int J Parasitol. 2012;**42**:1049-1054.

[120] Ashley EA, Recht J, White NJ. Primaquine: the risks and the benefits. Malar J. 2014;**13**:418.

[121] Gomez-Manzo S, Marcial-Quino J, Vanoye-Carlo A, et al. Glucose-6-Phosphate Dehydrogenase: Update and Analysis of New Mutations around the World. Int J Mol Sci. 2016;**17**.

[122] Minucci A, Moradkhani K, Hwang MJ, et al. Glucose-6-phosphate dehydrogenase (G6PD) mutations database: review of the "old" and update of the new mutations. Blood cells, molecules & diseases. 2012;**48**:154-165.

[123] Luzzatto L, Nannelli C, Notaro R. Glucose-6-Phosphate Dehydrogenase Deficiency. Hematol Oncol Clin North Am. 2016;**30**:373-393.

[124] Howes RE, Dewi M, Piel FB, et al. Spatial distribution of G6PD deficiency variants across malaria-endemic regions. Malar J. 2013;**12**:418.

[125] Ruwende C, Khoo SC, Snow RW, et al. Natural selection of hemi- and heterozygotes for G6PD deficiency in Africa by resistance to severe malaria. Nature. 1995;**376**:246-249.

[126] Shah SS, Rockett KA, Jallow M, et al. Heterogeneous alleles comprising G6PD deficiency trait in West Africa exert contrasting effects on two major clinical presentations of severe malaria. Malar J. 2016;**15**:13.

[127] Guindo A, Fairhurst RM, Doumbo OK, et al. X-linked G6PD deficiency protects hemizygous males but not heterozygous females against severe malaria. PLoS Med. 2007;**4**:e66.

[128] Bienzle U, Ayeni O, Lucas AO, et al. Glucose-6-phosphate dehydrogenase and malaria. Greater resistance of females heterozygous for enzyme deficiency and of males with non-deficient variant. Lancet. 1972;**1**:107-110.

[129] Louicharoen C, Patin E, Paul R, et al. Positively selected G6PD-Mahidol mutation reduces *Plasmodium vivax* density in Southeast Asians. Science. 2009;**326**:1546-1549.

[130] Yi H, Li H, Liang L, et al. The glucose-6-phosphate dehydrogenase Mahidol variant protects against uncomplicated *Plasmodium vivax* infection and reduces disease severity in a Kachin population from northeast Myanmar. Infect Genet Evol. 2019;**75**:103980.

[131] Howes RE, Dewi M, Piel FB, et al. Spatial distribution of G6PD deficiency variants across malaria-endemic regions. Malaria journal. 2013;**12**:418.

[132] Nkhoma ET, Poole C, Vannappagari V, et al. The global prevalence of glucose-6-phosphate dehydrogenase deficiency: a systematic review and meta-analysis. Blood Cells Mol Dis. 2009;**42**:267-278.

[133] Howes RE, Piel FB, Patil AP, et al. G6PD deficiency prevalence and estimates of affected populations in malaria endemic countries: a geostatistical model-based map. PLoS Med. 2012;**9**:e1001339.

[134] Chu CS, Bancone G, Nosten F, et al. Primaquine-induced haemolysis in females heterozygous for G6PD deficiency. Malar J. 2018;**17**:101.

[135] Chu CS, Bancone G, Moore KA, et al. Haemolysis in G6PD heterozygous females treated with primaquine for *Plasmodium vivax* malaria: a nested cohort in a trial of radical curative regimens. PLoS Med. 2017;**14**:e1002224.

[136] Karwacki JJ, Shanks GD, Kummalue T, et al. Primaquine induced hemolysis in a Thai soldier. Southeast Asian J Trop Med Public Health. 1989;**20**:555-556.

[137] Chen X, He Y, Miao Y, et al. A young man with severe acute haemolytic anaemia. BMJ. 2017;**359**:j4263.

[138] Domingo GJ, Satyagraha AW, Anvikar A, et al. G6PD testing in support of treatment and elimination of malaria: recommendations for evaluation of G6PD tests. Malar J. 2013;**12**:391.

[139] Baird JK. Management of *Plasmodium vivax* risk and illness in travelers. Trop Dis Travel Med Vaccines. 2017;**3**:7.

[140] Commons RJ, McCarthy JS, Price RN. Tafenoquine for the radical cure and prevention of malaria: the importance of testing for G6PD deficiency. Med J Aust. 2020;**212**:152-153 e151.

[141] Devine A, Howes RE, Price DJ, et al. Cost-effectiveness analysis of sex-stratified *Plasmodium vivax* treatment strategies using available G6PD diagnostics to accelerate access to radical cure. Am J Trop Med Hyg. 2020;**103**:394-403.

[142] Bennett JW, Pybus BS, Yadava A, et al. Primaquine failure and cytochrome P-450 2D6 in *Plasmodium vivax* malaria. N Engl J Med. 2013;**369**:1381-1382.

[143] Pybus BS, Marcsisin SR, Jin X, et al. The metabolism of primaquine to its active metabolite is dependent on CYP 2D6. Malar J. 2013;**12**:212.

[144] Pybus BS, Sousa JC, Jin X, et al. CYP450 phenotyping and accurate mass identification of metabolites of the 8-aminoquinoline, anti-malarial drug primaquine. Malar J. 2012;**11**:259.

[145] Baird JK, Louisa M, Noviyanti R, et al. Association of Impaired Cytochrome P450 2D6 Activity Genotype and Phenotype With Therapeutic Efficacy of Primaquine Treatment for Latent *Plasmodium vivax* Malaria. JAMA Netw Open. 2018;**1**:e181449.

[146] Brasil LW, Rodrigues-Soares F, Santoro AB, et al. CYP2D6 activity and the risk of recurrence of *Plasmodium vivax* malaria in the Brazilian Amazon: a prospective cohort study. Malar J. 2018;**17**:57.

[147] Silvino ACR, Kano FS, Costa MA, et al. Novel insights into *Plasmodium vivax* therapeutic failure: CYP2D6 activity and time of exposure to malaria modulate the risk of recurrence. Antimicrob Agents Chemother. 2020;**64**.

[148] Ingram RJ, Crenna-Darusallam C, Soebianto S, et al. The clinical and public health problem of relapse despite primaquine therapy: case review of repeated relapses of *Plasmodium vivax* acquired in Papua New Guinea. Malar J. 2014;**13**:488.

[149] He X, Pan M, Zeng W, et al. Multiple relapses of *Plasmodium vivax* malaria acquired from West Africa and association with poor metabolizer CYP2D6 variant: a case report. BMC Infect Dis. 2019;**19**:704.

[150] Goncalves BP, Pett H, Tiono AB, et al. Age, weight, and CYP2D6 genotype are major determinants of primaquine pharmacokinetics in african children. Antimicrob Agents Chemother. 2017;**61**:e02590-02516.

[151] Pett H, Bradley J, Okebe J, et al. CYP2D6 polymorphisms and the safety and gametocytocidal activity of single dose primaquine for *P. falciparum*. Antimicrob Agents Chemother. 2019.

[152] Marcsisin SR, Reichard G, Pybus BS. Primaquine pharmacology

in the context of CYP 2D6 pharmacogenomics: Current state of the art. Pharmacol Ther. 2016.

[153] Zhou SF, Liu JP, Lai XS. Substrate specificity, inhibitors and regulation of human cytochrome P450 2D6 and implications in drug development. Curr Med Chem. 2009;**16**:2661-2805.

[154] Zhou SF. Polymorphism of human cytochrome P450 2D6 and its clinical significance: Part I. Clin Pharmacokinet. 2009;**48**:689-723.

[155] Gaedigk A, Simon SD, Pearce RE, et al. The CYP2D6 activity score: translating genotype information into a qualitative measure of phenotype. Clin Pharmacol Ther. 2008;**83**:234-242.

[156] Baird JK, Battle KE, Howes RE. Primaquine ineligibility in anti-relapse therapy of *Plasmodium vivax* malaria: the problem of G6PD deficiency and cytochrome P-450 2D6 polymorphisms. Malar J. 2018;**17**:42.

[157] Spring MD, Lon C, Sok S, et al. Prevalence of CYP2D6 genotypes and predicted phenotypes in a cohort of cambodians at high risk for infections with *Plasmodium vivax*. Am J Trop Med Hyg. 2020;**103**:756-759.

[158] Nelwan EJ, Ekawati LL, Tjahjono B, et al. Randomized trial of primaquine hypnozoitocidal efficacy when administered with artemisinin-combined blood schizontocides for radical cure of *Plasmodium vivax* in Indonesia. BMC Med. 2015;**13**:294.

[159] Alving AS, Arnold J, Hockwald RS, et al. Potentiation of the curative action of primaquine in vivax malaria by quinine and chloroquine. J Lab Clin Med. 1955;**46**:301-306.

[160] Dembele L, Franetich JF, Soulard V, et al. Chloroquine potentiates primaquine activity against active and latent hepatic plasmodia ex vivo: potentials and pitfalls. Antimicrob Agents Chemother. 2021;**65**:e01416-20.

[161] Baird JK, Hoffman SL. Primaquine therapy for malaria. Clin Infect Dis. 2004;**39**:1336-1345.

[162] Thomas D, Tazerouni H, Sundararaj KG, et al. Therapeutic failure of primaquine and need for new medicines in radical cure of *Plasmodium vivax*. Acta Trop. 2016;**160**:35-38.

[163] Imwong M, Snounou G, Pukrittayakamee S, et al. Relapses of *Plasmodium vivax* infection usually result from activation of heterologous hypnozoites. J Infect Dis. 2007;**195**:927-933.

[164] Chen N, Auliff A, Rieckmann K, et al. Relapses of *Plasmodium vivax* infection result from clonal hypnozoites activated at predetermined intervals. J Infect Dis. 2007;**195**:934-941.

[165] Sutanto I, Tjahjono B, Basri H, et al. Randomized, open-label trial of primaquine against vivax malaria relapse in Indonesia. Antimicrob Agents Chemother. 2013;**57**:1128-1135.

[166] Vallejo AF, Garcia J, Amado-Garavito AB, et al. *Plasmodium vivax* gametocyte infectivity in sub-microscopic infections. Malar J. 2016;**15**:48.

[167] Almeida ACG, Kuehn A, Castro AJM, et al. High proportions of asymptomatic and submicroscopic *Plasmodium vivax* infections in a peri-urban area of low transmission in the Brazilian Amazon. Parasit Vectors. 2018;**11**:194.

[168] Tadesse FG, Slater HC, Chali W, et al. The Relative Contribution of Symptomatic and Asymptomatic *Plasmodium vivax* and *Plasmodium falciparum* Infections to the Infectious Reservoir in a Low-Endemic

Setting in Ethiopia. Clin Infect Dis. 2018;**66**:1883-1891.

[169] Collins WE, Sullivan JS, Nace D, et al. Experimental infection of *Anopheles farauti* with different species of Plasmodium. J Parasitol. 2002;**88**:295-298.

[170] Sattabongkot J, Tsuboi T, Zollner GE, et al. *Plasmodium vivax* transmission: chances for control? Trends Parasitol. 2004;**20**:192-198.

[171] Battle KE, Gething PW, Elyazar IR, et al. The global public health significance of *Plasmodium vivax*. Adv Parasitol. 2012;**80**:1-111.

[172] Hemingway J. The role of vector control in stopping the transmission of malaria: threats and opportunities. Philos Trans R Soc Lond B Biol Sci. 2014;**369**:20130431.

[173] Bhatt S, Weiss DJ, Cameron E, et al. The effect of malaria control on *Plasmodium falciparum* in Africa between 2000 and 2015. Nature. 2015;**526**:207-211.

[174] Killeen GF. Control of malaria vectors and management of insecticide resistance through universal coverage with next-generation insecticide-treated nets. Lancet. 2020;**395**:1394-1400.

[175] Smithuis FM, Kyaw MK, Phe UO, et al. Entomological determinants of insecticide-treated bed net effectiveness in Western Myanmar. Malar J. 2013;**12**:364.

[176] Smithuis FM, Kyaw MK, Phe UO, et al. The effect of insecticide-treated bed nets on the incidence and prevalence of malaria in children in an area of unstable seasonal transmission in western Myanmar. Malar J. 2013;**12**:363.

[177] Edwards HM, Chinh VD, Le Duy B, et al. Characterising residual malaria transmission in forested areas with low coverage of core vector control in central Viet Nam. Parasit Vectors. 2019;**12**:454.

[178] Edwards HM, Sriwichai P, Kirabittir K, et al. Transmission risk beyond the village: entomological and human factors contributing to residual malaria transmission in an area approaching malaria elimination on the Thailand-Myanmar border. Malar J. 2019;**18**:221.

[179] Chareonviriyaphap T, Bangs MJ, Suwonkerd W, et al. Review of insecticide resistance and behavioral avoidance of vectors of human diseases in Thailand. Parasit Vectors. 2013;**6**:280.

[180] Van Bortel W, Trung HD, Thuan le K, et al. The insecticide resistance status of malaria vectors in the Mekong region. Malar J. 2008;**7**:102.

[181] Verhaeghen K, Van Bortel W, Trung HD, et al. Absence of knockdown resistance suggests metabolic resistance in the main malaria vectors of the Mekong region. Malar J. 2009;**8**:84.

[182] Derua YA, Kweka EJ, Kisinza WN, et al. Bacterial larvicides used for malaria vector control in sub-Saharan Africa: review of their effectiveness and operational feasibility. Parasit Vectors. 2019;**12**:426.

[183] Geissbuhler Y, Kannady K, Chaki PP, et al. Microbial larvicide application by a large-scale, community-based program reduces malaria infection prevalence in urban Dar es Salaam, Tanzania. PLoS One. 2009;**4**:e5107.

[184] Chaccour CJ, Kobylinski KC, Bassat Q, et al. Ivermectin to reduce malaria transmission: a research agenda for a promising new tool for elimination. Malar J. 2013;**12**:153.

[185] Kobylinski KC, Ubalee R, Ponlawat A, et al. Ivermectin

susceptibility and sporontocidal effect in Greater Mekong Subregion Anopheles. Malar J. 2017;**16**:280.

[186] Sluydts V, Durnez L, Heng S, et al. Efficacy of topical mosquito repellent (picaridin) plus long-lasting insecticidal nets versus long-lasting insecticidal nets alone for control of malaria: a cluster randomised controlled trial. Lancet Infect Dis. 2016;**16**:1169-1177.

[187] Gryseels C, Uk S, Sluydts V, et al. Factors influencing the use of topical repellents: implications for the effectiveness of malaria elimination strategies. Sci Rep. 2015;**5**:16847.

[188] Wang S, Jacobs-Lorena M. Genetic approaches to interfere with malaria transmission by vector mosquitoes. Trends Biotechnol. 2013;**31**:185-193.

[189] Barreaux P, Barreaux AMG, Sternberg ED, et al. Priorities for broadening the malaria vector control tool kit. Trends Parasitol. 2017;**33**:763-774.

[190] WHO. Malaria-free Maldives. 2016.

[191] Premaratne R, Ortega L, Janakan N, et al. Malaria elimination in Sri Lanka: what it would take to reach the goal. WHO South East Asia J Public Health. 2014;**3**:85-89.

[192] WHO. Turkmenistan certified malaria-free. Weekly epidemiological record. 2010;**85**:461-472.

[193] Feng J, Zhang L, Huang F, et al. Ready for malaria elimination: zero indigenous case reported in the People's Republic of China. Malar J. 2018;**17**:315.

[194] Cao J, Sturrock HJ, Cotter C, et al. Communicating and monitoring surveillance and response activities for malaria elimination: China's "1-3-7" strategy. PLoS Med. 2014;**11**:e1001642.

[195] Feng J, Liu J, Feng X, et al. Towards malaria elimination: monitoring and evaluation of the "1-3-7" approach at the China-Myanmar border. Am J Trop Med Hyg. 2016;**95**:806-810.

[196] Yang H, Wang J, Liu H, et al. Randomized, double-blind, placebo-controlled studies to assess safety and prophylactic efficacy of naphthoquine-azithromycin combination for malaria prophylaxis in Southeast Asia. Antimicrob Agents Chemother. 2018;**62**:e00793-00718.

[197] Yang H, Wang J, Liu H, et al. Efficacy and safety of a naphthoquine-azithromycin co-formulation for malaria prophylaxis in Southeast Asia: A phase 3, double-blind, randomized, placebo-controlled trial. Clin Infect Dis. 2020.

[198] Song J, Socheat D, Tan B, et al. Rapid and effective malaria control in Cambodia through mass administration of artemisinin-piperaquine. Malar J. 2010;**9**:57.

[199] Landier J, Kajeechiwa L, Thwin MM, et al. Safety and effectiveness of mass drug administration to accelerate elimination of artemisinin-resistant falciparum malaria: A pilot trial in four villages of Eastern Myanmar. Wellcome open research. 2017;**2**:81.

[200] Zhou S, Li Z, Cotter C, et al. Trends of imported malaria in China 2010-2014: analysis of surveillance data. Malar J. 2016;**15**:39.

[201] Sleigh AC, Liu XL, Jackson S, et al. Resurgence of vivax malaria in Henan Province, China. Bull World Health Organ. 1998;**76**:265-270.

[202] Cohen JM, Smith DL, Cotter C, et al. Malaria resurgence: a systematic review and assessment of its causes. Malar J. 2012;**11**:122.

[203] Mendis K. Eliminating malaria should not be the end of vigilance. Nature. 2019;**573**:7.

[204] Bahk YY, Lee HW, Na BK, et al. Epidemiological characteristics of re-emerging vivax malaria in the Republic of Korea (1993-2017). Korean J Parasitol. 2018;**56**:531-543.

[205] Fernando SD, Booso R, Dharmawardena P, et al. The need for preventive and curative services for malaria when the military is deployed in endemic overseas territories: a case study and lessons learned. Mil Med Res. 2017;**4**:19.

[206] Karunasena VM, Marasinghe M, Koo C, et al. The first introduced malaria case reported from Sri Lanka after elimination: implications for preventing the re-introduction of malaria in recently eliminated countries. Malar J. 2019;**18**:210.

Chapter 11

Plasmodium vivax and *Plasmodium ovale* in the Malaria Elimination Agenda in Africa

Isaac K. Quaye and Larysa Aleksenko

Abstract

In recent times, several countries in sub-Saharan Africa have reported cases of *Plasmodium vivax (Pv)* with a considerable number being Duffy negative. Current efforts at malaria elimination are focused solely on *Plasmodium falciparum (Pf)* excluding non-falciparum malaria. *Pv* and *Plasmodium ovale (Po)* have hypnozoite forms that can serve as reservoirs of infection and sustain transmission. The burden of these parasites in Africa seems to be more than acknowledged, playing roles in migrant and autochthonous infections. Considering that elimination and eradication is a current aim for WHO and Roll Back Malaria (RBM), the inclusion of *Pv* and *Po* in the elimination agenda cannot be over-emphasized. The biology of *Pv* and *Po* are such that the same elimination strategies as are used for *Pf* cannot be applied so, going forward, new approaches will be required to attain elimination and eradication targets.

Keywords: *Plasmodium vivax* transmission, *Plasmodium ovale*, asymptomatic transmission, sub-Saharan Africa

1. Introduction

Malaria elimination is defined as interruption of local transmission of malaria in a defined area [1, 2]. Within a geographical demarcation, malaria transmission is heterogenous ranging between high, intermediate or low [3, 4]. This means that elimination efforts must be defined with respect to the geographical area, and interventions targeted to specified strata to achieve elimination goals [5, 6]. Data for such targeted intervention can come from the use of sensitive and specific surveillance diagnostic tools that can discriminate between species, including asymptomatic infections. In Africa, current efforts of intervention by National Malaria Control Programs and recommendation by WHO and Roll Back Malaria (RBM) are focused mainly on *Plasmodium falciparum* (*Pf*) with little to no attention on non-falciparum species although the latter are established to be present in all of Africa [7, 8]. Clearly if elimination is envisaged based on the target of RBM, then inclusion of all human *Plasmodium* species in the elimination agenda is relevant. Non- falciparum *Plasmodial* species are more complicated in their transmission than *Pf* [9–11]. Especially, *Plasmodium vivax (Pv),* that is the most prevalent in the world and the two sympatric species of *Plasmodium ovale* (*Po*), *Plasmodium ovale curtisi* and *Plasmodium ovale wallikeri* both of which cause severe disease and have hypnozoite stages in their transmission cycle as *Pv* [12–15]. The inclusion of all species should be well planned in such a way that it does not take away from the efforts being made to reduce *Pf* transmission but to go hand in hand. The transmission dynamics of these species must be well understood so that measures tailored to them are put in place. Here aspects of the biology of the parasites are elaborated so they are put in perspective with regards to elimination.

2. Biology of *Pv* and *Po*

Plasmodium species are obligate intracellular parasites that infect *Anopheles* mosquitoes in the sexual life cycle and humans in their asexual life cycle [16]. In humans, replication takes place in the liver hepatocytes, following inoculation by an infected *Anopheles* mosquito into the skin, and migration of the parasite through the capillaries into the blood stream and then to the liver parenchyma cells [17]. This pattern of infection is similar in all known human *Plasmodium* parasites which currently are *P. falciparum*, *P. vivax*, *P. ovale curtisi*, *P. ovale wallikeri*, *P. malariae* and *P. knowlesi* [18].

Outside of Africa, *Pv* is the predominant parasite, but even so the phenotypic characteristic from individuals infected with the parasite from different populations appear to differ. One of the most important differences between plasmodial species infecting humans is the ability of *Pv* and *Po* to relapse after the cure of the original infection [9, 12]. A proportion of sporozoites do not undergo immediate development in the invaded hepatocytes. Instead, they remain dormant in the liver as hypnozoites for prolonged periods of time before developing and causing recurrent infection [19]. *P. vivax* strains from different geographical areas show widely different relapse patterns, reflecting evolutionary adaptation to local environmental conditions that optimize transmission potential of the parasite [20]. In Africa, it had previously been generally accepted that because of the high prevalence of ACKR1 polymorphism, individuals of African descent are resistant to infection by the parasite [21]. Recent evidence of *Pv* presence in nearly the whole of Africa, indicates that *Pv* may have other mechanisms for invasion [22]. Advancing research into the parasites' biology and mechanism of invasion is necessary for elimination and eradication. Although *Po* is not limited by the Duffy antigen polymorphism, the shared biology of hypnozoites and their relapse makes it of equal concern in malaria elimination. What is palpably clear is that reporting of these two parasites from countries in Africa, appears not to reflect the true prevalence rate as reporting is largely passive and not active.

2.1 Parasite transmission

Transmission of the parasite defines the processes that the parasite takes to complete a life cycle [1]. The process in the *Anopheles* vector is referred to as sporogony while that in humans is referred to as schizogony. Schizogony begins when liver schizonts which contain multiples of merozoites mature and burst with subsequent release of the merozoites into the blood stream [23]. The merozoites invade young reticulocytes that have the surface marker CD71(CD71$^+$) [24] where they mature into trophozoites. The trophozoites mature into blood stage schizonts containing multiples of merozoites, burst the reticulocytes and initiate a new cycle of blood stage transmission. Some of the merozoites mature into male and female gametocytes that are picked by female *Anopheles* mosquitoes when mature, to begin the sporogonic cycle [1]. In *Pv* and *Po* some of the liver schizonts remain dormant for weeks, months or years and then get activated to initiate a new infection in the reticulocytes [16]. It is not clear what exactly triggers the reactivation, although new *Plasmodium* and other infections and inflammation, have been suggested as contributory [9, 25]. The subsets that remain in the liver are the hypnozoites, and the reactivation process is called 'relapse'. The activation of hypnozoites is reported to cause most of the blood stage infections [26]. It is not clear whether the under-reporting of *Pv* and *Po* infections in Africa is attributed to hypnozoites relapsing or lack of tools or focus for targeting these species for detection.

It has been reported that the hypnozoites are not only derived from liver parenchyma cells, but also from bone marrow parenchyma that abounds in young and $CD71^+$ reticulocytes [24]. It has been shown that the bone marrow is enriched in gametocytes extravascularly, while the liver is enriched with tissue schizonts in the sinusoids compared to peripheral blood [24]. In addition, a small number of parasites are seen in the vasculature of the lungs as opposed to those in the bone marrow and liver which are extravascular [27]. The hypnozoite stages are particularly troubling because chemotherapy against them with the use of primaquine is restrictive due to glucose-6-phosphate dehydrogenase deficiency and CYP2D6 polymorphism [28]. Also, it has been reported that primaquine may not be efficacious against some strains of the hypnozoite stages [29]. Nevertheless, radical cure with primaquine at least can go a long way in the agenda towards elimination.

2.2 Hypnozoite stages

Previously there was no direct evidence of hypnozoite stages of *Po*, however recent reports have clearly shown that such stages indeed exist for both *Po curtisi* and *Po wallikeri* [30]. The sub-species of the parasite contribute to the transmission dynamics and need to be fully interrogated for markers and drug targeting. Another unique biology of the parasite is the early emergence and maturation of gametocytes in the blood. While gametocytes for *Pf*, *Pm* mature in about 10–12 days, for *Pv and Po*, gametocytes are seen between 3 to 5 days following the first documentation of parasites in the peripheral blood [1, 16, 23]. This means even before any symptoms of infection are seen the parasite would have been transmitted if female Anopheles mosquitoes fed within the period. In this case an intervention in the transmission process can be missed. It maybe that these traditionally unseen parasites, contribute to the low parasitemia usually seen with these infections and why *Pv* and *Po* infections are characterized as benign although they can cause as much severe disease as in *Pf* infections.

2.3 Transmission dynamics

In regions outside of sub-Saharan Africa (SSA) where *Pf* and *Pv* coexist, mixed-species infections are common [31]. In such situations, there are observed shifts in the dominant parasite towards *Pv* as *Pf* transmission declines. Surveys usually report rates less than 2% and yet careful clinical studies record rates of up to 30% and this figure is even higher when PCR detection methods are used. This trend means that in a couple of years to come, without effective and necessary interventions, when the *Pf* burden has been significantly reduced in Africa, *Pv* and *Po* infections could constitute the most dominant *Plasmodium* species on the continent. We observe that countries that were on course for *Pf* elimination such as Botswana, eSwatini, and South Africa have seen changes recently, part of which is due to *Pv* and *Po*. Concurrent infections with different *Plasmodium* species may have important implications on the host response and development of cross-species immunity. The potential for *Pv* to attenuate *Falciparum* malaria obviously requires further characterization and has significant implications for vivax-only vaccination strategies, and the deployment of drugs such as chloroquine, which has lost efficacy against *Pf* but still retain it against *Pv*. The transmission of the parasite in Duffy negative individuals raises serious concern as essentially *Pf* is the only targeted species in the elimination agenda in Africa, with minimal consideration for *Pv and Po*.

2.4 What is needed currently on *Pv* and *Po* transmission?

As noted previously, *Pv* and *Po* can cause severe disease [13, 15]. The most characteristic of *Pv* are acute respiratory distress syndrome (ARDS), anemia and decreased oxygen saturation in both children and adults [32, 33]; clinical conditions which are also seen in *Po* infections [34–36]. The respiratory illnesses are associated with high mortality, with a higher risk in women. In the cited *Po* cases of ARDS, the patients were also HIV positive, so it is not clear if HIV facilitated development to full blown ARDS or not [32, 37]. The new tissue sequestration sites of *Pv* and *Po* mention previously, which are out of routine diagnostic procedures, means the task of eliminating *Pv* and *Po* is clearly not an easy one. When the unique biology of *Pv* and *Po* vis-à-vis the evidence of their presence in Africa are considered, there is a need for a paradigm shift regarding *Pv* and *Po* research by putting in place the following:

1. Sensitization of National Malaria Control Programs (NMCPs) to the menace of the two parasites in asymptomatic and symptomatic infections

2. Provision of baseline and standardized tools for sample collection, detection and assays for *Pv* and *Po* towards the elimination of the parasites.

3. Measures for all individuals irrespective of age in Africa to be at reduced risk to *Pv* and *Po* infections

4. De-escalation of the burden of *Pv and Po,* through the utilization of novel and available tools that can be integrated into malaria control and elimination agenda in sub-Saharan Africa.

5. Crosstalk between NMCPs and researchers as well as institutions engaged in malaria research.

6. Creation of fora for exchange of knowledge and resources between *Pv* and *Po* focused scientists in Africa and globally, to facilitate progress in control and elimination activities.

3. Conclusion and future perspectives

The presence of *Pv* and *Po* in Africa is certain. Malaria control programs generally focus on providing good vector control, early diagnosis, and access to effective antimalarial regimens, preferably with anti-gametocyte activity to reduce transmission. All these tools cannot be optimally employed without a knowledge of the transmission dynamics of all parasites within a community or country. Re-engaging the focus of NMCPs on non-falciparum malaria that harbor hypnozoites and that potentially could be a significant problem in the very near future is a necessity. Pooling of resources regionally and internationally are key elements for the fight against reducing the burden of non-falciparum malaria and their elimination. It is important that NMCPs and researchers from Universities and Research Institutions engage in crosstalk to facilitate accurate detection and surveillance, and generate the human resource required for sustaining these efforts.

Acknowledgements

The authors acknowledge the patience and support of the Intech Open team and our entire family in the write up.

Conflict of interest

The authors declare no conflict of interest.

Author details

Isaac K. Quaye[1*] and Larysa Aleksenko[2]

1 Department of Applied Health Sciences, Regent University College of Science and Technology, Accra, Ghana

2 Division of Obstetrics and Gynecology, Department of Clinical Sciences, Faculty of Medicine, Lund University, Lund, Sweden

*Address all correspondence to: isaac.quaye@regent.edu.gh

References

[1] S.K. Nilsson, L.M. Childs, C. Buckee, M. Marti, Targeting Human Transmission Biology for Malaria Elimination, PLoS Pathog. 11 (2015) e1004871.

[2] J.M. Cohen, B. Moonen, R.W. Snow, D.L. Smith, How absolute is zero? An evaluation of historical and current definitions of malaria elimination, Malar J. 9 (2010) 213-2875-9-213.

[3] M.E. Woolhouse, Patterns in parasite epidemiology: the peak shift, Parasitol. Today. 14 (1998) 428-434.

[4] T. Bousema, J.T. Griffin, R.W. Sauerwein, D.L. Smith, T.S. Churcher, W. Takken, A. Ghani, C. Drakeley, R. Gosling, Hitting hotspots: spatial targeting of malaria for control and elimination, PLoS Med. 9 (2012) e1001165.

[5] T. Bousema, G. Stresman, A.Y. Baidjoe, J. Bradley, P. Knight, W. Stone, V. Osoti, E. Makori, C. Owaga, W. Odongo, P. China, S. Shagari, O.K. Doumbo, R.W. Sauerwein, S. Kariuki, C. Drakeley, J. Stevenson, J. Cox, The Impact of Hotspot-Targeted Interventions on Malaria Transmission in Rachuonyo South District in the Western Kenyan Highlands: A Cluster-Randomized Controlled Trial, PLoS Med. 13 (2016) e1001993.

[6] T. Bousema, B. Kreuels, R. Gosling, Adjusting for heterogeneity of malaria transmission in longitudinal studies, J. Infect. Dis. 204 (2011) 1-3.

[7] A.A. Lover, J.K. Baird, R. Gosling, R.N. Price, Malaria Elimination: Time to Target All Species, Am. J. Trop. Med. Hyg. 99 (2018) 17-23.

[8] K.A. Twohig, D.A. Pfeffer, J.K. Baird, R.N. Price, P.A. Zimmerman, S.I. Hay, P.W. Gething, K.E. Battle, R.E. Howes, Growing evidence of Plasmodium vivax across malaria-endemic Africa, PLoS Negl Trop. Dis. 13 (2019) e0007140.

[9] N.J. White, Determinants of relapse periodicity in *Plasmodium vivax* malaria, Malar J. 10 (2011) 297-2875-10-297.

[10] B.M. Greenwood, Asymptomatic malaria infections--do they matter? Parasitol. Today. 3 (1987) 206-214.

[11] C. Doderer-Lang, P.S. Atchade, L. Meckert, E. Haar, S. Perrotey, D. Filisetti, A. Aboubacar, A.W. Pfaff, J. Brunet, N.W. Chabi, C.D. Akpovi, L. Anani, A. Bigot, A. Sanni, E. Candolfi, The ears of the African elephant: unexpected high seroprevalence of Plasmodium ovale and Plasmodium malariae in healthy populations in Western Africa, Malar J. 13 (2014) 240-2875-13-240.

[12] M. Groger, H.S. Fischer, L. Veletzky, A. Lalremruata, M. Ramharter, A systematic review of the clinical presentation, treatment and relapse characteristics of human Plasmodium ovale malaria, Malar J. 16 (2017) 112-017-1759-2.

[13] S. Amireh, H. Shaaban, G. Guron, Severe Plasmodium vivax cerebral malaria complicated by hemophagocytic lymphohistiocytosis treated with artesunate and doxycycline, Hematol. Oncol. Stem Cell. Ther. 11 (2018) 34-37.

[14] W.A. Krotoski, W.E. Collins, R.S. Bray, P.C. Garnham, F.B. Cogswell, R.W. Gwadz, R. Killick-Kendrick, R. Wolf, R. Sinden, L.C. Koontz, P.S. Stanfill, Demonstration of hypnozoites in sporozoite-transmitted Plasmodium vivax infection, Am. J. Trop. Med. Hyg. 31 (1982) 1291-1293.

[15] A. D'Abramo, S. Gebremeskel Tekle, M. Iannetta, L. Scorzolini, A. Oliva, M.G. Paglia, A. Corpolongo, E. Nicastri,

Severe Plasmodium ovale malaria complicated by acute respiratory distress syndrome in a young Caucasian man, Malar J. 17 (2018) 139-018-2289-2.

[16] J.H. Adams, I. Mueller, The Biology of *Plasmodium vivax*, Cold Spring Harb Perspect. Med. 7 (2017) 10.1101/cshperspect.a025585.

[17] L.M. Yamauchi, A. Coppi, G. Snounou, P. Sinnis, Plasmodium sporozoites trickle out of the injection site, Cell. Microbiol. 9 (2007) 1215-1222.

[18] B. Singh, L. Kim Sung, A. Matusop, A. Radhakrishnan, S.S. Shamsul, J. Cox-Singh, A. Thomas, D.J. Conway, A large focus of naturally acquired Plasmodium knowlesi infections in human beings, Lancet. 363 (2004) 1017-1024.

[19] T.N. Wells, J.N. Burrows, J.K. Baird, Targeting the hypnozoite reservoir of Plasmodium vivax: the hidden obstacle to malaria elimination, Trends Parasitol. 26 (2010) 145-151.

[20] L.J. Robinson, R. Wampfler, I. Betuela, S. Karl, M.T. White, C.S. Li Wai Suen, N.E. Hofmann, B. Kinboro, A. Waltmann, J. Brewster, L. Lorry, N. Tarongka, L. Samol, M. Silkey, Q. Bassat, P.M. Siba, L. Schofield, I. Felger, I. Mueller, Strategies for understanding and reducing the *Plasmodium vivax* and Plasmodium ovale hypnozoite reservoir in Papua New Guinean children: a randomised placebo-controlled trial and mathematical model, PLoS Med. 12 (2015) e1001891.

[21] L.H. Miller, S.J. Mason, D.F. Clyde, M.H. McGinniss, The resistance factor to *Plasmodium vivax* in blacks. The Duffy-blood-group genotype, FyFy, N. Engl. J. Med. 295 (1976) 302-304.

[22] P.A. Zimmerman, Plasmodium vivax Infection in Duffy-Negative People in Africa, Am. J. Trop. Med. Hyg. 97 (2017) 636-638.

[23] E. Meibalan, M. Marti, Biology of Malaria Transmission, Cold Spring Harb Perspect. Med. 7 (2017) 10.1101/cshperspect.a025452.

[24] B. Malleret, A. Li, R. Zhang, K.S. Tan, R. Suwanarusk, C. Claser, J.S. Cho, E.G. Koh, C.S. Chu, S. Pukrittayakamee, M.L. Ng, F. Ginhoux, L.G. Ng, C.T. Lim, F. Nosten, G. Snounou, L. Renia, B. Russell, Plasmodium vivax: restricted tropism and rapid remodeling of CD71-positive reticulocytes, Blood. 125 (2015) 1314-1324.

[25] I. Mueller, M.R. Galinski, J.K. Baird, J.M. Carlton, D.K. Kochar, P.L. Alonso, H.A. del Portillo, Key gaps in the knowledge of Plasmodium vivax, a neglected human malaria parasite, Lancet Infect. Dis. 9 (2009) 555-566.

[26] A.I. Adekunle, M. Pinkevych, R. McGready, C. Luxemburger, L.J. White, F. Nosten, D. Cromer, M.P. Davenport, Modeling the dynamics of Plasmodium vivax infection and hypnozoite reactivation in vivo, PLoS Negl Trop. Dis. 9 (2015) e0003595.

[27] A. Mayor, A. Bardaji, E. Macete, T. Nhampossa, A.M. Fonseca, R. Gonzalez, S. Maculuve, P. Cistero, M. Ruperez, J. Campo, A. Vala, B. Sigauque, A. Jimenez, S. Machevo, L. de la Fuente, A. Nhama, L. Luis, J.J. Aponte, S. Acacio, A. Nhacolo, C. Chitnis, C. Dobano, E. Sevene, P.L. Alonso, C. Menendez, Changing Trends in *P. falciparum* Burden, Immunity, and Disease in Pregnancy, N. Engl. J. Med. 373 (2015) 1607-1617.

[28] J.K. Baird, K.E. Battle, R.E. Howes, Primaquine ineligibility in anti-relapse therapy of *Plasmodium vivax* malaria: the problem of G6PD deficiency and cytochrome P-450 2D6 polymorphisms, Malar J. 17 (2018) 42-018-2190-z.

[29] D. Thomas, H. Tazerouni, K.G. Sundararaj, J.C. Cooper, Therapeutic failure of primaquine and need for new

medicines in radical cure of Plasmodium vivax, Acta Trop. 160 (2016) 35-38.

[30] M. Groger, L. Veletzky, A. Lalremruata, C. Cattaneo, J. Mischlinger, R. Manego Zoleko, J. Kim, A. Klicpera, E.L. Meyer, D. Blessborn, M. Winterberg, A.A. Adegnika, S.T. Agnandji, P.G. Kremsner, B. Mordmuller, G. Mombo-Ngoma, H.P. Fuehrer, M. Ramharter, Prospective Clinical and Molecular Evaluation of Potential Plasmodium ovale curtisi and wallikeri Relapses in a High-transmission Setting, Clin. Infect. Dis. 69 (2019) 2119-2126.

[31] P.A. Zimmerman, R.K. Mehlotra, L.J. Kasehagen, J.W. Kazura, Why do we need to know more about mixed Plasmodium species infections in humans? Trends Parasitol. 20 (2004) 440-447.

[32] E. Tjitra, N.M. Anstey, P. Sugiarto, N. Warikar, E. Kenangalem, M. Karyana, D.A. Lampah, R.N. Price, Multidrug-resistant Plasmodium vivax associated with severe and fatal malaria: a prospective study in Papua, Indonesia, PLoS Med. 5 (2008) e128.

[33] N.M. Anstey, B. Russell, T.W. Yeo, R.N. Price, The pathophysiology of vivax malaria, Trends Parasitol. 25 (2009) 220-227.

[34] K.K. Dayananda, R.N. Achur, D.C. Gowda, Epidemiology, drug resistance, and pathophysiology of Plasmodium vivax malaria, J. Vector Borne Dis. 55 (2018) 1-8.

[35] Y.L. Lau, W.C. Lee, L.H. Tan, A. Kamarulzaman, S.F. Syed Omar, M.Y. Fong, F.W. Cheong, R. Mahmud, Acute respiratory distress syndrome and acute renal failure from Plasmodium ovale infection with fatal outcome, Malar J. 12 (2013) 389-2875-12-389.

[36] S. Eiam-Ong, Malarial nephropathy, Semin. Nephrol. 23 (2003) 21-33.

[37] M.V. Lacerda, S.C. Fragoso, M.G. Alecrim, M.A. Alexandre, B.M. Magalhaes, A.M. Siqueira, L.C. Ferreira, J.R. Araujo, M.P. Mourao, M. Ferrer, P. Castillo, L. Martin-Jaular, C. Fernandez-Becerra, H. del Portillo, J. Ordi, P.L. Alonso, Q. Bassat, Postmortem characterization of patients with clinical diagnosis of Plasmodium vivax malaria: to what extent does this parasite kill? Clin. Infect. Dis. 55 (2012) e67–e74.

Chapter 12

Progress in Parasite Genomics and Its Application to Current Challenges in Malaria Control

Cheikh Cambel Dieng, Colby T. Ford, Jennifer Huynh, Linda E. Amoah, Yaw A. Afrane, Daniel A. Janies and Eugenia Lo

Abstract

A wide deployment of malaria control tools have significantly reduced malaria morbidity and mortality across Africa. However, in the last five to seven years, there has been a resurgence of malaria in several African countries, raising the questions of whether and why current control mechanisms are failing. Since the first *Plasmodium falciparum* reference genome was published in 2002, few thousands more representing a broad range of geographical isolates have been sequenced. These advances in parasite genomics have improved our understanding of mutational changes, molecular structure, and genetic mechanisms associated with diagnostic testing, antimalarial resistance, and preventive measures such as vaccine development. In this chapter, we summarize the current progress on: (1) genomic characteristics of *P. falciparum*; (2) novel biomarkers and revolutionary techniques for diagnosing malaria infections; and (3) current vaccine targets and challenges for developing efficacious and long-lasting malaria vaccines.

Keywords: genomics, *Plasmodium falciparum*, malaria diagnosis, bioinformatics, antimalarial resistance, malaria vaccines, biomarkers, genetic diversity

1. Introduction

Malaria remains a serious public health problem in several developing countries. Globally, there are about 3.2 billion people at risk of malaria and 435,000 malaria-related deaths, most of which happening in West Africa [1, 2]. Malaria is a complicated disease caused by the genus *Plasmodium* in the protozoan phylum Apicomplexa. While *P. falciparum* is the most prevalent form of malaria, *P. vivax* is most widespread around the world. *Plasmodium* has a complicated life cycle that reproduces asexually in human and sexually in mosquito hosts. The parasite is transmitted by the female *Anopheles* mosquitoes. *Anopheles* mosquitoes thrive in warm, tropical climates as the temperature allows for quicker breeding and hatching [3]. The abundance of vectors is positively correlated with the transmission rate of malaria [4]. People infected with malaria normally experience fever, chills, diarrhea, vomiting, and anemia [5]. If remain untreated, the disease can progress to a severe form and result in death [6].

A wide deployment of malaria control tools in the past few decades have significantly reduced malaria morbidity and mortality worldwide. The number of countries with fewer than 100 clinical malaria cases increased from six to 27. Countries including Iran, Malaysia, Timor-Leste Belize, Cabo Verde, China, and El Salvador reported zero malaria cases in 2019 and malaria cases dropped by 90% in the Greater Mekong subregion (GMS) [7]. However, in the last five to seven years, there has been a resurgence of malaria in several African countries, raising the questions of whether and why current control mechanisms are failing. A number of factors has limited malaria control and elimination efforts. First, *Plasmodium* isolates may respond differently to antimalarial drugs, with some evolved to become more resistant than the others due to prolonged drug use. Second, multiplicity of infection (MOI), i.e., the number of *Plasmodium* isolates co-infecting a single host, has made molecular characterization of the parasites and understanding of disease severity difficult [8]. Third, diagnostic inaccuracy related to false negative results by rapid diagnostic tests (RDTs) is becoming a more widespread phenomenon [9]. Other factors such as asymptomatic reservoirs leading to transmission, lack of effective vaccine, and warmer climates and changing environments caused by human activities [10] have also hampered malaria elimination efforts. Thus, it is critically important to create new tools that allow us to monitor parasite changes and use that information to improve existing control strategies. In this chapter, we will summarize the current progress on: (1) genomic characteristics of *P. falciparum*; (2) novel biomarkers and revolutionary techniques for diagnosing malaria infections; and (3) current vaccine targets and challenges for developing efficacious and long-lasting malaria vaccines.

2. Genomic characteristics of *Plasmodium falciparum*

Knowledge of the evolution and genetic variation of the *Plasmodium* genome offers incredible insights into novel means of malaria diagnosis and treatment. The advances in parasite genomics have improved our understanding of mutational changes, molecular structure, and genetic mechanisms associated with failure in diagnostic testing [11], antimalarial resistance [12], and preventive measures such as vaccine development [13]. Since the first reference genome of *P. falciparum* was published in 2002 [14], several thousand DNA sequences have been collected and deposited in public databases. *Plasmodium falciparum* genome is approximately 23.7 Mb with 14 chromosomes, a plasmid of about 35 kb, and lots of mitochondrial DNA copies of about 6 kb [15]. There are currently 5,438 genes that have been predicted/discovered within the genome with 33% uncertainty of their functions [16]. The genome contains many rich AT regions in both exons and introns (80% and 90%, respectively), which has some advantages and disadvantages when learning more about the genetic architecture of the parasites [17]. The advantage associated with the genomic data would be using its rich polymorphic AT content as biomarkers to map out the evolutionary structure of the parasites and correlating it with any drug resistant genes [15]. Although having a rich AT genome has contributed to a high yield in microsatellites or simple sequence repeats, there are some disadvantages when using the genome in genetic studies [15]. For example, within CRISPR-Cas9, the high AT content resulted in a decrease in the amount of gRNA target sites needed [18]. A deeper knowledge of the genome's polymorphic and conserved genes are therefore essential towards understanding the evolutionary timeline of various *P. falciparum* lineages.

Compared to other eukaryotic organisms, whole genome sequencing (WGS) showed that the genome of *P. falciparum* contains fewer genes for enzymes and transporters, but more genes for immune evasion to support host–parasite interactions [14]. With an average length of 2.4 Kb, *P. falciparum* genes are considerably larger than many organisms. *P. falciparum*'s genome contains a full set of transfer RNA (tRNA) ligase genes with minimal redundancy. 43 tRNAs have been identified to bind all codons except TGT and TGC, which code for cysteine, thus giving *P. falciparum* a slightly different amino acid translation than is seen in humans and other eukaryotes. By contrast, the mitochondrial genome of *P. falciparum* is only about 6Kb and does not contain any genes that encode for tRNAs, implying that the mitochondrion must import tRNAs from elsewhere into the cells [19, 20]. Polymorphic genes in the *P. falciparum* genome are useful in creating linkage maps to monitor mutational changes and genetic diversity of the parasites in response to malaria interventions and control efforts [21]. Polymorphic genes are variations in genes at higher frequencies that can be advantageous, neutral, or disadvantageous [22]. The role of polymorphic genes is to influence coding regions, alter protein sequences and gene expression, and eventually the metabolic pathway and function [23]. For example, remarkable polymorphisms observed in the merozoite surface proteins (*MSP*), *PfAMA1*, *PfEBA*, and *PfRHs* genes that involved in merozoite evasion have been shown to increase the evasion ability of *P. falciparum* to the host immune system [24].

In comparison, conserved genes are genes that have not been altered. They contribute to important biological processes and fitness [25]. Information of conserved genes allow us to infer phylogenetic relatedness and trace the genetic origin of different lineages, determine new targets for therapeutic treatment, and serve as a guide when determining functions of unknown genes [18]. The processes that determine the polymorphisms of the parasitic genome include both selective pressures and recombination frequencies. Selective pressures on conserved genes allow certain important genes to remain unmodified for normal metabolic activities, whereas polymorphic genes diversify through frequent recombination allow for better evasion of antimalarial drug treatments and escape detection from diagnostic tests [26]. For example, the *PfHRP2* gene has shown with partial deletions and/or mutations over the past few years due to the usage of *HRP2*-specific Rapid Diagnostic tests (RDTs) [27, 28]. More specifically, the histidine-rich repeats in the *PfHRP2* gene drastically change the length of the gene and the ability of the parasites to evade RDTs. Therefore, novel genes that encode for parasite specific function might be potential new targets for malaria diagnosis and/or treatment [14]. It is important to distinguish metabolic pathways that the parasites use for invasion of the host cells as well as evasion of the host immune system.

P. falciparum is clearly genetically distinct by geographical regions [29, 30]. Given the complex life cycle of *Plasmodium*, genomic data coupled with Genome-Wide Association Studies can offer deep insights into the tangled relationships among humans, mosquitoes, and the parasites. To date, databases such as PlasmoDB have integrated sequence information, functional genomics, and annotation of data emerging from the *P. falciparum* genome sequencing consortium [31]. These databases provide an important platform to retrieve biological meaning from new 'omic' data and enhance diagnosis and treatment of infections caused by this dreadful malaria pathogen.

3. Conventional and novel methods for malaria diagnosis

One of the challenges to malaria elimination is the burden of submicroscopic asymptomatic infections that contribute to malaria transmission [7]. The gold standard for malaria diagnosis is microscopy [32]. Microscopy can differentiate malaria species and quantify parasite density, but only has a detection threshold of 10 to 50 parasites μl of blood (approximately 0.001% parasitemia, assuming an erythrocyte count of 5 × 106 cells μl) [33]. However, it requires well trained microscopists and is labor-intensive and time-consuming [32]. Previous studies have reported higher prevalence of asymptomatic parasitemia (6–7 times higher) using PCR compared to microscopy [5]. Nested PCR of the *18 s* rRNA genes has been commonly used to detect submicroscopic infections. PCR-based methods are also more sensitive than microscopy at detecting gametocytes particularly in asymptomatic individuals with low-density infections [34]. However, recent studies indicated a relatively high number of misdiagnosed infections [9], possibly due to low parasite density being less detectable by conventional PCR. The *18 s* rRNA gene has a reported detection thresholds of 0.5–5 parasites μl [35], but parasite density of asymptomatic infections especially in low transmission settings could be well below this threshold. As a result, many of these infections remain undetected in the general populations of several malaria-endemic countries [10, 36, 37] and provide perfect reservoirs for transmission at any time. Therefore, it is crucial to identify new gene targets or novel tools that are convenient and affordable for detecting asymptomatic infections, particularly in countries approaching elimination phase. Below are comparisons of various conventional and novel detection methods.

3.1 Rapid diagnostic test (RDT)

Rapid Diagnostic Test (RDT) is a lateral flow immunochromatographic test that can detect the presence of *Plasmodium* parasites by using blood from patients. The blood samples collected from patients must be lysed before the *Plasmodium* antigens being stained. RDT will indicate if the patient has malaria or not [38]. This diagnostic method is useful in rural areas as it is inexpensive and does not require expertise to perform the test [38]. There are various types of RDTs that can detect different antigens of *Plasmodium* parasites including *P. falciparum* and *P. vivax*, namely *P. falciparum* histidine-rich protein 2 (*PfHRP2*) and lactate dehydrogenase (*PfLDH*). However, recent studies indicated that parasites lacking the *pfhrp2/pfhrp3* genes could result in false-negative *PfHRP2*-RDT results, and these *pfhrp2/pfhrp3* variants have been spreading in many East and West African countries [39–42]. Reports of deletion of *HRP2* and *HRP3* genes was first reported in 2010 within the Peruvian Amazon [43] and the number of false negative RDTs has substantially increased in late 2014 [44]. Prevalence of false negative cases related to *HRP2* deletions in South America (with the exception of Peru) is lower than Asia and Sub-Saharan Africa [45]. The highest prevalence (50% *pfhrp2* deletions among all positive cases) were reported in Cambodia, Peru, and Eritrea [46]. Such a high prevalence could be explained by technical errors, mutations, selection and spread of the *pfhrp2* and 3 variants [47] from South America to Africa and Asia [41]. Recently, a novel HRP2-based Alere™ Malaria Ag P.f RDT (uRDT) was developed specifically for the detection of asymptomatic infections. Compared to the existing RDTs, the uRDT showed a greater than 10-fold improvement in diagnosing clinical and asymptomatic cases [48]. However, the sensitivities of the uRDT were inconsistent among different transmission settings [49]. Thus, although very promising for the detection of asymptomatic infections, the performance of uRDT must be further evaluated especially in areas with a already high prevalence of *pfhrp2* and *pfhrp3* gene deletions.

3.2 Enzyme-linked immunosorbent assay (ELISA)

ELISA is an enzyme-linked immunosorbent assay that is used to detect antigens and antibodies by utilizing a highly specific antibody–antigen interaction and their bonding affinity to proteins on a solid surface [50]. Samples, including and positive and negative controls are inserted on a 96 well plate which enables the possibility to analyze multiple samples simultaneously, then samples get incubated and detection of the signal is generated directly or indirectly via secondary tag on the specific antibody [51]. ELISA can be very efficient diagnostic tool for *Plasmodium* because it is highly specific and sensitive and therefore can be used to screen blood donors and pregnant women who may or may not have been exposed to the parasite [1]. However there are some limitations associated with using ELISA, as it is unable to detect antibodies in patients with acute infections, patients with different *Plasmodium* species, and various antigens within the different life stages of the parasite [52]. A recent study showed a lower detection threshold (3 parasites/μl) by ELISA test of the *Plasmodium* lactate dehydrogenase (*pLDH*) as compared to RDT (50–60 parasites/μl) [53]. However, ELISA has a lower sensitivity (69.9%) to antigens than RDT (88%) [53], and can be expensive and require a trained technician to operate and interpret the results [53].

3.3 Lateral flow immunoassay (LFIA)

One of the current diagnostic tests in development is an antibody-based lateral flow immunoassay (LFIA). Unlike ELISA that requires repeated incubation and washing steps, LFIA is considered to be a simple, user-friendly and cost-effective method for front-line diagnosis [54]. LFIA is versatile enough to detect target genes in sample matrices including whole blood, saliva, and urine. This method is primarily applied to detecting gametocytes in malaria-infected samples. Gametocytes are the sexual form of the parasite that gets transmitted to the mosquito host. They play a very important role in malaria transmission, and can contribute to up to 80% [55] of the infectious reservoirs. Previous studies have shown that infections with parasitemia as low as 4 gametocytes/μl can sustain transmission [56]. LFIA targets *Pfs25* in infected blood samples, which is a glycophosphatidylinositol-linked protein expressed on the surface of *P. falciparum* zygotes and ookinetes but only found on female gametocytes in the human hosts [57]. The detection limit of *Pfs25* LFIA is 0.02 gametocytes/μl, much more sensitive than *pfhrp2* RDT with a detection limit of 50–100 parasites per μL of blood [35, 58]. Another protein at the surface of the female gametocyte *PSSP17*, which is presumably more abundant in saliva samples, was also investigated in Cameroon, Zambia and Sierra Leone with an estimated sensitivity of 83% (95% CI, 61 to 95) in symptomatic patients when compared to PCR as the gold standard [58]. Detection of *pfhrp2* in saliva have been reported recently using LFIA, but the sensitivity was only shown to be improved in severe to moderate form of infections with parasitemia >60,000 parasites/μL [59]. Although convenient, *pfhrp2*-based LFIA could be less useful in detecting asymptomatic infections.

3.4 PCR-based methods

The combination of PCR-based assays and sequencing technologies have revolutionized malaria diagnosis since their introduction in the early 2000s. Various gene targets have be used to monitor genetic and/or mutational changes in the parasites that cause the disease. PCR is a very common technique used in malaria diagnoses in laboratory settings. The main advantage of this technique is that it enables us to identify individuals with low parasitemia (**Table 1**). There are multiple versions of this technique including nested conventional PCR, real-time quantitative PCR and reverse transcriptase PCR. Nested PCR is the easiest and least expensive methods among the others. It only requires a thermocycler, set of primers, reagents and visualization after gel electrophoresis. It is mostly a qualitative method as it is fairly difficult to estimate parasite density on a agarose gel. Unlike conventional PCR that uses gel electrophoresis to visualize PCR products, real-time PCR or qPCR detects and quantifies the amount of amplified DNA usually by SYBR green or a fluorogenic probe designed based on a target gene segment (TaqMan). The standard cycle threshold (Ct) value is inversely proportional to the amount of target DNA in the sample [66] and allows estimation of parasite density even in submicroscopic samples. Different from nested and qPCRs, reverse transcriptase PCR uses RNA as template and transcribes RNA into complementary DNA. This method has been widely used to detect and quantify gametocyte density in malaria samples. Though PCR-based methods are undoubtedly more sensitive than microscopic diagnosis, the level of sensitivity is highly dependent on the gene targets (**Table 1**).

3.4.1 18 s rRNA

The *18 s* rRNA genes have been the main gene target for molecular screening as it contains 5–8 copies per genome [62] in *Plasmodium*, but recent studies indicated a relatively high level of misdiagnosed infections [45]. The advantage of using the *18 s* rRNA is that it is highly specific compared to microscopy or RDT diagnoses. The primer sequences and protocols for both nested and qPCRs have been readily established. However, it fails to reveal infections with low parasite density (0.5–5 parasites/μL of blood) [35]. Thus, new target genes have been examined in the past few years with the goal to achieve an ultra-sensitive biomarker with higher sensitivity and specificity compared to the *18 s* rRNA.

3.4.2 Mitochondrial cytochrome c oxidase III (COX3)

The cytochrome c oxidase III (*COX3*) gene plays a very important role in cellular respiration [67]. It is a mitochondrial gene that inherited solely from the female gametocyte and less likely to undergo genetic recombination, making it an ideal candidate for identifying the origin and transmission of the parasites [68].

Type	Target	Sensitivity (%)	Specificity (%)	Application	Detection Limit	Refs
RDT	*HRP2/3*	57	99	Field	50–100 parasites/μL of blood	[35]
RDT	*LDH*	58	93	Field	50–100 parasites/μL of blood	[35]
PCR	*18 s* rRNA	64	92	Laboratory	0.5–5 parasites/μL of blood	[60]
PCR	*COX3*	—	—	Laboratory	0.6–2 parasites/μL blood	[60]
PCR	*TARE-2*	81	49	Laboratory	6–24 parasites in 200 μL whole blood	[61]
PCR	*var*ATS	—	—	Laboratory	12–30 parasites in 200 μL whole blood	[62]
PCR	*Pfs25*	—	—	Laboratory	0.3 mature females/μL blood	[63]
ELISA	*LDH*	69.9	100	Laboratory	3 parasites/μL blood	[53, 64]
LFIA	*Pfs25*	—	—	Laboratory	0.02 gametocytes/μl blood	[58]
SERS	Hemozoin	—	—	Laboratory	30 parasites/μL of blood	[65]

— Denotes that the sensitivity or specificity is not reported.

Table 1.
Existing malaria diagnostic tests and their respective performance.

More importantly, there are around 20 to 150 copies of the *COX3* gene in the *Plasmodium* genome [62] and PCR analysis of this gene indicated a detection limit of 0.6–2 parasites/μL, much more sensitive than the *18 s*-rRNA [60].

3.4.3 Telomere associated repetitive element 2 (TARE-2)

The recently discovered Telomere Associated Repetitive Element 2 (*TARE-2*) has demonstrated better performance than the conventional *18 s* rRNA marker in detecting low density parasite infections. There are about 250 copies of the *TARE-2* gene in the *Plasmodium* genome and this gene is highly specific to *P. falciparum* [69]. *TARE-2* has been previously shown to be useful for detecting ultra-low density *P. falciparum* infections in Papua New Guinea and Tanzania [62]. A recent study in Ghana showed a slightly higher sensitivity of *TARE-2* compared to *18 s* rRNA (81.2% vs. 80.9%) using microscopy as a gold standard, but with a lower specificity reduced by almost two-fold [37], making this gene less desirable for active case surveillance.

3.4.4 Var. gene acidic terminal sequence (varATS)

The *var* gene family is located primarily in the subtelomeric region of the *Plasmodium* genome. It is a family of genes known to be highly polymorphic. For instance, the genome of the 3D7 culture strain harbors 59 different *var* genes with an estimated 50–150 copies per genome [14]. One of the main gene in the *var* gene family encodes the *P. falciparum* erythrocyte membrane protein 1 (*PfEMP1*) that contains a highly variable extracellular part and a well conserved intracellular *var* gene acidic terminal sequence (*var*ATS) [61]. The *var*ATS has a detection limit of 12–30 parasites in 200 μL whole blood. Though more sensitive *18 s* rRNA, *var*ATS employs a qPCR approach that could be less feasible for routine case detection in rural areas or developing countries [62].

3.5 Raman spectroscopy

Raman spectroscopy is a relatively novel technique that can be used to diagnose the presence of *Plasmodium*. This technique measures the amount of wavelength and light intensity of scattered light reflected from the target molecule of *Plasmodium* present in an infected sample either in liquid, gas, or solid form [70]. Raman spectroscopy can be used specifically to characterize hemozoin, a pigment produced by infected erythrocytes and can be used to track the progression of the disease and efficacy of drug treatment [71]. A specific type of Raman spectroscopy known as Surface Enhanced Raman Spectroscopy (SERS) has been utilized to detect early signs of erythrocytic infections and was shown with a detection limit of 30 parasites/μL [65]. Tip-enhanced Raman spectroscopy (TERS), on the other hand, can enhance *Plasmodium*'s hemozoin vacuole from 10^6 to 10^7 [71]. While Raman spectroscopy is more cost effectiveness than PCR and microscopy [71], this technique cannot detect hemozoin in early ring stage nor differentiate hemozoin from active and previous infections [71]. Further investigations are needed to refine Raman signals in order to enhance the technique's detection abilities.

4. Revolutionized techniques and genomics tools for monitoring parasite changes

Extensive level of genetic diversity observed in *Plasmodium* is a major threat to the eradication of the disease. Previous studies used sanger sequencing of the merozoite surface protein (MSP) or microsatellite genotyping methods to assess parasite genetic diversity. Though affordable, these methods are time-consuming and labor-intensive for large scale genetic studies. Moreover, differentiating or phasing clonal genotypes for samples with more than two clones can be difficult. Restriction enzyme cutting followed by gel electorphoresis of the MSP gene has been conventionally used to assess parasite diversity and define multiplicity of infections (MOI) based on the number of distinct bands present on a gel. MSP is the most abundant protein at the surface of the merozoite and play a critical role in the *Plasmodium* invasion mechanism to the erythrocyte [72]. It is an informative gene for resolving clonal relationships and depicting population structure of *Plasmodium* given its size polymorphisms [73]. However, in high transmission areas where parasites are highly variable and different by single nucleotide polymorphisms (SNPs), gel electorphoresis of the MSP gene would underestimate the levels of diversity and polyclonality [74]. Microsatellite genotyping has also extensively been used for *Plasmodium* population structure and genetic diversity study [75]. While this marker has the advantages of being polymorphic, evolutionary neutrally, and are abundant in the *Plasmodium* genome [76], polyclonal samples with more than two alleles detected from two or more genetic loci are usually discarded in the analyses. Thus, next-generation sequencing (NGS) technologies offer a novel, alternative approach to shed light on the polyclonal and complex nature of *Plasmodium* infections [77].

4.1 Amplicon deep sequencing

In regions in high malaria endemicity, individuals typically harbor multiple *Plasmodium falciparum* isolates due to repeated exposure to mosquitoes infected with multiple parasite isolates [78]. Polyclonal infections have become a growing concern as some parasite isolates may be resistant to antimalarial drugs and/or more pathogenic [79]. Identification of genetically distinct clones is necessary to critically evaluate the causation of resistance to drugs and any other therapeutic treatments. Recently, due to reduced cost of high throughput NGS technology, other types of molecular tools have emerged to address the complex issue related to MOI. MOI is defined as the number of parasite clones within an infected sample. Deep sequencing of a targeted gene amplicon coupled with bioinformatic analyses allow differentiation of various *P. falciparum* strains based on SNPs [75] and discrimination of major from minor clones [80]. It also provides an increased capability to detect the genetic relatedness among clones within and between hosts as well as minor *P. falciparum* variants [81]. This technique can be applied to different gene regions such as Circumsporozoite (CSP), MSP1/2, and Apical membrane antigen (AMA) to monitor changes as well as selection pressure acting on the parasite populations [82].

4.2 Molecular inversion probe

Molecular inversion probes (MIPs) are another deep sequencing technique that targets several short gene regions across the genome. MIPs are single stranded DNA molecules that contain flanking regions of the targeted gene regions up to several hundred base pairs long [83]. MIPs can hybridize with the target sequence and undergo gap filling ligation to form circular DNA. The target sequence will also contain adaptors and barcodes to be further amplified by PCR [83]. The advantages of this technique include low rate of errors, small amount of DNA samples, high throughput, and cost-effective for several hundreds of samples. It is scalable to the number of targeted gene regions and samples, requires minimal costs in terms of reagents and labor, and allows efficient capture of DNA extracted from dried blood spots [84]. The latter advantage would make large-scale population studies feasible. MIPs have been used for monitoring SNP mutations associated with drug

Anti-malarial	Chloroquine	Amodiaquine	Sulfadoxine	Pyrimethamine	Artemisinin
Gene	Crt	Mdr1	Dhps	Dhfr	K13
Mutation(s)	K76T	N86Y, Y184F	A437G, K540E	N51I, C59R, S108N	M476I, Y493H, R539T, I543T, C580Y

Table 2.
Gene mutations associated with antimalarial drug resistance.

resistance, such as *crt*, *mdr1*, *dhps*, *dhfr*, and *K13* (**Table 2**) [84]. For example, a recent study based on MIPs analysis found that the *PfDHPS* gene associated with Sulfadoxine resistance has been rapidly spread from east to west of the Democratic Republic of Congo [84]. Apart from drug-resistant mutations, a number of microsatellite loci have also been added to the MIP panel to estimate genetic structure and diversity of *P. falciparum*. This technique allows multiple loci to be genotyped simultaneously. However, the design of the MIP panel would require prior information of the gene regions of interest.

5. From parasite genes to malaria vaccines

Genetic information of *P. falciparum* has allowed a careful selection of gene targets for vaccine development [85]. Vaccines can offer protection against clinical malaria especially in young children and reduce transmission in a population. However, there are several challenges in developing a highly effective malaria vaccine, mostly due to the complexity in the parasite life cycle and host immune system. *Plasmodium* parasites reproduce asexually in human hosts. They can be found throughout the body's bloodstream and liver in various stages. There are numerous potential parasite antigens that elicit different levels of host immune response [86], but the protective response towards a particular antigen or one parasite life-stage is not effective in conferring protection against other stages [87]. One solution for that is to choose an immunogenic antigen/epitope that can elicit a strong immune response and potentially confer the highest efficacy. Conjugating the target antigen or epitope with an adjuvant or better drug delivery system can help elicit a stronger and safer immune response [88]. Alternatively, it is also possible to activate other immune cells such as natural killer cells and neutrophils that can elicit a long-lasting immune response [89]. Natural killer cells act faster than T cells while neutrophils can activate either a humoral or cell mediated immunity [90]. Both natural killer cells and neutrophils in response to *P. falciparum* invasion have not been studied in depth compared to antibodies and T cells [90]. To date, there are three types of malarial vaccines that are being studied and tested in clinical trials: pre-erythrocytic, erythrocytic, and transmission blocking vaccines (**Table 3**).

5.1 Pre-erythrocytic vaccines

Pre-erythrocytic vaccines aim to kill infected hepatocytes and prevent sporozoites from reaching the liver [101]. There are various gene targets currently being investigated and in clinical trials.

5.1.1 RTS,S/AS01E

RTS,S/AS01E is a well-known pre-erythrocytic vaccine that has successfully completed phase III of clinical testing. It is currently distributed by World Health

Name of Vaccine	Type of Vaccine	Target of Vaccine	Malarial Life Cycle Stage	Phase of Vaccine	Efficacy	Refs
RTS,S/ AS01E	Recombinant protein vaccine	Circumsporozoite protein (CSP)	Pre-Erythrocytic	Phase III	35.2% in Children 20.3% in Infants	[91]
PfSPZ	Live, radiation-attenuated vaccine	Sporozoite (SPZ)	Pre-Erythrocytic	Phase III	Homologous challenge: 64% Heterologous challenge: 83%	[92]
PfLSA Vaccine	Recombinant protein vaccine	Liver-stage antigen 1 (*LSA-1*)	Pre-Erythrocytic	Phase I	Efficacy has yet to be found in humans	[93]
MSP1 Vaccine	Subunit based Vaccine	MSP1	Erythrocytic	Phase I	Efficacy has yet to be found in humans	[94]
AMA-1 Vaccine	Recombinant protein vaccine?	*AMA-1*	Erythrocytic	Phase II	Efficacy has yet to be found in humans	[95]
R21 Vaccine	Recombinant protein vaccines	Illicit a higher anti-CSP antibody count	Erythrocytic	Phase I/IIa	Efficacy has yet to be found in humans	[96]
Pfs 230 & *Pfs48/45*	Potential new target	*Pfs230* and *Pfs48/45* combined with a FAB fragment of a monoclonal antibody, 4F12, can act on parasitic gametes by forming a membrane-bound protein complex and increase the vaccine activity	Transmission Blocking Vaccine	None	Efficacy has yet to be found in humans	[97]
Pfs25	Recombinant conjugated vaccines	Antibodies against the *Pfs25* antigen in the human host to stop the development and transmission of the parasite when the vector feeds on the host.	Transmission Blocking Vaccine	Phase I	Efficacy has yet to be found in humans	[98]
PfGARP	Potential new target	Glutamic acid rich protein	Erythrocytic	None	Efficacy has yet to be found in humans	[99]
PfRH5-PfCyRPA-PfRipr (RCR) complex	Potential new target	Induce strain-transcending neutralizing antibodies against blood-stage *P. falciparum*	Erythrocytic	Phase I/II	Efficacy has yet to be found in humans	[100]

Table 3.
Overview of current vaccines candidates against Plasmodium falciparum.

Organization (WHO) in Malawi, Ghana, and Kenya to further investigate vaccine efficacy [96]. RTS,S is a vaccine that targets circumsporozoite proteins (CSP) from

P. falciparum. CSP are surface proteins that is important in hepatocyte invasion. Interactions between CSP and heparin sulfate proteoglycans (HSPGs) allows the sporozoite to attach to the surface of hepatocytes and triggers a signaling cascade that allows for the sporozoite to invade liver cells [102]. Subsequent to invasion, the sporozoites will mature, multiply, and feed on the hepatocytes until the hepatocytes lyse and release merozoites into the bloodstream. Preventing the invasion of sporozoites will inhibit the progression and severity of the disease. Using the C-terminus and central tandem repeat (NANP) of *PfCSP*, Hepatitis B surface membrane antigen (HSbAg), and an AS01 adjuvant system, the vaccine will elicit a strong, stable immune response [91]. After vaccination, the host immune system will response to *PfCSP* antigen by producing anti-CSP antibodies and activating CD4+ T cells [103]. RTS,S/AS01E is given on a three-dose schedule within three months followed by a fourth dose at 20 months [91]. It has been shown across clinical malarial studies that the vaccine has an 39–50% efficacy in children ages 5–17 months and 23–30% efficacy in children ages 6–12 months [104–106]. Efficacy warned rapidly from 35.2% and 20.3% to 19.1% and 12.7%, respectively, in children and infants within 20–32 months without a booster [91]. Such a decay in vaccine efficacy could be due to reduced IgG and IgM antibodies against CSP antigen. Anti-CSP antibodies were shown to increase by almost 10-fold from 318.2 EU/mL to 34.2 EU/mL in children one month after a booster was given [96]. Apart from the short-lived nature of the vaccine, older children who were vaccinated showed an increased risk of malarial infections, likely due to RTS,S/AS01E interference with naturally acquired immunity [96]. Another similar vaccine R21 is currently testing in Phase 1/2a clinical trials [107]. This vaccine aims to elicit a high anti-CSP antibody content similar to the mechanisms of RTS,S vaccine. R21 comprises particles from CSP-HBsAg protein infused with an adjuvant, matrix-M [107]. It has been shown to increase the production of T cells and is still in the process of development [96]. Further studies should investigate alternative antigens that can elicit stronger and long-lasting efficacy as well as the mechanisms of the cell-mediated immune response against malaria in humans.

5.1.2 PfSPZ

Plasmodium falciparum sporozoites (PfSPZ) is another pre-erythrocytic vaccine target. As aforementioned, sporozoites transferred from the infected Anopheles mosquito to the human host. They enter the bloodstream and reach the liver before invading the hepatocytes using the sporozoite proteins P36 and P52. P36 interacts with hepatocyte's extracellular receptor EphA2 to create a protective parasitophorous vacuole that facilitates hepatocyte invasion [108]. *PfSPZ* vaccine prevents the sporozoites reaching the liver and infecting hepatocytes [109], and is currently undergoing phase III clinical trial [92]. *PfSPZ* vaccine was designed to have a live, whole sporozoite that is radiated-attenuated. It is injected intravenously and given in 3–5 doses. Recent studies using controlled human malaria infection (CHMI) showed that this vaccine provided about 33 weeks of stabilized protection in 50% of the vaccinated subjects [110]. The vaccine induced interferon gamma (IFN-γ) that can recruit and activate CD8+ and CD4+ T cells against homologous and heterologous parasitic strains [110]. Subjects who received the *PfSPZ* vaccine also developed IgM antibodies that can help inhibit proliferation of the parasites [111]. However, the vaccine requires specific storage in ultra-cold condition and trained medical workers to inject the vaccine intravenously [96]. Furthermore, efficacy varied by locations. For example, in Mali, 29% efficacy was reported in subject who were exposed to heterologous strain; whereas in CHMI, 83% of subjects were found to be protected from exposure to heterologous strains [92]. Further studies are needed to compare efficacy among different geographical or transmission settings.

5.1.3 PfLSA-1 and PfLSA-3

Liver surface antigen (LSA) is another pre-erythrocytic vaccine target. LSA is essential for the survival of the parasites during the late liver schizogony stage [93]. Schizonts are asexual stage of *Plasmodium* that developed from sporozoites and matured in infected hepatocytes. Once the infected hepatocytes are filled up with mature schizonts, they rupture and release merozoites into the bloodstream to invade erythrocytes. LSA vaccine prevents the maturation of schizonts and rupture of infected hepatocytes. There are two liver stage antigens, LSA-1 and LSA-3, that are used as vaccine targets. *PfLSA-1* is high conserved in *P. falciparum* and is found in parasitophorous vacuole in the liver stage of the parasites. *PfLSA-1* contains 17 amino acids repeats and is associated with the late liver schizont stage [93, 112]. LSA-1 can induce IgG and IgM antibodies as well as CD4+ T cell production [93, 113]. LSA-1 vaccine is currently in phase I clinical trial and is still unclear its efficacy in humans. LSA-3, on the other hand, is found in dense granules in the blood stage of the parasites and the protein is about 175 kDa [114]. LSA-3 appears to play a role in the parasitic growth in infected hepatocytes and erythrocytes [114]. A recent study indicated that LSA-3 provided full protect to chimpanzees from heterologous *P. falciparum* sporozoites [93]. Like LSA-1, LSA-3 is also in phase I clinical trial and its efficacy and immunogenicity in humans remain unclear.

5.2 Erythrocytic vaccines

Erythrocytic vaccines aim to kill and terminate the asexual reproduction and invasion of the parasite within red blood cells (RBC). Infected individuals typically experience symptoms when the parasites invade a threshold number of RBCs and disrupt their normal functions. Preventing the parasites developed into blood stage will inhibit progression of malaria symptoms such as chills, aches, and fevers.

5.2.1 PfMSP1

Merozoite surface protein 1 (MSP1) is one of the targets used for erythrocytic vaccine. MSP1 is a glycosylphosphatidylinositol-anchored protein found in abundance on the surface of the merozoites [115]. MSP1 plays an important role in the invasion of erythrocytes as it binds and recruits other peripheral merozoite surface proteins to form a complex [115]. MSP1 starts off as a precursor of about 196 kDa and then cleave into four subunits before invading the erythrocytes [94]. The four subunits are held non-covalently forming a complex attached to the merozoite's GPI anchor [94]. Once the MSP1 complex is formed, it binds with the receptors on erythrocytes and activates a spectrin-binding function to enter the erythrocytes [94]. MSP1 has been shown to elicit both humoral (IgM and IgG antibodies) and cell-mediated immune responses (memory T cells) that lasted about 6 months after immunization [94]. These results are promising as MSP1 vaccine will also activate antibodies for complement fixation, induce opsonizing antibodies, and initiate secretion of reactive oxygen species by other immune cells [94]. To date, MSP1 vaccine is in phase I clinical trial. Further investigation is needed to evaluate efficacy.

5.2.2 PfAMA-1

The erythrocytic vaccine based on Apical Membrane Antigen 1 (AMA1) is currently in phase II clinical trial [116]. The AMA1 protein is approximately 83 kDa and can be found in both the merozoite and sporozoite stages of *P. falciparum* [116]. The complex AMA1 and another parasite protein namely the rhoptry neck protein 2 (RON2), is essential for merozoite invasion during the blood stage of infection, and initiates the parasite traversal into the RBCs [117]. The AMA1 vaccine has been shown to elicit high levels of antibodies that can block the invasion of the erythrocytes, despite high polymorphisms observed in the AMA1 protein [117]. The AMA1-Diversity Covering (DiCo) vaccine was thus designed to include three recombinant variants of AMA1 and this vaccine is currently testing in phase Ia/Ib clinical trial [118]. To increase efficacy of the AMA1 vaccine, AMA1 was paired with the RON2 receptor and vaccinated in eight *Aotus* monkeys [117]. Half of the monkeys were able to achieve complete immunity from the *P. falciparum* infection when vaccinated with AMA1 and RON2 [117]. The vaccine with AMA1 and RON2 induced a higher level of antibodies than the AMA1 vaccine. Further investigation is needed to examine other potential AMA1 variants or merozoite structures that can be paired up with the AMA1 protein to increase efficacy.

5.2.3 PfGARP

Plasmodium falciparum glutamic acid rich protein (PfGARP) is an 80 kDa antigen commonly expressed on the surface of infected erythrocytes during the late trophozoite stage [119]. The *PfGARP* gene is relatively conserved. Antibodies against the *PfGARP* antigen protein have been shown to confer protection against severe malaria and reduce parasite densities by 3.5 folds [99]. Further, anti-*PfGARP* antibodies were able to successfully induce apoptosis in ring-stage parasite cultures, resulting in full loss of their mitochondrial function within a 24 hour period [99]. In addition, the size of food vacuoles in the parasites was decreased or condensed tightly around the hemozoin crystals, making them inaccessible and parasite growth was reduced by 76–87% *in vitro* [99].

5.2.4 PfRH5-PfCyRPA-PfRipr (RCR) complex

The *PfRH5-PfCyRPA-PfRipr* (RCR) complex is a protein trimer composed of three different proteins *PfRH5*, *PfCyRPA*, and *PfRipr* that are found on the surface of merozoites [100]. *P. falciparum* Reticulocyte-binding Protein Homolog 5 (*PfRH5*) is a 63 kDa protein commonly expressed during the schizont stage. After *PfRH5* binds with basigin (a receptor found on human erythrocytes), a large amount of calcium is released to initiate invasion [100]. Monoclonal antibodies against *PfRH5* has been found to disrupt the binding between basigin and *PfRH5* [100]. *P. falciparum* Cysteine-rich Protective Antigen (*PfCyRPA*) is a highly conserved 43 kDa protein [100]. It plays an important role in erythrocyte invasion by interacting with *PfRH5* to bind to the receptor basigin [56]. Although *PfCyRPA* is not immunogenic compared to *PfRipr* and *PfRH5*, monoclonal antibodies produced against this protein can cause cross strain neutralization [100]. *P. falciparum* RH5-interacting Protein (*PfRipr*) is a highly conserved 120 kDa protein found in the schizont stage [100]. It is composed of 87 cysteines and 10 epidermal growth factor-like (EGF) domains [100]. Prior to erythrocyte invasion, *PfRipr* cleaves into two different fragments including the N-terminus and C-terminus. The N-terminus contains EGF domains 1 and 2 while the C-terminus contains EGF domains 3–10 [100]. Antibodies against *PfRipr* EGF domains 6–8 have been shown to neutralize the parasites [100]. Combining the anti-PfCyRPA c12 mAb with anti-RH5 BS1.2 mAbr will inhibit parasite growth *in vitro* from 21–31% to 59%. Thus, this antigen protein complex is expected to elicit a strong immune response against blood stage *P. falciparum* [120].

5.3 Transmission blocking vaccine (TBV)

TBV aims to prevent and kill the sexual stages of the *Plasmodium* parasites before transferring into the mosquito hosts. This vaccine offers protection against infection and transmission.

5.3.1 Pfs25

Pfs25 is an important glycophosphatidylinositol-linked protein expressed on the surface of ookinetes. It is found only within the *Anopheles* host and is approximately 25 kDa with 11 disulfie bonds [121]. The parasites require *Pfs25* to survive in the *Anopheles*'s midgut and develop into oocysts [122]. *Pfs25* is a conserve protein with low diversity. *Pfs25* vaccine was designed to elicit antibodies against the *Pfs25* antigen in humans and prohibit the development and transmission of gametocytes [98]. However, a recent study based on an adjuvant of *Pfs25* and a non-enveloped virus like protein (VLP) indicated weak IgG antibody responses in healthy individuals [123]. In another study, the antibody response of *Pfs25* proteins combined with four different adjuvants including alum, Toll-like receptor 4 (TLR-4) agonist glucopyranosal lipid A (GLA) plus alum, squalene–oil-in-water emulsion, and GLA plus squalene–oil-in-water emulsion were compared in mice. *Pfs25* combined with GLA plus squalene–oil-in-water emulsion was shown to induce the highest amounts of IgG antibodies [124]. Further studies should examine the formulation of this vaccine for better efficacy.

5.3.2 Pfs230 and Pfs48/45

Pfs230 and *Pfs48/45*-based vaccines are antigens rich in cysteine produced by the sexual stage gametocytes [97]. *Pfs48/45* can be found on the plasma membrane surface of both male and female gametocytes and are bounded to a GPI anchor that form a complex with *Pfs230* [125]. *Pfs230* is a 230 kDa protein that contains 14 6-cysteine rich domains [97]. *Pfs48/45*, on the other hand, contains three 6-cysteine rich domains [125]. The 6-cysteine rich domains of these antigens are essential for the formation of disulfide bonds on epitopes needed for antibody elicitation [125]. A recent study showed that mice injected with fragments of *Pfs48/45* and *Pfs230* prodomain produced higher levels of antibodies that induced complement fixation [125]. *Pfs230* and *Pfs48/45* combined with a FAB fragment of a monoclonal antibody 4F12 have been shown to further increase vaccine efficacy [97]. This vaccine is currently in early clinical development phase [97, 125].

6. Conclusion

WHO aims to achieve malaria elimination in at least 35 countries, reduce incidence and mortality rates by 90%, and prevent resurgence in malaria-free countries by 2030. This ambitious goal has been challenged by the emergence and spread of antimalarial resistance, inaccurate diagnostic testing, asymptomatic transmission, and lack of effective vaccines [126]. Information of the *Plasmodium* genomes allow us to improve and reinvent tools/techniques for monitoring parasite changes as well as tracking and stopping transmission of the disease. Several hundreds of *P. falciparum* genomes have been generated in the past two decades. Genetic variation and function of various genes have improved our understanding of mutational changes, molecular structure, and evolutionary mechanisms in *Plasmodium*. There is an urgent need to retrieve utmost biological meaning from the available genomic data and translate such into tools that help resolve epidemiological challenges. This includes the identification of novel antigens for accurate and affordable diagnostic assays and vaccines, informative biomarkers that can distinguish different isolates and pinpoint the source of infections at fine geographical scale, and sensitive tool(s) for large-scale screening of asymptomatic infections in both high and low transmission areas. Future studies should examine how climate/environmental changes and selective pressure from interventions mediate genetic changes in the parasites, how host immune system responses to parasite changes, and how to uncover hidden parasite reservoirs and effectively control transmission.

Acknowledgements

We thank our colleagues at the University of North Carolina at Charlotte and the University of Ghana for the inspiration and discussion that lead to the conceptualization of this paper. We also thank the reviewers for their insightful comments.

Conflict of interest

The authors declare no conflict of interest.

Author contributions

Conceptualization, C.C.D. and E.L.; resources, D.A.J. and E.L.; writing—original draft preparation, C.C.D., C.T.F., J.H., and E.L.; writing—review and editing, C.C. D., C.T.F., L.E.A, Y.A.A., D.A.J., and and E.L.; funding acquisition, E.L. All authors have read and agreed to the published version of the manuscript.

Funding

This research was funded by NIH/NIAID, grant number R15 AI138002.

Author details

Cheikh Cambel Dieng[1*], Colby T. Ford[2], Jennifer Huynh[1], Linda E. Amoah[3,4], Yaw A. Afrane[5], Daniel A. Janies[2] and Eugenia Lo[1*]

1 Department of Biological Sciences, University of North Carolina at Charlotte, Charlotte, USA

2 Department of Bioinformatics and Genomics, University of North Carolina at Charlotte, Charlotte, USA

3 Department of Immunology, Noguchi Memorial Institute for Medical Research, University of Ghana, Accra, Ghana

4 West Africa Center for Cell Biology of Infectious Pathogens, University of Ghana, Accra, Ghana

5 Department of Medical Microbiology, University of Ghana Medical School, University of Ghana, Accra, Ghana

*Address all correspondence to: cdieng@uncc.edu and eugenia.lo@uncc.edu

References

[1] Talapko J, Škrlec I, Alebić T, Jukić M, Včev A. Malaria: The Past and the Present. Microorganisms. 2019 Jun;7(6). [PubMed Central:PMC6617065] [DOI: 10.3390/microorganisms7060179] [PubMed:30760324].

[2] Abossie A, Yohanes T, Nedu A, Tafesse W, Damitie M. Prevalence of Malaria and Associated Risk Factors Among Febrile Children Under Five Years: A Cross-Sectional Study in Arba Minch Zuria District, South Ethiopia. Infect Drug Resist. 2020;13:363–372. [PubMed Central:PMC7012238] [DOI: 10.2147/IDR.S223873] [PubMed: 27137913].

[3] Ahmed T, Hyder MZ, Liaqat I, Scholz M. Climatic Conditions: Conventional and Nanotechnology-Based Methods for the Control of Mosquito Vectors Causing Human Health Issues. Int J Environ Res Public Health. 2019 08;16 (17). [PubMedCentral:PMC6747303] [DOI:10.3390/ijerph16173165] [PubMed:23688176].

[4] Castro MC. Malaria Transmission and Prospects for Malaria Eradication: The Role of the Environment. Cold Spring Harb Perspect Med. 2017 Oct;7 (10). [PubMedCentral:PMC5629986] [DOI:10.1101/cshperspect.a025601] [PubMed:7907685].

[5] Kimenyi KM, Wamae K, Ochola-Oyier LI. Understanding P. falciparum Asymptomatic Infections: A Proposition for a Transcriptomic Approach. Front Immunol. 2019;10:2398. [PubMed Central:PMC6803459] [DOI:10.3389/fimmu.2019.02398] [PubMed: 10450423].

[6] Milner DA. Malaria Pathogenesis. Cold Spring Harb Perspect Med. 2018 01;8(1). [PubMed Central: PMC5749143] [DOI:10.1101/cshperspect.a025569] [PubMed: 24854175].

[7] Organization WH. World malaria report 2020: 20 years of global progress and challenges. World Health Organization; 2020.

[8] Mahdi Abdel Hamid M, Elamin AF, Albsheer MM, Abdalla AA, Mahgoub NS, Mustafa SO, et al. Multiplicity of infection and genetic diversity of *Plasmodium falciparum* isolates from patients with uncomplicated and severe malaria in Gezira State, Sudan. Parasit Vectors. 2016 06;9(1):362. [PubMed Central:PMC4924276] [DOI:10.1186/s13071-016-1641-z] [PubMed:16879742].

[9] Koita OA, Doumbo OK, Ouattara A, Tall LK, Konar'e A, Diakité M, et al. False-negative rapid diagnostic tests for malaria and deletion of the histidine-rich repeat region of the hrp2 gene. Am J Trop Med Hyg. 2012 Feb;86(2):194–198. [PubMed Central:PMC3269266] [DOI: 10.4269/ajtmh.2012.10-0665] [PubMed: 20565816].

[10] Chaumeau V, Kajeechiwa L, Fustec B, Landier J, Naw Nyo S, Nay Hsel S, et al. Contribution of Asymptomatic Plasmodium Infections to the Transmission of Malaria in Kayin State, Myanmar. J Infect Dis. 2019 04;219(9): 1499–1509. [PubMed Central: PMC6467188] [DOI:10.1093/infdis/jiy686] [PubMed:3227404].

[11] von Seidlein L. The failure of screening and treating as a malaria elimination strategy. PLoS Med. 2014 Jan;11(1):e1001595. [PubMed Central: PMC3904824] [DOI:10.1371/journal.pmed.1001595] [PubMed:11075770].

[12] White NJ. Antimalarial drug resistance. J Clin Invest. 2004 Apr;113 (8):1084–1092. [PubMed Central: PMC385418] [DOI:10.1172/JCI21682] [PubMed:14688565].

[13] Hill AV. Vaccines against malaria. Philos Trans R Soc Lond B Biol Sci. 2011

Oct;366(1579):2806–2814. [PubMed Central:PMC3146776] [DOI:10.1098/rstb.2011.0091] [PubMed:21237715].

[14] Gardner MJ, Hall N, Fung E, White O, Berriman M, Hyman RW, et al. Genome sequence of the human malaria parasite *Plasmodium falciparum*. Nature. 2002 Oct;419(6906):498–511. [PubMed Central:PMC3836256] [DOI:10.1038/nature01097] [PubMed:11069183].

[15] Su XZ, Lane KD, Xia L, Sá JM, Wellems TE. Plasmodium Genomics and Genetics: New Insights into Malaria Pathogenesis, Drug Resistance, Epidemiology, and Evolution. Clin Microbiol Rev. 2019 09;32(4). [PubMed Central:PMC6750138] [DOI:10.1128/CMR.00019-19] [PubMed:28213434].

[16] Bohme U, Otto TD, Sanders M, Newbold CI, Berriman M. Progression of the canonical reference malaria parasite genome from 2002–2019. Wellcome Open Res. 2019;4:58. [PubMed Central:PMC6484455] [DOI:10.12688/wellcomeopenres.15194.2] [PubMed:20562415].

[17] Hamilton WL, Claessens A, Otto TD, Kekre M, Fairhurst RM, Rayner JC, et al. Extreme mutation bias and high AT content in *Plasmodium falciparum*. Nucleic Acids Res. 2017 02;45(4):1889–1901. [PubMed Central:PMC5389722] [DOI:10.1093/nar/gkw1259] [PubMed:351412].

[18] Zhang M, Wang C, Otto TD, Oberstaller J, Liao X, Adapa SR, et al. Uncovering the essential genes of the human malaria parasite *Plasmodium falciparum* by saturation mutagenesis. Science. 2018 05;360(6388). [PubMed Central:PMC6360947] [DOI:10.1126/science.aap7847] [PubMed:9002517].

[19] Vaidya AB, Akella R, Suplick K. Sequences similar to genes for two mitochondrial proteins and portions of ribosomal RNA in tandemly arrayed 6-kilobase-pair DNA of a malarial parasite. Molecular and biochemical parasitology. 1989;35(2):97–107.

[20] Vaidya AB, Lashgari MS, Pologe LG, Morrisey J. Structural features of Plasmodium cytochrome b that may underlie susceptibility to 8-aminoquinolines and hydroxynaphthoquinones. Molecular and biochemical parasitology. 1993;58 (1):33–42.

[21] Zhang CL, Zhou HN, Liu Q, Yang YM. Genetic polymorphism of merozoite surface proteins 1 and 2 of *Plasmodium falciparum* in the China-Myanmar border region. Malar J. 2019 Nov;18(1):367. [PubMed Central: PMC6862846] [DOI:10.1186/s12936-019-3003-8] [PubMed:19706922].

[22] Karki R, Pandya D, Elston RC, Ferlini C. Defining "mutation" and "polymorphism" in the era of personal genomics. BMC Med Genomics. 2015 Jul;8:37. [PubMed Central: PMC4502642] [DOI:10.1186/s12920-015-0115-z] [PubMed:11237011].

[23] Jin Y, Wang J, Bachtiar M, Chong SS, Lee CGL. Architecture of polymorphisms in the human genome reveals functionally important and positively selected variants in immune response and drug transporter genes. Hum Genomics. 2018 09;12(1):43. [PubMed Central:PMC6139121] [DOI:10.1186/s40246-018-0175-1] [PubMed:26888265].

[24] Belachew EB. Immune Response and Evasion Mechanisms of Plasmodium falciparum Parasites. J Immunol Res. 2018;2018:6529681.

[25] Dimonte S, Bruske EI, Enderes C, Otto TD, Turner L, Kremsner P, et al. Identification of a conserved var gene in different *Plasmodium falciparum* strains. Malar J. 2020 May;19(1):194. [PubMed Central:PMC7260770] [DOI:10.1186/s12936-020-03257-x] [PubMed:22004584].

[26] Miles A, Iqbal Z, Vauterin P, Pearson R, Campino S, Theron M, et al. Indels, structural variation, and recombination drive genomic diversity in *Plasmodium falciparum*. Genome Res. 2016 09;26(9):1288–1299. [PubMed Central:PMC5052046] [DOI:10.1101/gr.203711.115] [PubMed:17325376].

[27] Baker J, McCarthy J, Gatton M, Kyle DE, Belizario V, Luchavez J, et al. Genetic diversity of Plasmodium falciparum histidine-rich protein 2 (PfHRP2) and its effect on the performance of PfHRP2-based rapid diagnostic tests. J Infect Dis. 2005 Sep; 192(5):870–877.

[28] Baker J, Ho MF, Pelecanos A, Gatton M, Chen N, Abdullah S, et al. Global sequence variation in the histidine-rich proteins 2 and 3 of *Plasmodium falciparum*: implications for the performance of malaria rapid diagnostic tests. Malaria Journal. 2010 May;9(1):129. Available from: https: // doi.org/10.1186/1475-2875-9-129.

[29] Miotto O, Amato R, Ashley EA, MacInnis B, Almagro-Garcia J, Amaratunga C, et al. Genetic architecture of artemisinin-resistant Plasmodium falciparum. Nature genetics. 2015;47(3):226–234.

[30] Miotto O, Almagro-Garcia J, Manske M, MacInnis B, Campino S, Rockett KA, et al. Multiple populations of artemisinin-resistant Plasmodium falciparum in Cambodia. Nature genetics. 2013;45(6):648–655.

[31] Bahl A, Brunk B, Crabtree J, Fraunholz MJ, Gajria B, Grant GR, et al. PlasmoDB: the Plasmodium genome resource. A database integrating experimental and computational data. Nucleic Acids Res. 2003 Jan;31(1):212–215. [PubMed Central:PMC165528] [DOI:10.1093/nar/gkg081] [PubMed: 17040811].

[32] Ayogu EE, Ukwe CV, Nna EO. Assessing the reliability of microscopy and rapid diagnostic tests in malaria diagnosis in areas with varying parasite density among older children and adult patients in Nigeria. J Postgrad Med. 2016;62(3):150–156.

[33] Mathison BA, Pritt BS. Update on Malaria Diagnostics and Test Utilization. J Clin Microbiol. 2017 07;55 (7):2009–2017. [PubMed Central: PMC5483902] [DOI:10.1128/JCM.02562-16] [PubMed:22550113].

[34] Ballard E, Wang CYT, Hien TT, Tong NT, Marquart L, Pava Z, et al. A validation study of microscopy versus quantitative PCR for measuring Plasmodium falciparum parasitemia. Trop Med Health. 2019;47:49.

[35] Mbanefo A, Kumar N. Evaluation of Malaria Diagnostic Methods as a Key for Successful Control and Elimination Programs. Trop Med Infect Dis. 2020 Jun;5(2). [PubMed Central: PMC7344938] [DOI:10.3390/tropicalmed5020102] [PubMed: 29078786].

[36] Hassanpour G, Mohebali M, Zeraati H, Raeisi A, Keshavarz H. Asymptomatic Malaria and its Challenges in the Malaria Elimination Program in Iran: a Systematic Review. J Arthropod Borne Dis. 2017 Jun;11(2): 172–181.

[37] Dieng CC, Gonzalez L, Pestana K, Dhikrullahi SB, Amoah LE, Afrane YA, et al. Contrasting Asymptomatic and Drug Resistance Gene Prevalence of *Plasmodium falciparum* in Ghana: Implications on Seasonal Malaria Chemoprevention. Genes (Basel). 2019 07;10(7).

[38] Iwuafor AA, Ita OI, Ogban GI, Udoh UA, Amajor CA. Evaluation of Diagnostic Accuracy of Rapid Diagnostic Test for Malaria Diagnosis among Febrile Children in Calabar, Nigeria. Niger Med J. 2018;59(6):64–69. [PubMed Central:PMC6668302] [DOI:

10.4103/nmj.NMJ 165 18] [PubMed: 9988333].

[39] Golassa L, Messele A, Amambua-Ngwa A, Swedberg G. High prevalence and extended deletions in Plasmodium falciparum hrp2/3 genomic loci in Ethiopia. PLoS One. 2020;15(11): e0241807.

[40] Thomson R, Beshir KB, Cunningham J, Baiden F, Bharmal J, Bruxvoort KJ, et al. pfhrp2 and pfhrp3 Gene Deletions That Affect Malaria Rapid Diagnostic Tests for *Plasmodium falciparum*: Analysis of Archived Blood Samples From 3 African Countries. J Infect Dis. 2019 09;220(9):1444–1452.

[41] Watson OJ, Slater HC, Verity R, Parr JB, Mwandagalirwa MK, Tshefu A, et al. Modelling the drivers of the spread of Plasmodium falciparum hrp2 gene deletions in sub-Saharan Africa. Elife. 2017 08;6.

[42] Grignard L, Nolder D, Sepúlveda N, Berhane A, Mihreteab S, Kaaya R, et al. A novel multiplex qPCR assay for detection of *Plasmodium falciparum* with histidine-rich protein 2 and 3 (pfhrp2 and pfhrp3) deletions in polyclonal infections. EBioMedicine. 2020 May;55. Available from: https://doi.org/10.1016/j.ebiom.2020.102757.

[43] Li P, Xing H, Zhao Z, Yang Z, Cao Y, Li W, et al. Genetic diversity of *Plasmodium falciparum* histidine-rich protein 2 in the China-Myanmar border area. Acta Trop. 2015 Dec;152:26–31. [PubMed Central:PMC4918506] [DOI: 10.1016/j.actatropica.2015.08.003] [PubMed:24086328].

[44] Berhane A, Russom M, Bahta I, Hagos F, Ghirmai M, Uqubay S. Rapid diagnostic tests failing to detect *Plasmodium falciparum* infections in Eritrea: an investigation of reported false negative RDT results. Malar J. 2017 03;16(1):105. [PubMed Central: PMC5339986] [DOI:10.1186/s12936-017-1752-9] [PubMed:16407339].

[45] Kojom LP, Singh V. Prevalence of *Plasmodium falciparum* field isolates with deletions in histidine-rich protein 2 and 3 genes in context with sub-Saharan Africa and India: a systematic review and meta-analysis. Malar J. 2020 Jan;19 (1):46. [PubMed Central:PMC6986054] [DOI:10.1186/s12936-019-3090-6] [PubMed:30170596].

[46] Thomson R, Parr JB, Cheng Q, Chenet S, Perkins M, Cunningham J. Prevalence of Plasmodium falciparum lacking histidine-rich proteins 2 and 3: a systematic review. Bull World Health Organ. 2020 Aug;98(8):558–568.

[47] Amoah LE, Abuaku B, Bukari AH, Dickson D, Amoako EO, Asumah G, et al. Contribution of P. falciparum parasites with Pfhrp 2 gene deletions to false negative PfHRP 2 based malaria RDT results in Ghana: A nationwide study of symptomatic malaria patients. PLoS One. 2020;15(9):e0238749.

[48] Das S, Peck RB, Barney R, Jang IK, Kahn M, Zhu M, et al. Performance of an ultra-sensitive Plasmodium falciparum HRP2-based rapid diagnostic test with recombinant HRP2, culture parasites, and archived whole blood samples. Malar J. 2018 Mar;17(1):118.

[49] Unwin VT, Ahmed R, Noviyanti R, Puspitasari AM, Utami RAS, Trianty L, et al. Use of a highly-sensitive rapid diagnostic test to screen for malaria in pregnancy in Indonesia. Malar J. 2020 Jan;19(1):28.

[50] Waritani T, Chang J, McKinney B, Terato K. An ELISA protocol to improve the accuracy and reliability of serological antibody assays. MethodsX. 2017;4:153–165. [PubMed Central: PMC5387895] [DOI:10.1016/j.mex.2017.03.002] [PubMed:9013990].

[51] Dewasurendra RL, Dias JN, Sepulveda N, Gunawardena GS, Chandrasekharan N, Drakeley C, et al. Effectiveness of a serological tool to

predict malaria transmission intensity in an elimination setting. BMC Infect Dis. 2017 01;17(1):49. [PubMed Central: PMC5223541] [DOI:10.1186/s12879-016-2164-0] [PubMed:26770994].

[52] Ruiz Moreno Y, Donato ST, Nogueira F, Sousa Silva M. Comparative Analysis of the Serological Reactivity of Individuals with Clinical History of Malaria using Two Different ELISA Tests. Diagnostics (Basel). 2019 Oct;9 (4). [PubMed Central:PMC6963549] [DOI:10.3390/diagnostics9040168] [PubMed:22561398].

[53] Kwenti TE, Njunda LA, Tsamul B, Nsagha SD, Assob NJ, Tufon KA, et al. Comparative evaluation of a rapid diagnostic test, an antibody ELISA, and a pLDH ELISA in detecting asymptomatic malaria parasitaemia in blood donors in Buea, Cameroon. Infect Dis Poverty. 2017 Aug;6(1):103. [PubMed Central:PMC5537946] [DOI: 10.1186/s40249-017-0314-2] [PubMed: 22550113].

[54] Koczula KM, Gallotta A. Lateral flow assays. Essays Biochem. 2016 06;60 (1):111–120.

[55] Bousema T, Okell L, Felger I, Drakeley C. Asymptomatic malaria infections: detectability, transmissibility and public health relevance. Nat Rev Microbiol. 2014 12;12(12):833–840.

[56] Favuzza P, Blaser S, Dreyer AM, Riccio G, Tamborrini M, Thoma R, et al. Generation of Plasmodium falciparum parasite-inhibitory antibodies by immunization with recombinantly-expressed CyRPA. Malar J. 2016 Mar;15:161.

[57] Santolamazza F, Avellino P, Siciliano G, Yao FA, Lombardo F, Ouédraogo JB, et al. Detection of Plasmodium falciparum male and female gametocytes and determination of parasite sex ratio in human endemic populations by novel, cheap and robust RTqPCR assays. Malar J. 2017 Nov;16 (1):468.

[58] Tao D, McGill B, Hamerly T, Kobayashi T, Khare P, Dziedzic A, et al. A saliva-based rapid test to quantify the infectious subclinical malaria parasite reservoir. Sci Transl Med. 2019 01;11 (473). [PubMed Central:PMC6441545] [DOI:10.1126/scitranslmed.aan4479] [PubMed:21871864].

[59] Aninagyei E, Abraham J, Atiiga P, Antwi SD, Bamfo S, Acheampong DO. Evaluating the potential of using urine and saliva specimens for malaria diagnosis in suspected patients in Ghana. Malar J. 2020 Sep;19(1):349. [PubMed Central:PMC7526349] [DOI: 10.1186/s12936-020-03427-x] [PubMed: 24906879].

[60] Echeverry DF, Deason NA, Davidson J, Makuru V, Xiao H, Niedbalski J, et al. Human malaria diagnosis using a single-step direct-PCR based on the Plasmodium cytochrome oxidase III gene. Malar J. 2016 Feb;15: 128.

[61] Hofmann N, Mwingira F, Shekalaghe S, Robinson LJ, Mueller I, Felger I. Ultra-sensitive detection of *Plasmodium falciparum* by amplification of multi-copy subtelomeric targets. PLoS Med. 2015 Mar;12(3):e1001788. [PubMed Central:PMC4348198] [DOI: 10.1371/journal.pmed.1001788] [PubMed:15635001].

[62] Lloyd YM, Esemu LF, Antallan J, Thomas B, Tassi Yunga S, Obase B, et al. PCR-based detection of Plasmodium falciparum in saliva using mitochondrial cox3 and varATS primers. Trop Med Health. 2018;46:22.

[63] Schneider P, Reece SE, van Schaijk BC, Bousema T, Lanke KH, Meaden CS, et al. Quantification of female and male Plasmodium falciparum gametocytes by reverse transcriptase quantitative PCR. Mol Biochem Parasitol. 2015;199(1–2):

29–33. [DOI:10.1016/j.molbiopara.2015.03.006] [PubMed:25827756].

[64] Noedl H, Yingyuen K, Laoboonchai A, Fukuda M, Sirichaisinthop J, Miller RS. Sensitivity and specificity of an antigen detection ELISA for malaria diagnosis. Am J Trop Med Hyg. 2006 Dec;75(6):1205–1208.

[65] Chen F, Flaherty BR, Cohen CE, Peterson DS, Zhao Y. Direct detection of malaria infected red blood cells by surface enhanced Raman spectroscopy. Nanomedicine. 2016 08;12(6):1445–1451. [PubMed Central:PMC4955673] [DOI:10.1016/j.nano.2016.03.001] [PubMed:23563168].

[66] Haanshuus CG, Mørch K, Blomberg B, Strøm GEA, Langeland N, Hanevik K, et al. Assessment of malaria real-time PCR methods and application with focus on low-level parasitaemia. PLoS One. 2019;14(7):e0218982. [PubMed Central: PMC6611585] [DOI:10.1371/journal.pone.0218982] [PubMed:20925928].

[67] Fontanesi F, Soto IC, Barrientos A. Cytochrome c oxidase biogenesis: new levels of regulation. IUBMB Life. 2008 Sep;60(9):557–568.

[68] Schmedes SE, Patel D, Kelley J, Udhayakumar V, Talundzic E. Using the Plasmodium mitochondrial genome for classifying mixed-species infections and inferring the geographical origin of P. falciparum parasites imported to the U. S. PLoS One. 2019;14(4):e0215754.

[69] Figueiredo LM, Pirrit LA, Scherf A, Pirritt LA. Genomic organisation and chromatin structure of Plasmodium falciparum chromosome ends. Mol Biochem Parasitol. 2000 Feb;106(1):169–174.

[70] Gitta B, Kilian N. Diagnosis of Malaria Parasites Plasmodium spp. in Endemic Areas: Current Strategies for an Ancient Disease. Bioessays. 2020 01;42(1):e1900138. [DOI:10.1002/bies.201900138] [PubMed:31830324].

[71] Chen K, Yuen C, Aniweh Y, Preiser P, Liu Q. Towards ultrasensitive malaria diagnosis using surface enhanced Raman spectroscopy. Sci Rep. 2016 Feb;6:20177. [PubMed Central: PMC4746575] [DOI:10.1038/srep20177] [PubMed:18165483].

[72] Baldwin MR, Li X, Hanada T, Liu SC, Chishti AH. Merozoite surface protein 1 recognition of host glycophorin A mediates malaria parasite invasion of red blood cells. Blood. 2015 Apr;125(17):2704–2711.

[73] Zhong D, Afrane Y, Githeko A, Yang Z, Cui L, Menge DM, et al. Plasmodium falciparum genetic diversity in western Kenya highlands. Am J Trop Med Hyg. 2007 Dec;77(6):1043–1050.

[74] Somé AF, Bazié T, Zongo I, Yerbanga RS, Nikiéma F, Neya C, et al. Plasmodium falciparum msp1 and msp2 genetic diversity and allele frequencies in parasites isolated from symptomatic malaria patients in Bobo-Dioulasso, Burkina Faso. Parasit Vectors. 2018 May;11(1):323.

[75] Carter TE, Malloy H, Existe A, Memnon G, St Victor Y, Okech BA, et al. Genetic Diversity of Plasmodium falciparum in Haiti: Insights from Microsatellite Markers. PLoS One. 2015;10(10):e0140416.

[76] Fola AA, Kattenberg E, Razook Z, Lautu-Gumal D, Lee S, Mehra S, et al. SNP barcodes provide higher resolution than microsatellite markers to measure Plasmodium vivax population genetics. Malar J. 2020 Oct;19(1):375.

[77] Havryliuk T, Orjuela-Sánchez P, Ferreira MU. Plasmodium vivax: microsatellite analysis of multiple-clone infections. Exp Parasitol. 2008 Dec;120(4):330–336.

[78] Das S, Muleba M, Stevenson JC, Pringle JC, Norris DE. Beyond the entomological inoculation rate: characterizing multiple blood feeding behavior and *Plasmodium falciparum* multiplicity of infection in Anopheles mosquitoes in northern Zambia. Parasit Vectors. 2017 01;10(1):45. [PubMed Central:PMC5267472] [DOI:10.1186/s13071-017-1993-z] [PubMed:15619515].

[79] Abukari Z, Okonu R, Nyarko SB, Lo AC, Dieng CC, Salifu SP, et al. The Diversity, Multiplicity of Infection and Population Structure of P. falciparum Parasites Circulating in Asymptomatic Carriers Living in High and Low Malaria Transmission Settings of Ghana. Genes (Basel). 2019 06;10(6). [PubMed Central:PMC6628376] [DOI:10.3390/genes10060434] [PubMed:28070005].

[80] Lin JT, Hathaway NJ, Saunders DL, Lon C, Balasubramanian S, Kharabora O, et al. Using Amplicon Deep Sequencing to Detect Genetic Signatures of Plasmodium vivax Relapse. J Infect Dis. 2015 Sep;212(6):999–1008.

[81] Tessema SK, Raman J, Duffy CW, Ishengoma DS, Amambua-Ngwa A, Greenhouse B. Applying next-generation sequencing to track falciparum malaria in sub-Saharan Africa. Malar J. 2019 Sep;18(1):268. [PubMed Central:PMC6720407] [DOI:10.1186/s12936-019-2880-1] [PubMed:31298657].

[82] Miller RH, Hathaway NJ, Kharabora O, Mwandagalirwa K, Tshefu A, Meshnick SR, et al. A deep sequencing approach to estimate *Plasmodium falciparum* complexity of infection (COI) and explore apical membrane antigen 1 diversity. Malar J. 2017 Dec;16(1):490. [PubMed Central:PMC5732508] [DOI:10.1186/s12936-017-2137-9] [PubMed:21565059].

[83] Niedzicka M, Fijarczyk A, Dudek K, Stuglik M, Babik W. Molecular Inversion Probes for targeted resequencing in non-model organisms. Sci Rep. 2016 Apr;6:24051. [PubMed Central:PMC4820773] [DOI:10.1038/srep24051] [PubMed:21565059].

[84] Aydemir O, Janko M, Hathaway NJ, Verity R, Mwandagalirwa MK, Tshefu AK, et al. Drug-Resistance and Population Structure of *Plasmodium falciparum* Across the Democratic Republic of Congo Using High-Throughput Molecular Inversion Probes. J Infect Dis. 2018 08;218(6):946–955. [PubMed Central:PMC6093412] [DOI:10.1093/infdis/jiy223] [PubMed:25061906].

[85] Bettencourt P. Current Challenges in the Identification of Pre-Erythrocytic Malaria Vaccine Candidate Antigens. Front Immunol. 2020;11:190. [PubMed Central:PMC7046804] [DOI:10.3389/fimmu.2020.00190] [PubMed:9252123].

[86] Palacpac NMQ, Horii T. Malaria vaccines: facing unknowns. F1000Res. 2020;9. [PubMed Central:PMC7194457] [DOI:10.12688/f1000research.22143.1] [PubMed:23613845].

[87] Hoffman SL, Vekemans J, Richie TL, Duffy PE. The march toward malaria vaccines. Vaccine. 2015 Nov;33 Suppl 4:13–23. [PubMed Central:PMC5634526] [DOI:10.1016/j.vaccine.2015.07.091] [PubMed:24872326].

[88] Draper SJ, Sack BK, King CR, Nielsen CM, Rayner JC, Higgins MK, et al. Malaria Vaccines: Recent Advances and New Horizons. Cell Host Microbe. 2018 07;24(1):43–56.

[89] Tannous S, Ghanem E. A bite to fight: front-line innate immune defenses against malaria parasites. Pathog Glob Health. 2018 02;112(1):1–12.

[90] Beeson JG, Kurtovic L, Doba̴no C, Opi DH, Chan JA, Feng G, et al. Challenges and strategies for developing efficacious and long-lasting malaria

vaccines. Sci Transl Med. 2019 01;11 (474). [DOI:10.1126/scitranslmed.aau1458] [PubMed:30626712].

[91] Sánchez L, Vidal M, Jairoce C, Aguilar R, Ubillos I, Cuamba I, et al. Erratum: Author Correction: Antibody responses to the RTS,S/AS01E vaccine and *Plasmodium falciparum* antigens after a booster dose within the phase 3 trial in Mozambique. NPJ Vaccines. 2020;5:63. [PubMed Central: PMC7371631] [DOI:10.1038/s41541-020-00213-3] [PubMed:32704386].

[92] Molina-Franky J, Cuy-Chaparro L, Camargo A, Reyes C, Gómez M, Salamanca DR, et al. *Plasmodium falciparum* pre-erythrocytic stage vaccine development. Malar J. 2020 Feb; 19(1):56. [PubMed Central: PMC6998842] [DOI:10.1186/s12936-020-3141-z] [PubMed:24992338].

[93] Skwarczynski M, Chandrudu S, Rigau-Planella B, Islam MT, Cheong YS, Liu G, et al. Progress in the Development of Subunit Vaccines against Malaria. Vaccines (Basel). 2020 Jul;8(3). [PubMed Central: PMC7563759] [DOI:10.3390/vaccines8030373] [PubMed:30219621].

[94] Blank A, Furle K, Jaschke A, Mikus G, Lehmann M, Husing J, et al. Immunization with full-length *Plasmodium falciparum* merozoite surface protein 1 is safe and elicits functional cytophilic antibodies in a randomized first-in-human trial. NPJ Vaccines. 2020;5:10. [PubMed Central: PMC6994672] [DOI:10.1038/s41541-020-0160-2] [PubMed:26468747].

[95] Duffy PE, Patrick Gorres J. Malaria vaccines since 2000: progress, priorities, products. NPJ Vaccines. 2020;5:48. [PubMed Central:PMC7283239] [DOI:10.1038/s41541-020-0196-3] [PubMed:24133188].

[96] Laurens MB. RTS,S/AS01 vaccine (Mosquirixâ¡U+0084¿¢): an overview. Hum Vaccin Immunother. 2020 03;16 (3):480–489. [PubMed Central: PMC7227679] [DOI:10.1080/21645515.2019.1669415] [PubMed:30376866].

[97] Singh K, Burkhardt M, Nakuchima S, Herrera R, Muratova O, Gittis AG, et al. Structure and function of a malaria transmission blocking vaccine targeting Pfs230 and Pfs230-Pfs48/45 proteins. Commun Biol. 2020 Jul;3(1):395. [PubMed Central:PMC7381611] [DOI:10.1038/s42003-020-01123-9] [PubMed:24179220].

[98] Scally SW, McLeod B, Bosch A, Miura K, Liang Q, Carroll S, et al. Molecular definition of multiple sites of antibody inhibition of malaria transmission-blocking vaccine antigen Pfs25. Nat Commun. 2017 11;8(1):1568.

[99] Raj DK, Das Mohapatra A, Jnawali A, Zuromski J, Jha A, Cham-Kpu G, et al. Anti-PfGARP activates programmed cell death of parasites and reduces severe malaria. Nature. 2020 06;582 (7810):104–108. [PubMed Central: PMC7372601] [DOI:10.1038/s41586-020-2220-1] [PubMed:32427965].

[100] Ragotte RJ, Higgins MK, Draper SJ. The RH5-CyRPA-Ripr Complex as a Malaria Vaccine Target. Trends Parasitol. 2020 06;36(6):545–559. [PubMed Central:PMC7246332] [DOI:10.1016/j.pt.2020.04.003] [PubMed:26458807].

[101] Zheng J, Pan H, Gu Y, Zuo X, Ran N, Yuan Y, et al. Prospects for Malaria Vaccines: Pre-Erythrocytic Stages, Blood Stages, and Transmission-Blocking Stages. Biomed Res Int. 2019; 2019:9751471. [PubMed Central: PMC6794966] [DOI:10.1155/2019/9751471] [PubMed:29700348].

[102] Zhao J, Bhanot P, Hu J, Wang Q. A Comprehensive Analysis of Plasmodium Circumsporozoite Protein Binding to Hepatocytes. PLoS One. 2016;11(8):

e0161607. [PubMed Central: PMC4999272] [DOI:10.1371/journal.pone.0161607] [PubMed:8876233].

[103] White MT, Verity R, Griffin JT, Asante KP, Owusu-Agyei S, Greenwood B, et al. Immunogenicity of the RTS,S/AS01 malaria vaccine and implications for duration of vaccine efficacy: secondary analysis of data from a phase 3 randomised controlled trial. Lancet Infect Dis. 2015 Dec;15(12):1450–1458. [PubMed Central:PMC4655306] [DOI:10.1016/S1473-3099(15)00239-X] [PubMed:25012228].

[104] Mahmoudi S, Keshavarz H. Efficacy of phase 3 trial of RTS, S/AS01 malaria vaccine: The need for an alternative development plan. Hum Vaccin Immunother. 2017 09;13(9):2098–2101.

[105] authors listed N. Efficacy and safety of RTS,S/AS01 malaria vaccine with or without a booster dose in infants and children in Africa: final results of a phase 3, individually randomised, controlled trial. Lancet. 2015 Jul;386(9988):31–45. [PubMed Central: PMC5626001] [DOI:10.1016/S0140-6736(15)60721-8] [PubMed:21816029].

[106] van den Berg M, Ogutu B, Sewankambo NK, Biller-Andorno N, Tanner M. RTS,S malaria vaccine pilot studies: addressing the human realities in large-scale clinical trials. Trials. 2019 May;20(1):316. [PubMed Central: PMC6544944] [DOI:10.1186/s13063-019-3391-7] [PubMed:30035349].

[107] Collins KA, Snaith R, Cottingham MG, Gilbert SC, Hill AVS. Enhancing protective immunity to malaria with a highly immunogenic virus-like particle vaccine. Sci Rep. 2017 04;7:46621.

[108] Kaushansky A, Douglass AN, Arang N, Vigdorovich V, Dambrauskas N, Kain HS, et al. Malaria parasites target the hepatocyte receptor EphA2 for successful host infection. Science. 2015 Nov;350(6264):1089–1092. [PubMed Central:PMC4783171] [DOI:10.1126/science.aad3318] [PubMed:19625622].

[109] Richie TL, Billingsley PF, Sim BK, James ER, Chakravarty S, Epstein JE, et al. Progress with *Plasmodium falciparum* sporozoite (PfSPZ)-based malaria vaccines. Vaccine. 2015 Dec;33(52):7452–7461. [PubMed Central: PMC5077156] [DOI:10.1016/j.vaccine.2015.09.096] [PubMed:21514658].

[110] Lyke KE, Ishizuka AS, Berry AA, Chakravarty S, DeZure A, Enama ME, et al. Attenuated PfSPZ Vaccine induces strain-transcending T cells and durable protection against heterologous controlled human malaria infection. Proc Natl Acad Sci U S A. 2017 03;114(10):2711–2716.

[111] Zenklusen I, Jongo S, Abdulla S, Ramadhani K, Lee Sim BK, Cardamone H, et al. Immunization of Malaria-Preexposed Volunteers With PfSPZ Vaccine Elicits Long-Lived IgM Invasion-Inhibitory and Complement-Fixing Antibodies. J Infect Dis. 2018 04;217(10):1569–1578.

[112] Halbroth BR, Sebastian S, Salman AM, Ulaszewska M, Gola A, Longley RJ, et al. Preclinical Development and Assessment of Viral Vectors Expressing a Fusion Antigen of *Plasmodium falciparum* LSA1 and LSAP2 for Efficacy against Liver-Stage Malaria. Infect Immun. 2020 01;88(2). [PubMed Central:PMC6977128] [DOI:10.1128/IAI.00573-19] [PubMed:18159254].

[113] Pratt-Riccio LR, De Souza Perce-Da-Silva D, Da Costa Lima-Junior J, Pratt Riccio EK, Ribeiro-Alves M, Santos F, et al. Synthetic Antigens Derived from *Plasmodium falciparum* Sporozoite, Liver, and Blood Stages: Naturally Acquired Immune Response and Human Leukocyte Antigen Associations in Individuals Living in a

Brazilian Endemic Area. Am J Trop Med Hyg. 2017 Nov;97(5):1581–1592. [PubMed Central:PMC5817778] [DOI: 10.4269/ajtmh.17-0359] [PubMed: 16111789].

[114] Morita M, Takashima E, Ito D, Miura K, Thongkukiatkul A, Diouf A, et al. Immunoscreening of *Plasmodium falciparum* proteins expressed in a wheat germ cell-free system reveals a novel malaria vaccine candidate. Sci Rep. 2017 04;7:46086. [PubMed Central: PMC5380959] [DOI:10.1038/srep46086] [PubMed:19874576].

[115] Lin CS, Uboldi AD, Marapana D, Czabotar PE, Epp C, Bujard H, et al. The merozoite surface protein 1 complex is a platform for binding to human erythrocytes by Plasmodium falciparum. J Biol Chem. 2014 Sep;289 (37):25655–25669.

[116] Wang YN, Lin M, Liang XY, Chen JT, Xie DD, Wang YL, et al. Natural selection and genetic diversity of domain I of *Plasmodium falciparum* apical membrane antigen-1 on Bioko Island. Malar J. 2019 Sep;18(1):317. [PubMed Central:PMC6751645] [DOI: 10.1186/s12936-019-2948-y] [PubMed: 8910611].

[117] Srinivasan P, Baldeviano GC, Miura K, Diouf A, Ventocilla JA, Leiva KP, et al. A malaria vaccine protects Aotus monkeys against virulent Plasmodium falciparum infection. NPJ Vaccines. 2017;2.

[118] Sirima SB, Durier C, Kara L, Houard S, Gansane A, Loulergue P, et al. Safety and immunogenicity of a recombinant *Plasmodium falciparum* AMA1-DiCo malaria vaccine adjuvanted with GLA-SE or AlhydrogelÂ® in European and African adults: A phase 1a/1b, randomized, double-blind multi-centre trial. Vaccine. 2017 10;35(45): 6218–6227.

[119] Wrighton KH. A novel vaccine target for malaria. Nat Rev Drug Discov. 2020 06;19(6):386. [DOI:10.1038/d41573-020-00082-4] [PubMed: 32355320].

[120] Favuzza P, Guffart E, Tamborrini M, Scherer B, Dreyer AM, Rufer AC, et al. Structure of the malaria vaccine candidate antigen CyRPA and its complex with a parasite invasion inhibitory antibody. Elife. 2017 02;6.

[121] Huang WC, Deng B, Mabrouk MT, Seffouh A, Ortega J, Long C, et al. Particle-based, Pfs230 and Pfs25 immunization is effective, but not improved by duplexing at fixed total antigen dose. Malar J. 2020 Aug;19(1): 309.

[122] McLeod B, Miura K, Scally SW, Bosch A, Nguyen N, Shin H, et al. Potent antibody lineage against malaria transmission elicited by human vaccination with Pfs25. Nat Commun. 2019 09;10(1):4328. [PubMed Central: PMC6760140] [DOI:10.1038/s41467-019-11980-6] [PubMed:31551421].

[123] Chichester JA, Green BJ, Jones RM, Shoji Y, Miura K, Long CA, et al. Safety and immunogenicity of a plant-produced Pfs25 virus-like particle as a transmission blocking vaccine against malaria: A Phase 1 dose-escalation study in healthy adults. Vaccine. 2018 09;36 (39):5865–5871.

[124] Patra KP, Li F, Carter D, Gregory JA, Baga S, Reed SG, et al. Alga-produced malaria transmission-blocking vaccine candidate Pfs25 formulated with a human use-compatible potent adjuvant induces high-affinity antibodies that block Plasmodium falciparum infection of mosquitoes. Infect Immun. 2015 May;83(5):1799–1808.

[125] Singh SK, Thrane S, Chourasia BK, Teelen K, Graumans W, Stoter R, et al.

Pfs230 and Pfs48/45 Fusion Proteins Elicit Strong Transmission-Blocking Antibody Responses Against Plasmodium falciparum. Front Immunol. 2019;10:1256.

[126] World Health Organization. Global targets; 2019. Available from: https://www.who.int/malaria/areas/global targets/en/.

Chapter 13

Using an Educational Training Module to Increase Knowledge, Attitudes and Practices of Malaria among Medicine Vendors in Yobe, Nigeria

Yahaya Mohammed Katagum, Hayati Binti Kadir Shahar, Faisal Bin Ibrahim, Anisah Baharom and Rafee Baharudin

Abstract

This training module focuses on providing basic guidance on the current recommended approaches regarding malaria basic information, signs/symptoms, case detection, treatment, referral, and effective prevention strategies. The module can be used for in-service training programs on malaria or to assist in improving other health educator's work as well as serve as referral handbook for practicing health professionals. It can thus be used as a stand-alone training or together with modules dealing with other aspects of malaria control, prevention and elimination. The module uses a problem-solving approach to facilitate understanding and thereby motivate trainees on improved malaria case management. In essence, the training aims to generally improve the knowledge, attitudes and practices (KAP) of the most common handlers of malaria cases in this part of the world, the training module is then expected to improve services obtained by the majority of patients on malaria. On completion of training using this module, trainees will have acquired appreciable knowledge and skills on malaria basic-information, signs/symptoms, case detection/differentials, recommended drug treatment/appropriate dosing, indication for referral of complicated cases, effective prevention methods and the need to sensitise communities to stand up against malaria.

Keywords: malaria KAP training, case detection, management and prevention, medicine vendors

1. Introduction

Malaria remains a major global public health and development challenge over the years and in its World Malaria Report 2019, the World Health Organisation's (WHOs) global tally of malaria in 2018 alone was estimated at 228 million cases and 405,000 deaths [1]. Malaria is holo-endemic in many parts of sub-Saharan Africa thereby infecting citizens all year round and hence impacting the most devastation in this region. Worldwide, about 88 countries still remain at risk of malaria, with the types of species, severity and disease trends depending on the geographical location.

One of the greatest challenges facing malaria endemic countries with regards to malaria containment efforts is the lack of proper basic information, poor diagnosis and hence lacking early treatment of uncomplicated cases which progresses to the deadly severe stages, poor treatment and referral practices and poor preventive strategies [2].

Problems of malaria endemicity cannot be unconnected to the widely claimed inadequately trained health manpower and hence poor practices of the health personnel, these health personnel comprise mostly of Patent Medicine Vendors (PMVs) in most rural areas of sub-Saharan Africa. It has been reported that up to 60% of all malaria cases in this sub-region are preferentially first treated by the PMVs and these services leaves much to be desired [3], a situation which informed the development of this training in an attempt to give a more pragmatic approach to PMV the training program. Patent Medicine Vendors are individuals that usually engage in the stocking and sale of Over-the-Counter (OTC) drugs as well as provision of other basic healthcare services and as such, they assume the most common sources of antimalarial treatment throughout Sub-Saharan Africa as they also play a potentially critical role in the struggle against malaria [4].

To facilitate learning by all participants, the training strategies will encourage participants to learn from each other as well as from the researcher / facilitators, particularly in the form of lecture sessions, group discussions, demonstration exercises, role plays, brainstorming exercises and collectively tackling case studies. Each participant will therefore be expected to take part actively throughout the course. In working through the modules, there will be opportunities to put into practice, individually or collectively, what has been learnt. Various strategies were then implored to achieve this objective.

Presentations: Formal presentations such as lectures from the facilitators will be limited to a minimum and this will be presented in the form of explanation to the principles, basic knowledge, and then practical experiences with the class in session. All information provided in sessions are contained in the modules and participants need not to take much notes. Lectures will be combined with a demonstration (physically or on slides). The participants will be asked frequently to present their work in plenary session. This will provide experience on how to tackle arising issues, both by presenting and by learning from the observations and suggestions made during discussion. Posters and slides will be used to enhance learning.

Demonstrations / Practical Sessions: Demonstrations will be used to illustrate some procedures for the diagnosis, treatment and prevention of malaria that will be carried out. The program will include demonstration sessions so as to provide as much practical experience in all aspects of malaria to be studied. In some sessions, the facilitator will work with smaller sub-groups of not more than ten participants; by limiting the size of the groups, the participants will receive extensive individual attention and increased opportunities for learning and practice.

Group discussions / Small group discussions: Discussions will be based on topics and cases taken from the modules which will take place during small group exercises and in general plenary sessions. In these exercises, the facilitator will lead the discussions on the selected subjects with emphasis on participation of group members. These sessions provide opportunities for the participants to give their individual opinions and experiences, to develop ideas, learn from one another, to discuss issues with respective colleagues, to share ideas, opinions and useful experiences, and to finally make efforts towards drawing their own conclusions from intensive discussions. Small group discussions are usually considered to form a valuable component of the courses taken. Participants are also encouraged to take full advantage of these useful sessions and to partake freely and actively in all the discussions. At each session in the group work, there will be changes in the moderator and also the reporter so as to ensure that every participant gains experience in such roles and this will also ensure that tasks are shared equitably. Solving case studies, role plays and quiz sessions will also encourage sharing ideas.

This program is designed to employ the use of various motivational enhancement techniques. Motivational Enhancements can be thought of as processes encouraging 'the probability that a person will enter into, continue to, and adhere to specific change strategies'. It is the responsibility of a facilitator to increase the probabilities that participants will follow a recommended course of action towards changes. Thus, motivation is a key part of a facilitators tasks.

For facilitators, five general principles guides behaviour during sessions. They include:

1. Express Empathy: use skillful reflective listening to understand and accept the participant's contributions without judging, criticising, or blaming.

2. Develop Discrepancy: Raise / draw the participant's consciousness and awareness of the consequences of unhealthy, unethical practices. Remember that participants should lead group discussions and present the need for changes in their attitudes and practices.

3. Avoid Arguments: Arguments are counter-productive and increases participant's resistance to change, as such facilitators should be diplomatic.

4. Support Self-Efficacy: Facilitators must always convey to participants a feeling of 'You can do it, and you will succeed' message. In essence, imparting a belief in the ability for change is an important motivator. Hope is usually found in the range of different approaches available. If one does not work, the facilitator can try others.

5. Elicit self-motivational statements: this strategy helps participant's move beyond ambivalence.

It is important to understand the community culture and traditions. These are the basis of community members' values, which shape community members' attitudes on topics like malaria control. Often, these local beliefs influence community members' actions (or non-actions) more than any other source of information. Community members are likely to trust what they hear from family, friends and community leaders. Often they hear a mix of information, including local beliefs and messages that are passed down from health workers. Some myths / local beliefs about malaria will be reviewed in sections 4 and 6. These mix of messages can be very confusing, so informed participants could use the opportunity to impact on their community's health.

The use of drugs for malaria treatment and prevention involves only drugs recommended by the World Health Organisation (WHO) and employed by the Nigerian government for malaria treatment within the region, this is so because recommended drugs vary depending on region of the world due to the particular specie of malaria infesting the region and the pattern of resistance there.

2. Malaria basic information

Table 1 below describes the training module on malaria basic information, which comprises the session objectives, learning objectives, time duration for the

Session Objectives	To understand the basic information on malaria	
	To understand the cause and how malaria can be transmitted	
	To understand the malaria cycle in man and in vector	
	To understand who is most vulnerable to malaria	
Duration	25 mins	
Learning objectives At the end of the session, participants should be able to:	Know what uncomplicated malaria is	
	Know what complicated malaria is	
	Be able to differentiate what causes and what does not cause malaria	
	Be able to differentiate what transmits and what does not transmit malaria	
	Be able to differentiate between suspected and confirmed malaria	
	Be able to differentiate between uncomplicated and severe malaria	
Training Materials	Participant's manual	Pens & Notebook
	Slides	Laptop computer
	LCD projector	Flip chart and markers
Methods used	Lecture	
	Demonstration classes	
	Question & Answer sessions (Brainstorming exercise)	
	Group discussions	
	Reflection on the module	
Instructions for the facilitator	1. Begin the session by explaining the objectives of the session	
	2. Get the participants to discuss what they understand by malaria and their experiences	
	3. Give a lecture on the general information about malaria using Lecture 2.1 below. (Notes below each slide explain what points need to be made)	
	4. Think about sections which the participants might find difficult and common questions they may ask	
	5. Ask the series of questions (at end of this module) and discuss the answers	
	6. Ask the group questions to be discussed	

	7. Try to find out if the participants did understood the lecture by making the class participatory since everyone knows at-least something on malaria

Table 1.
Summary of session on malaria basic information.

module, training materials needed, methods used and other relevant instructions that will assist the facilitators.

2.1 General facts about malaria

You may be wondering why the emphasis on improving knowledge, treatment and prevention. The main reason is because malaria, being a life-threatening parasitic disease affects parts of the world we live in and remains the major public health problem in Nigeria. It is an avoidable cause of death and illness in children and adults. In Nigeria, malaria continues to be endemic and is the first major cause of morbidity and mortality among the most vulnerable groups- children under 5 years, pregnant women and people living with HIV/Aids. Malaria is characterised by a stable, perennial, transmission in all parts of the country. Transmission is higher in the wet season than in the dry season. This seasonal difference is more striking in the northern part of the country.

According to the World Malaria Report (2013), there was a worldwide estimate of 207 million cases of malaria and an estimated 627 000 deaths in 2012 alone. 81% of these cases and 91% of the deaths were from sub-Saharan Africa [5], and Nigeria alone bears up to 25% of the burden [6]. Again, about 63% of hospital attendance in the Nigerian health care facilities are caused by malaria which is also the cause of absence in workplace / schools, in addition to a huge health expenditure to households leading to a total estimated economic loss to the country of up to 132 billion Naira per year [6].

Note that, in the absence of an effective vaccine, malaria treatment and prevention still remains the vital strategies of malaria control, especially to you PMVs, who are usually the first place of call to the bulk of community residents.

- What is Malaria?

□ Malaria is a serious and sometimes fatal disease caused by a parasite called plasmodium which infects human blood cells. (A parasite is an organism that can only exist in the body of another organism for all or part of their life)

□ There are 4 main kinds of plasmodium parasites that cause malaria in humans. These are:

- *Plasmodium falciparum* (Pf).
- *Plasmodium vivax* (Pv).
- Plasmodium malariae (Pm).
- Plasmodium ovale (Po).

In Nigeria 98% of malaria infections are due to *P. falciparum*. This parasite causes the most deadly form of malaria, known as severe malaria. Other forms of malaria present in Nigeria include *P. ovale* and *P. malariae* which play a minor role with the latter being quite common as a double infection in children.

Note THAT:

☐ Malaria is NOT caused by body contact, drinking contaminated water or eating any kind of food as is the assumption in some localities.

☐ Neither is malaria caused by staying under the sun, exposure to cold weather or living in a dirty environment. Though, these conditions can aggravate malaria.

2.2 Types of vector mosquitoes

There are three common types of Mosquito Vectors:

1. Anopheline mosquito

☐ wings with dark spots

☐ sits at an angle of 45 degree with the resting surface

☐ breeds in clean water

☐ bites at late night

☐ transmits malaria

2. Culex mosquito

☐ usually are referred to as nuisance mosquitoes

☐ usually found to breed in dirty waters

☐ no unique dark spots found on the wings (usually plane dark wings)

☐ appears with a hunchback when in sitting position

☐ usually transmits filariasis

3. Aedes mosquito

☐ are usually dark ornamental mosquito with unique white spots

☐ usually breeds in clean waters found in containers / overhead tanks and wells

☐ usually bites during the day time

☐ bite from this specie is usually very painful

☐ transmits Dengue/DHF/Chikungunia which are viral diseases

2.3 Life cycle of malaria parasite and the malaria transmission cycle

The vectors that carry malaria parasites (mosquito) prefer to feed on humans rather than other animals. Another unique characteristic is that the vectors prefer to feed indoors. While taking a blood meal, the female mosquito injects saliva into the person's blood vessels to stop the blood from clotting to make it easier to suck in. While injecting saliva, if she is infected with malaria parasites, she injects them as sporozoites into the person's blood as seen in **Figure 1**. On the other hand, if the person is infected, when the mosquito draws up the blood it will also take up

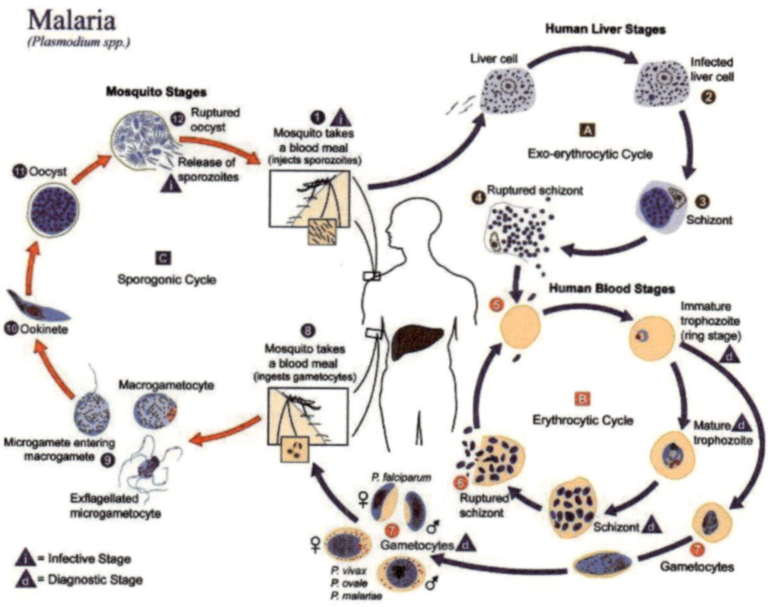

Figure 1.
Life cycle of plasmodium parasites illustrating stages of the cycle.

malaria parasites as gametocytes, the sexual forms of the malaria parasite. After a blood meal, the female mosquito usually finds a place to rest (usually the wall of the house) to digest her meal, and to develop her eggs. The malaria parasites which have been sucked up from the blood as gametocytes develop inside the mosquito over a period of 8 to 25 days to become sporozoites in the salivary glands. At this stage the female Anopheles mosquito becomes infective to the next person it feeds on.

Once the sporozoites get into a person with no or little immunity to malaria, they undergo various stages of development to cause disease about 7 to 12 days later as seen in **Figure 1**. Specifically, the sporozoites travel rapidly to the liver where they enter the liver cells and divide rapidly, forming merozoites. When a liver cell is full of merozoites, it bursts and discharges the merozoites into the blood where they quickly enter the red blood cells. In the red blood cells, the merozoites grow and divide again until the red blood cell bursts to release them into the blood stream to attack other red blood cells. This is what causes the person to experience symptoms such as fever, sweating and shivering. Some merozoites, however, change into the male and female forms of the parasite, called gametocytes, which are taken in by the mosquito when she sucks the blood to get her blood meal (**Figure 2**). The gametocytes enter the mosquito's stomach and mate to form eggs, which then in turn become sporozoites and move to the mosquitoe's salivary glands where they are ready to be injected into another person. Once the mosquito bites a person and infects him or her with sporozoites, it takes about 8 to 11 days for gametocytes to appear in the blood. In this way and under suitable conditions, one female Anopheles mosquito can transmit malaria parasites to many susceptible people during its average life span of 20 to 25 days [7]. This transmission cycle is illustrated in **Figure 2** below. In this way, this cycle of transmission continues unless interventions are used to break it.

2.3.1 The malaria transmission cycle

Key factors necessary for the process of transmission are:

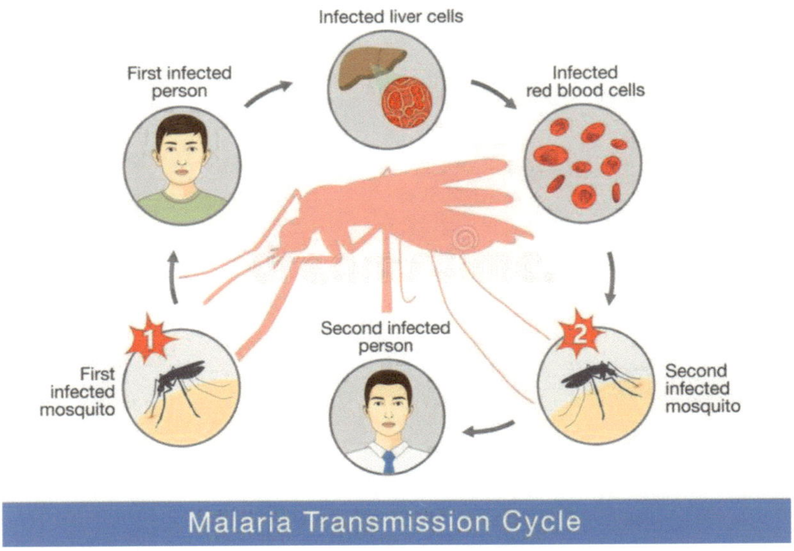

Figure 2.
Malaria transmission cycle showing how malaria parasites are carried by a female Anopheles mosquito from an infected person to a healthy one.

☐ The malaria parasite itself
☐ The vector / transmitting agent (i.e. the mosquito)
☐ The disease reservoir which refers to the total number of the subjects in the area carrying the malaria parasites. Their blood reservoir is where the vector obtains the infection.

- Malaria is transmitted by the bite of an infected female anopheles mosquito of which there are at least 400 different species. The common species are *Anopheles gambiae*, *A. funestus*, A.arabiensis and *A. melas*

- Within the *Anopheles gambiae* complex *A. gambiae* s.s. is the dominant species with A. arabiensis found more often in the Northern part of the country and *A. melas* found only in the mangrove coastal zone.

2.4 Brainstorming exercises

Note: Facilitator will ask these questions and different opinions from participants discussed.
Why is malaria a major public health problem in Nigeria.
Answer: Because Malaria is a major cause of:
☐ Ill health (morbidity)
☐ Death (mortality)
☐ Impaired child development
☐ Absenteeism in school children and work places
☐ Lost productivity (estimated economic loss to Nigeria is 132 billion Naira per year)
☐ Lost opportunities for economic development, e.g. tourism and foreign investment.
How is this Anopheles mosquito specie different from other mosquitoes?
Answer: It is a large mosquito and when standing it is tilted with head downwards and tail upwards in the air.

Which people are most vulnerable to Malaria?

Answer:

☐ Pregnant women

☐ Children under 5 Years of age

☐ People living with HIV/AIDS

☐ People suffering from Sickle Cell disorders

☐ Travellers into malaria endemic areas

Note: The first two groups (Pregnant women & Children below 5 years) are most at risk within our communities because of their low immunity and the malaria endemic nature of Nigeria, as such malaria is even regarded as mainly a maternal, new-born and child health issue.

Why does only the female mosquito transmit the disease?

Answer: The female mosquito needs a blood meal for the nutrients to develop her eggs.

Do other biting insects such as flies transmit malaria?

Answer: No. Only the female mosquito transmit malaria.

List 3 factors or reasons why people who have malaria die.

Answer:

☐ Delay in starting treatment

☐ Inappropriate treatment (wrong drug, incorrect dosages, non-compliance)

☐ Failure to recognise and manage complications

What is the difference between Suspected Malaria and Confirmed Malaria?

Answer:

Suspected Malaria: A patient with a fever or history of fever in the last 24 hours who lives in, or has come from anywhere in Nigeria or any other endemic country. Previously, all patients with this definition of malaria were given treatment with an antimalarial. Now, however, the best practice is to test all patients with suspected malaria with a confirmatory test before giving treatment.

While Confirmed Malaria: A patient with suspected malaria who has been shown to have malaria parasites through a parasitological test such as microscopy (using a blood smear) or rapid diagnostic test (RDT).

What is the difference between uncomplicated malaria and severe malaria?

First: Ask participants to differentiate between the two.

Answer:

Uncomplicated Malaria is a situation where a patient presents with a history of fever, or a fever in the last 48 hours, with no signs of severity or evidence of vital organ dysfunction but with a positive confirmatory parasitological test;

While in severe malaria, a patient presents with a positive confirmatory parasitological test and presentation of one or even more symptoms of the severe disease state (see 3.1 below).

2.5 Reflections on this module

Think about the topics you have just been discussing. How will you use the new knowledge you have gained when you go back to your premises? Use the questions below to help you reflect on this. Record your thoughts on paper for discussions.

1. What is simple malaria?

2. What have I learned about malaria today that I did not know before I came to this training program?

3. How will this new information be useful when I go back to work?

4. What other questions do I now need to ask the trainer and get answers for?

5. What questions do I have about how I will use this information when I go back to my community?

3. Signs & symptom / diagnosis of malaria

Table 2 below describes the training module on signs and symptoms and the diagnosis of malaria. This comprises the session objectives, learning objectives, time duration for the module, training materials needed, methods used and other relevant instructions that will assist the facilitators to impact the training.

What is meant by Signs & Symptoms of a malaria?

First: Ask participants to assess their understanding.

Session Objectives	To understand the signs and symptoms of malaria (uncomplicated and severe)	
	To identify cases of suspected malaria	
	To understand that malaria can be diagnosed based on signs and symptoms, but this method has limitations	
	To understand the use of Rapid Diagnostic Tests (RDTs)	
Duration	25 mins	
Learning objectives At the end of the session, participants should be able to:	Know the signs and symptoms of uncomplicated & severe malaria	
	Know that not all fevers are caused by malaria; and know some diseases presenting with fevers	
	Appreciate the use the RDTs in malaria confirmation	
	Be able to conduct appropriate investigations of suspected malaria using RDTs	
Training Materials	Participant's manual	Pens & Notebook
	Slides	Laptop computer
	LCD projector	Flip chart and markers
	Rapid Diagnostic Test kits, pair of hand gloves, lancets, alcoholic pads	
Methods used	Lecture	
	Demonstration classes	
	Question & Answer sessions	
	Case Studies	
	Reflection exercise	

Instructions for the facilitator	1. Begin the session by explaining the objectives of the session
	2. Get the participants to mention the symptoms of uncomplicated malaria they know.
	3. Then give a lecture on the signs and symptoms of both uncomplicated and severe malaria using "Lecture 3.1"below.
	Note THAT each slide explain what points need to be made.
	4. Think about sections which the participants might find difficult and common questions they may ask.
	5. Ask a series of questions to find out if the participants did understood the lecture
	6. Try to simulate situations at the participants' place of work during discussions and while answering questions.

Table 2.
Summary of session on signs & symptoms/diagnosis.

Answer: There are varying approaches to defining the medical meanings of signs and symptoms. A symptom is generally subjective while a sign is objective. Any objective evidence of a disease, such as a convulsing patient or a skin rash is considered a sign. This can be recognised by the physician, nurse, PMV, family members and even the patient themselves. However, headache, pain and weakness, fatigue, and some others can only be detected by the patients themselves.

What is symptomatic diagnosis?

First: Ask participants to assess their understanding.

Answer: Symptomatic diagnosis of malaria as the name implies, is a diagnosis that is based on the patient's signs and symptoms which is also known as clinical diagnosis. Malaria can then be classified into two types depending on extent of the infection and the severity of the symptoms, they are: uncomplicated or simple malaria and severe or complicated malaria.

3.1 Signs and symptoms of malaria

Signs and symptoms of uncomplicated malaria

Fever is usually the main symptom of malaria. It can be reported by the patients themselves or parents of children (could be even when the temperature returns to normal when being examined) or ascertained by taking the temperature (equal to or higher than 37.5° under the armpit or up to 38° rectally).

The signs and symptoms that may occur in uncomplicated malaria include:

☐ Headache
☐ Fever
☐ Sweating
☐ fatigue and dizziness
☐ loss of appetite
☐ muscle and/or joint aches

□ chills / Rigours
□ perspiration
□ digestive disorder: such as diarrhoea, abdominal discomfort
□ nausea, vomiting
□ worsening malaise

These signs and symptoms can be identified by asking the patient or their caregiver what they have noticed since the patient started the episodes of illness. The PMV and other healthcare providers can also take the patient's vital signs, including their temperature. **Figure 3** shows presentations of a patient with malaria as it transits from shivering to profuse sweating.

Signs and symptoms of severe malaria

Malaria is said to be severe or complicated when a patient presents with one or several of the under listed signs and symptoms:

□ very high temperature (could be >40° C)
□ Prostration (i.e. generalised weakness that patient is unable to sit or walk)
□ severe anaemia (nomocytic type: a very common complication)
□ consciousness disorders (confusion, agitation, drowsiness and coma)
□ multiple convulsion (>2 in last 24 hrs)
□ repeated vomiting (hindering oral treatment),
□ dehydration (thirst, dry lips, sunken eyes and deep set fontanel),
□ icterus (jaundice),
□ dark (coca-cola) coloured urine
□ Renal failure
□ hypoglycaemia
□ breathing difficulties
□ spontaneous bleeding

Other clinical signs could also appear such as anaemia, acute renal injury, acute pulmonary oedema /Adult Respiratory Distress Syndrome (ARDS), circulatory collapse or shock, abnormal bleeding (e.g. bruising, bleeding gums, haemoglobinurea).

Cerebral Malaria is a common presentation of severe malaria and may cause residual problems. A patient with malaria and altered level of consciousness, confusion, delirium, hallucinations or frank coma with or without convulsion is said to have cerebral malaria.

Note that:

□ Malaria always causes fever and therefore any fever should be suspected to be due to malaria in endemic areas.

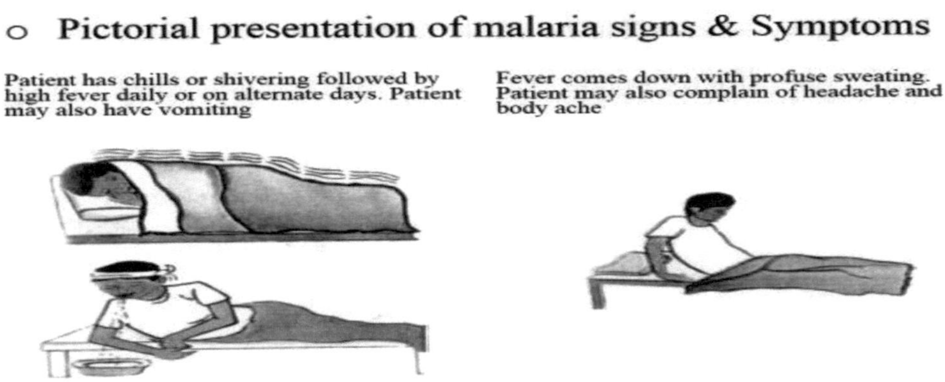

Figure 3.
Signs and symptoms of malaria.

☐ All cases of pregnant women and children below 5 years of age presenting with malaria are considered as severe malaria.

☐ All patients presenting with conditions listed above for complicated malaria or that which you do not fully understand, please REFER PATIENT IMMEDIATELY!

3.2 Diagnosis of malaria

3.2.1 Symptomatic malaria diagnosis

Symptomatic diagnosis of malaria is a diagnosis based on patient's signs and symptoms. This is also known as clinical diagnosis (suspected diagnosis). Remember that sign and symptoms of uncomplicated malaria are usually not only specific to malaria alone, with fever being a symptom to many illnesses. So if we take all fevers to be caused by malaria then this will certainly lead to over-diagnosis and hence an over-use of antimalarials.

The table below (**Table 3**) lists other possible reasons for fever including additional signs and symptoms. Noting that fever can be caused by other illnesses, it becomes of utmost importance to test and confirm if the fever is caused by malaria. Should any of the additional signs and symptoms be present, the patient should then be treated according to that disease.

3.2.2 Confirmatory malaria diagnosis

Diagnosing malaria on the basis of clinical features alone can be highly inaccurate and is likely to result in significant over-treatment. It is therefore important to establish capacity for confirmatory diagnostic testing. Effective confirmatory diagnostic testing can help to:

- identify patients who need antimalarial treatment;
- reduce unnecessary use of antimalarial drugs for patients without malaria;

Suspected disease	Additional signs and symptoms
Common cold	Running nostril, Cough
Gastroenteritis	Colicky pains, Diarrhoea (bloody or not), Vomiting
Hepatitis	Icterus, Enlarged spleen, Right hypochondriac pain
Meningitis	Stiff neck Bulging fontanel (young infants)
Mumps	Bilateral or unilateral swelling on the jaw
Pneumonia	Pneumonia Cough, Fast breathing Chest in-drawing
Tonsillitis sore throat	Pains in the throat Red inflamed throat with or without spots Painful cervical lymph nodes
Typhoid fever	Prolonged treatment not responding to appropriate antimalarial treatment. Dissociation between pulse rate and temperature.
Viral diseases Which include measles and varicella	Many cases in the neighbourhood with characteristic skin rash

Table 3.
Other diseases that fever presents as symptoms.

Note:

☐ Parasitological confirmation of suspected malaria before treatment is now recommended for all patients because not all fevers are due to malaria [8].

There are currently two widely available options for confirmatory diagnostic testing of malaria:

3.2.2.1 Light microscopy

Microscopy has been regarded as "gold standard" for a long time due to its effectiveness in malaria diagnosis. Microscopy is far more sensitive than RDTs for the detection of even low levels of *P. falciparum* parasitaemia (<100 parasites/μl) and the test can differentiate into the various malaria species. To achieve an effective microscopy for malaria parasites, we require: (i) good-quality reagents and equipment; (ii) skilled technicians with experience on how to prepare, stain films, in addition to identifying parasites and differentiate between the different Plasmodium species; and (iii) effective technical supervision and quality control of tests. However, these may not always be available in emergency situations, it is then easier and more beneficial for PMVs to establish a capacity for RDT.

3.2.2.2 Rapid diagnostic tests (RDTs)

In acute emergency phase of infections, limited time and resources make RDTs preferable to microscopy for confirmation of clinical diagnosis in low-transmission areas, and for confirming malaria in severely ill patients in moderate to high-transmission areas. RDTs found in Nigeria are usually only sensitive to *P. falciparum*. This is because *P. falciparum* is the most predominant species, accounting for about 98% of malaria cases in the country, and again, the majority of non-falciparum species within the country cause mixed infection with *P. falciparum*. The RDT differ from microscopic diagnosis of malaria through a number of ways. **Table 4** below is a comprehensive comparison between microscopy and RDTs.

3.3 Case studies

Activity 3.3.1

Instructions for the facilitator:

1. Divide the class into four groups, ask participants of each group to study the case studies below on the description of patient's signs & symptoms, diagnosis, misdiagnosis and appropriate suggestions from a trained PMV (allow 10 minutes to discuss & 5 minutes for each group to present).

2. Ask what the patient is suffering from.

3. Note the various points raised by participants and use them to discuss the various cases.

4. If the participants suspect that the patient has malaria, how do they arrive at such conclusions?

   NB. It is important to find out how they confirm this. Encourage them to emphasise the need to test.

5. Conclude the session by discussing each group's presentation

	Microscopy	RDTs
Requirements		
Equipment	Microscope	None
Electricity	Preferred, not necessary	None
Transport / storage conditions	Reagents stored out of direct sunlight	Avoid exposure to high temperature (4–30°C recommended)
Quality assurance	Periodic re-reading of percentage of slides by expert microscopist and supervision	Lot testing of kits, monitoring of storage temperature, supervision of workers
Performance		
Test duration	Usual minimum 60 minutes	15–20 minutes
Labour-intensiveness	High	Low
Dependence on individual competence	High	Low
Direct costs		
Cost per test	US$0.12–0.40	US$0.60–1.00
Technical specifications		
Detection of all 4 species	Yes	Some RDTs

Table 4.
Comparison between microscopy and RDTs.

Note that:

- RDTs are fast, convenient and can be handled by an incompetent hand. RDTs are fairly cheap and do not require electricity.

- They are thus convenient for use by PMVs where it will improve their services with resultant avoidance of unnecessary treatment and over-treatment with antimalarials.

Activity 3.3.2 Read and discuss the case studies below.

Case study 1: An unknown patient comes to your PMV shop and complains that he has fever, headache, and joint pains. He continued that the fever has been coming on and off for about three days but he usually feels fine during the day and in the evening he has fever.

What is he/she is suffering from and what is your line of action?

Case study 2: A mother comes to your premises with a 3 year old child that looks very weak. The child had vomited severally and on checking, you found the child had 40° C. discuss your actions.

3.4 Demonstration exercise

Demonstration of the use of RDT to show purple/red line in test and control windows on strip showing antigen–antibody reaction if positive. Discuss advantages of RDTs mentioned earlier.

3.5 Reflection on the module

Participants are asked to make think about the topics they have just discussed. How will they use the new knowledge gained when back to their premises? Also use the questions below to help reflect. Record the thoughts on paper for discussions.

1. What is RDT and how do you compare it to microscopy?

2. What have I learned about malaria today that I did not know before I came to this training program?

3. How will this new information be useful when I go back to work?

4. What other questions do I now need to ask the trainer and get answers for?

5. What questions do I have about how I will use this information when I go back to my community?

4. Treatment of malaria

Table 5 below describes the training module on malaria treatment. This module comprises the session objectives, learning objectives, time duration for the module, training materials needed, methods used and other relevant instructions that will assist facilitators to adequately explain malaria treatment approaches.

4.1 National treatment protocol

What is the National Malaria Treatment Protocol about?

Answer: The national treatment protocol contains recommendations on the most effective treatment that should be given for malaria. The current protocol recommends Artemisinin-based Combination Therapy (ACT) as the most effective treatment for uncomplicated malaria instead of Chloroquine and SP.

4.1.1 Treatment of uncomplicated malaria

- First line treatment:

To be given to a patients with malaria when ACT are not contra-indicated.

☐ **Artemether /lumefantrine (AL)**: as a fixed dose combination, given twice a day for (3) three consecutive days with the second dose being given 8 hours after the first [7–9].

OR

☐ Tabs **Artesunate + Amodiaquine (AA)**: Given once daily for three (3) consecutive days [7–9].

- Second line treatment:

To be given in the event of true treatment failure (defined as failure to clear parasites after the three days of a full treatment course). It can also be used in situations when ACT is not appropriate.

☐ **Oral Quinine**: 8 hourly for seven (7) days [8, 9].

Note: Details of treatment regimens are seen in Section 4.3 below.

Session Objectives	To understand the essence of the National Malaria Treatment Protocols	
	To understand the treatment of uncomplicated malaria	
	To understand the treatment of complicated malaria	
Duration	30 minutes	
Learning objectives At the end of the session, participants should be able to:	To appreciate why government changed its policy on malaria treatment (thereby appreciating the shortfalls associated with the use of Chloroquine which is still in use)	
	Know the treatment of uncomplicated malaria in children, adults & pregnant women	
	Know the treatment of complicated malaria for all categories of patients	
	To provide appropriate anti-malarial drugs to patients of all categories	
Training Materials	Participant's manual	Pens & Notebook
	Slides	Laptop computer
	LCD projector	Flip chart and markers
Methods used	Lecture	
	Quiz session	
	Group discussions	
	Demonstration Exercise	
	Role plays	
	Reflections on the module	
Instructions for the facilitator	1. Begin the session by explaining the learning objectives of this module	
	2. Give a lecture on the treatment of uncomplicated and severe malaria in various situations using "Lecture 4.1–4.6" below.	
	3. Think about and emphasise sections which the participants might find difficult and common questions they may ask.	
	4. Ask series of questions to find out if participants did understood the lecture	
	5. Divide the class into four groups for group discussions / Quiz	
	6. Try to simulate situations at the participants' place of work during discussions and while answering questions	

Table 5.
Summary of session on the treatment of malaria.

4.1.2 Management of uncomplicated Malaria in pregnancy

- First Trimester

Oral Quinine is used, or a combination of oral quinine and Clindamycin.

- Second and Third Trimesters

Oral Quinine is used or the combination of **AL or AA** is used [8].

Note THAT for pregnant women with co-morbidities of HIV and sickle cell anaemia, the above treatment shall be used.

4.1.3 Home management of uncomplicated malaria

AL is the combination drug of choice for treatment of uncomplicated malaria for children below five (5) years of age. Essential skills in behaviour change communication are thus necessary for community based agents such as the PMVs to effectively home manage uncomplicated malaria.

4.1.4 Treatment failure in uncomplicated malaria

Quinine shall remain the drug of choice for the management of malaria in the event of treatment failure.

When treatment fails in pregnancy, though ACTs are not recommended in the first trimester of pregnancy, their use shall however not be stopped in cases where they are considered to be life-saving and other antimalarials are not suitable.

For second and third trimesters in pregnancy, **Quinine or AL or AA** combination therapies shall be used depending on which drug was first given. Usually, a treatment option other than what was first given to the patient will be used where treatment failure is established.

4.1.5 Treatment of severe malaria

Management of severe/complicated malaria requires parenteral treatment to provide adequate blood-serum concentrations as quickly as possible initially; subsequently it is reverted to oral treatment as soon as the patient's condition permits.

IM/IV Quinine or I.M. Artemether shall be the drugs of choice for treating complicated malaria. The necessary support therapy shall be provided as and when appropriate.

The treatment of pregnant women with severe malaria shall be with Parenteral **Quinine (I.V. or I.M. in all trimesters)** until the patient can take oral preparations. I. M Artemether can be used for the second and third trimesters. Pregnant women with co-morbidities of HIV and sickle cell anaemia shall be treated as above.

Note that:

☐ Severe malaria is a Medical Emergency. So it should always be referred to secondary Healthcare facilities immediately!

☐ Severe malaria needs special attention because:

- It is associated with dangerous complications (See Section 2.1)

- It is a common cause of avoidable deaths from malaria

☐ The correct use of ACTs is essential for the success of treatment.

4.2 Why government changed 1st line malaria treatment from CQ to ACTs?

CQ and SP are no longer effective in treating malaria in Nigeria due to high treatment failures resulting from widespread resistance. Efficacy studies that test the ability of antimalarial medicines to kill and clear malaria parasites have shown that ACTs are better than chloroquine. **Table 6** below describes the two older drugs that are no longer indicated for malaria treatment.

S / No	Drug	Comments
1.	Sulphadoxine-Pyrimethamine (SP)	Not recommended for treatment of malaria. Reserved for intermittent preventive treatment (IPT) in pregnancy
2.	Chloroquine (CQ)	Inadequate efficacy and therefore no longer recommended for treatment of malaria in Nigeria

Table 6.
Older drugs for treatment of uncomplicated malaria.

Artemisinin derivatives are the most effective drugs against malaria in the world at the moment and yet if misused the parasites can potentially develop resistance to them. Already there are some signs from Far East Asia that improper use and use of poor quality ACTs is making the malaria parasites have some ability to withstand treatment with ACTs causing cure to take longer to achieve.

A technique to prevent resistance developing to Artemisinin derivatives is to combine them with other antimalarials so that as a combination there is less possibility of the parasites developing mechanisms to avoid both medicines.

Note that: The objective of prompt and effective malaria treatment is to:

- Cure the disease and eliminate the parasites from the body
- Prevent progression to severe disease or death
- Prevent transmission to others
- Prevent the parasites developing resistance to the malaria treatment
- Minimise adverse drug reactions

4.3 The first line treatment of malaria

Below are details of the treatments for malaria as recommended by the Government of Nigeria:

4.3.1 Artemether/Lumefantrine (AL)

This is a fixed dose combination of Artemether 20 mg and Lumefantrine 120 mg. It exists as several brands which have been registered by NAFDAC for use in the country. The combination is abbreviated sometimes as AM/LM. **Table 7** below describes the dosing for AL with respect to age and body weights.

NOTE: The tablets of Artemether/Lumefantrine can be in the form of plain tablets or dispersible tablets. The only difference is that the dispersible tablets dissolve when immersed in a liquid whereas the plain tablets have to be crushed to make a mixture for children that cannot swallow tablets. Only ACT 1 and 2 have dispersible tablets.

4.3.2 Artesunate + Amodiaquine (AA)

Artesunate + Amodiaquine is sometimes abbreviated as ASAQ. A fixed dose combination pre-pack and a co-packaged pre-pack exist as is seen in **Tables 8** and **9** below. There are three presentations of this combination, namely Infant, Child and Adult. These age and weight specific blister packs are colour coded.

		Number of tables and dosing times					
		Day 1		Day 2		Day 3	
Weight / Age	ACT pack	0 hOurs	8 hrs	24 hrs	36 hrs	48 hrs	60 hrs
5 to <15 kg / 6mths – 3 yrs	ACT1	1	1	1	1	1	1
15 to <25 kg /4 – 8 yrs	ACT2	2	2	2	2	2	2
25 to <35 kg /9 – 14 yrs	ACT3	3	3	3	3	3	3
≥ 35 kg /> 14 yrs	ACT4	4	4	4	4	4	`4

Table 7.
Dosage schedule for AL (AM 20 mg/LM 120 mg) showing the four weight and age categories.

Weight (kg)	Age	AS tablets (50 mg)			AQ tablets (153 mg)		
		Day 1	Day 2	Day 3	Day 1	Day 2	Day 3
6.5 to <10	4 to 11 months	½	½	½	½	½	½
10 to <22	1 year to <7 years	1	1	1	1	1	1
22 to <36	7 years to <14 years	2	2	2	2	2	2
36 and above	14 years and above	4	4	4	4	4	4

Table 8.
Dosage schedule for co-packaged pre-pack tables AS+AQ (AS 50 mg + AQ 153 mg) showing the four weight and age categories.

Weight/Age	Tablet strength	Dosage regimen
4.5 kg to <9 kg 2 months - 11 months	25 mg/67.5 mg	1 tablet once daily for three days
9 kg to <18 kg 1 year to 5 years	50 mg/135 mg	1 tablet once daily for three days (or 2 tabs of 25/67.5 mg)
18 kg to <36 kg 6 years to 13 years	100 mg/270 mg	1 tablet once daily for three days (or 2 tabs of 50/135 mg)
36 kg and above 14 years and above	100 mg/270 mg	2 tablets once daily for three days

Table 9.
Dosage schedule for tables AS/AQ fixed dose combination pre-pack (AS 50 mg + AQ 135 mg) showing the four weight and age categories.

When using the co-packaged tablets of AS+AQ, the client should be instructed that the.

Artesunate and Amodiaquine tablets must be taken together, at the same time. ASAQ fixed dose combination (FDC) should be used whenever possible.

Side effects of ACT:

☐ Artemisinins are generally well tolerated at the doses used to treat malaria.

☐ The side effects from the Artemisinin class of medicines are similar to the symptoms of malaria: nausea, vomiting, anorexia, and dizziness.

4.4 Second line treatment

The second line treatment for malaria in Nigeria is **Quinine** in tablet formulation. The indication for using Quinine is where a patient has confirmed malaria and has already taken a full course of the first line antimalarial treatment, i.e. AM / LM or AS+AQ, and has not recovered. Parasitological confirmation of the diagnosis should be done with microscopy before prescribing oral Quinine.

Dosage: Quinine tablets (300 mg salt) are given as a dose of 10 mg/kg body weight up to a maximum dose of 60 kg body weight, e.g., 600 mg every 8 hours for 7 days.

4.5 Good prescribing practices

NOTE THAT:

☐ Malaria can be 100% cured by ACTs, but ONLY when used appropriately

☐ The only ACTs recommended in the National Protocol are AM/LM and AS +AM.

☐ It is not advisable to use other non-recommended ACTs.

☐ Artemisinin monotherapies are not recommended as treatment for uncomplicated malaria.

☐ Use of antimalarials by patients that do not have malaria means patients are taking medicines that they do not need, which could be dangerous.

☐ Overuse of antimalarials also has economic consequences to patient & the nation

It is good practice to strongly encourage the client to take a full course of treatment and complete the dose, otherwise the patient will not get well. This means that you, as the health provider, need to counsel the client by providing health information and advice.

Clients need to know about:

☐ the type of treatment they are receiving

☐ how to take/give the medicine

☐ the dosage required

☐ importance of completing treatment

☐ details of how to watch out for adverse drug reactions

Dosing advice to healthcare providers regarding treatment of their clients:

☐ Always dispense the full 3-day course of medicines

☐ Show the client how to split the tablet (if necessary) to get the correct dose. This can be done by pressing a knife along the seam on the top of the tablet

☐ If possible, have client take the first dose in front of you, so you can supervise as needed

☐ Refer the client to health facility if they have any indications for referral.

Dosing advice to healthcare providers regarding treatment of their clients:

☐ They should always take the medicine with or right after meals with a full glass of water

☐ When using a co-packaged (two different drugs together) product, both medicines must be taken together in correct doses.

☐ To completely cure the illness, the full course of treatment (the correct number of tablets taken at the correct number of times each day for the correct number of days) must be taken.

☐ Symptoms may not disappear immediately after taking the first dose. Improvement may take up to two days.

☐ If the client vomits within half an hour, then the dose should be repeated.

☐ The client should take plenty of fluids to avoid dehydration and food to maintain strength. Fluids that contain sugar or glucose are an advantage.

☐ For small children, it helps to crush the tablets and mix it with fruit juices, or sugar and clean water to make a solution that is easier to swallow.

4.6 Demonstration exercise

Observe the commonly available ACTs and discuss dosage presentations, so also how to crush and split tablets for children (where necessary).

4.7 Group quiz

The facilitator will divide the class into four groups and each group will present their answers to the quiz question below:

1. What is the drug of choice used in the treatment of uncomplicated malaria in Nigeria excluding pregnant women?

Answer:
The anti-malarial drug of choice is: Artemeter - Lumefantrine (AL).
Alternatively: Artesunate + Amodiaquine (AA).

2. What drugs are used for severe malaria treatment?

Answer:
☐ Parenteral drugs (IM or IV route) are required
☐ IM or IV Quinine is the drug of choice.
☐ Injectable Artemether is an alternative choice
☐ Dosages are given in the treatment guidelines.

3. Which drug is used for treatment failure?

Answer:
☐ Oral Quinine (after laboratory confirmation and ruling out other causes of fever)
☐ In pregnancy depending on the alternatives available and the trimester of pregnancy (refer to Guidelines).

4. What drugs are used for treating uncomplicated malaria in pregnancy & What is the dose?

Answer: Artesunate-Amodiaquine or Artemether-Lumefantrine in the 2nd and 3rd trimesters; Quinine tablets or Quinine-Clindamycin in the first trimester of pregnancy. Refer to guidelines for dosage.

5. What drug is used for Intermittent Preventive treatment (IPT) of malaria in pregnancy?

Answer: Sulphadoxine - Pyrimethamine (SP) (Discuss why … ..Refer to treatment guidelines).

4.8 Role play

A volunteer from the class will be the health provider in a premises. Another volunteer pretended to be a client presenting with malaria symptoms. On provision of a complete ACT regimen, the client decides to take and pay for an incomplete treatment.

What will be your response in the situation and how will you convince the client?

4.9 Reflection on module

Think about the topics you have just been discussing. How will you use the new knowledge you have gained when you go back to your premises? Use the questions below to help you reflect on this. Record your thoughts on paper for discussions.

1. Outline the treatment of both uncomplicated and severe malaria?

2. What other treatments have you learnt today?

3. How will this new information be useful when you go back to work?

4. What other questions do you now need to ask the trainer and get answers for?

5. Indications for referral

Table 10 below describes the training module on referrals of malaria patients. This module comprises the session objectives, learning objectives, time duration for the module, training materials needed, methods used and other relevant instructions that will assist facilitators to adequately explain referrals and its approaches.

Emphasise that certain conditions require a patient to be referred from a primary health center to a higher level facility for treatment. These conditions are referred to in this module as indications for referral.

5.1 Conditions requiring referral

The indications for referral from a primary to a secondary or tertiary health facility are when:

☐ One or more danger signs are present

☐ The patient has features of severe malaria

☐ The patient is on recommended malaria treatment, but there is no improvement after 48 hours

☐ The client is not complying with treatment, because of vomiting or are otherwise unable to take drugs by mouth

☐ The client has adverse drug reactions to the ACT medicine that prevents him / her from taking / completing treatment

☐ You are unsure of the client's illness or condition

☐ The patient is having fever every day for seven or more days

Those patients who are not severely ill but have one or more indications for referral should be referred with a referral form / letter. Patients who are severely ill as shown by the presence of danger signs or features of severe malaria should be given pre-referral treatment.

5.2 Treatment failure

The recurrence of *P. falciparum* malaria usually results due to either a re-infection or recrudescence / failure. Failure in treatment is defined as the failure to effectively clear malaria parasites from the blood or can also be described as the

Session Objectives	To identify cases requiring referral from the signs and symptoms presented	
	To identify cases of treatment failure	
	To understand the causes of treatment failure	
	To understand and identify danger signs	
Duration	40 minutes	
Learning objectives At the end of the session, participants should be able to:	Know the conditions requiring referral	
	Applying the knowledge of conditions requiring referral to practice	
	Appreciate and identify when a treatment has failed	
	Be able to refer patients to the appropriate health facility	
	Be able to identify danger signs	
Training Materials	Participant's manual	Pens & Notebook
	Slides	Laptop computer
	LCD projector	Flip chart and markers
Methods used	Lecture	
	Case studies	
	Group discussions	
	Demonstration Exercise	
Instructions for the facilitator	1. Begin the session by explaining the learning objective of the session	
	2. Emphasise that reduction of death and disability from severe malaria is a public health priority for Nigeria. This can be achieved by prompt referrals of severe cases.	
	3. Give the lecture on Indications for referral, Treatment failure, Danger signs & Pre-referral treatment.	
	4. Think about sections which the participants might find difficult and common questions they may ask.	
	5. Ask a series of questions to find out if the participants did understood the lecture	
	6. Split the class into four groups to discuss and answer the case studies	
	7. Try to simulate situations at the participants' place of work during discussions and while answering questions	

Table 10.
Summary of session on indications for referral.

inability to resolve clinical symptoms despite administration of antimalarials. Treatment failure can result from so many causes.

- Vomiting or poor absorption of drug – the patient or the caregiver usually gets confused on what to do should the drug get vomited.

- Poor practices in prescribing – prescribing of incomplete course of treatment increases the risk of treatment failure in malaria. This is a common practice with PMVs. So always insist patients take home full / complete treatment regimen, with proper advice on need to complete dose.

- Poor adherence: which may be due to several factors, including:

  - information on correct regimen could be unclear to the patient or caregiver ab-initio;

  - some patients choose to stop taking treatment once the pressing symptoms have resolved (a common problem with drugs having a very rapid symptoms clearance), and some patients share the remaining treatment with their family / friends;

  - in cost-recovery systems, some patients cannot even afford a complete course of their treatment, this presents a big challenge;

  - Except for co-formulated products, patients may discard one of the components of the combination that is associated with side effects or taste hence its ineffectiveness.

- Drug quality – the use of substandard antimalarials with inadequate recommended amount of active ingredient is a particular risk for drug. So ACT quality must always be ensured by:

  - sourcing from reputable pharmaceutical outlets or their representatives;

  - proper storage all through the distribution system to avoid exposure to high temperatures; and

  - Avoiding administering expired drugs.

- Drug resistance in this case is the ability of a given parasite to survive or multiply despite drug administration and absorption in doses equal to or higher than the usually recommended, but within the tolerance of the subject.

Though treatment failure within 14 days of treatment with an ACT is very unusual, a good history and proper examination is necessary to confirm any non-malaria related causes of symptoms (refer to module 2). For instance, was a complete course of ACT really taken, accompanied by food or not where appropriate, and without vomiting in the first hour following any dose? So also, all treatment failures must be confirmed parasitologically, and preferably by taking blood slides for examination.

Note THAT, it is very important to keep good records of all confirmed treatment failures and this information forwarded to appropriate health authorities, as these failures need to be imputed into drug efficacy studies and these studies usually lead to the observed changes in first-line antimalarial treatment.

- Whenever the treatment failure is after 14 days of initial treatment, it should be considered to be a re-infections and another dose of ACT can be given.

- Treatment failures within 14 days of initial treatment should be treated with a second-line antimalarial such as Quinine (for a total of 7 days).

5.3 Danger signs

Generally, all danger signs are dangerous as the name indicates and emphasis is on the need for an immediate referral. The most common danger signs include:

- Convulsions or fits within the last two days or at present
- Not able to eat / drink or breastfeed (in children)
- Vomiting everything taken (severe vomiting) or severe diarrhoea
- Prostration indicated by extreme weakness, unable to sit or stand
- Altered mental state such as lethargy, drowsiness, confusion or unconsciousness
- Breathing difficulties
- Severe dehydration shown by sunken eyes or if skin is pinched
- Severe anaemia or lack of blood shown by pale lips or palms

Note that:
All patients who have danger signs need urgent treatment at a secondary or tertiary healthcare facility that has the equipment and expertise to handle emergency conditions. To save this patient, you need to refer immediately.

5.4 Pre-referral treatment

All patients especially children who do not respond to treatment (with AL within 24 hours) and the very ill (i.e., having any danger signs or features of severe malaria) shall be referred immediately to the nearest hospital. Time is important at this point and every hour of delay reduces the patient's chance of survival. Pre-referral treatment is used to increase the chance of the patient surviving long enough to get to the health facility for further treatment.

5.4.1 Rectal Artesunate (or Artemether)

10 mg/kg body weight rectal artesunate is the recommended minimum dose. Give a single dose as pre-referral treatment. The choices you have are artesunate or artemether suppositories. This is repeated after 8 hours if transfer is delayed.

5.4.2 IM quinine

IM quinine 10 mg/kg. This is an alternative to Rectal artesunate. OR.

5.4.3 IM Artesunate or Artemether

IM artesunate 2.4 mg/kg single dose, OR IM artemether 3.2 mg/kg single dose.

5.5 Demonstration exercises

- A sample of Artesunate Suppository is torn to show participants its presentation and the insertion process is described.
- Filling of Referral forms; done as a group work

Note that: Pre-referral treatment is not a replacement treatment for severe malaria.

6. Malaria prevention

Table 11 below describes the training module on malaria prevention. This module comprises the session objectives, learning objectives, time duration, training materials needed, methods used and other relevant instructions that will assist facilitators to adequately describe malaria prevention approaches.

6.1 Reasons for prevention

- Malaria can kill if it infects an individual, so we try to prevent it.
- Malaria will make you sick, and therefore make you unable to work, so people may lose jobs /miss school etc.
- Malaria leads to poverty because Malaria and poverty are connected, you cannot work and earn money or go to school for your future if you are ill with Malaria, and you will need to spend a lot of money for treatment.

Note that:

- The first step towards malaria control is prevention.
- It costs far less to prevent malaria than it costs to treat it.

What must you do as a healthcare provider to help your clients prevent malaria?

- Provide health education to your community. As a health care worker you can provide community members with information on prevention methods that are available so that they can take steps to prevent malaria.
- Be a good example to the community by using the preventive methods you are advocating, especially the ITNs.

What about the long awaited Vaccine for malaria?

An effective vaccine is not yet available for malaria, this is because of the different phases which the parasite does exist within the human body giving it different / contrasting properties. Although several vaccines are under development. So far, a prospective vaccine candidate known as RTS-S/AS01 has shown potentially promising results in clinical trials in Africa. Evidence-based policy recommendations on the issue are expected to be made this year (2015) depending on data that will become available. While this wait goes on, prevention will then depend on how to avoid parasites getting into the body.

Session Objectives	To understand reasons for emphasis on prevention	
	To understand the various prevention strategies	
	To identify reasons why many communities do not embrace malaria prevention and how best to encourage them	
Duration	60 minutes	
Learning objectives At the end of the session, participants should be able to:	Know the various prevention methods	
	Be able to appropriately treat and hang an ITN	
	Be able to appropriately advice clients on malaria prevention measures	
	Know the various locally circulated myths about malaria and how to address them	
	Understand the various excuses given by clients for not taking prevention and how to persuade them against such negative acts	
Training Materials	Participant's manual	Pens & Notebook
	Slides	Laptop computer
	LCD projector	Flip chart and markers
Methods used	Lecture	
	Case studies	
	Group discussions	
	Brainstorming exercise	
	Demonstration Exercise	
Notes to facilitators	1. Begin the session by explaining the objective of the session	
	2. Emphasise that reduction in death / disability from malaria and reduction in cost / stress of disease its treatment could be achieved by effective prevention strategies.	
	3. Think about sections which the participants might find difficult and common questions they may ask.	
	4. Give participants opportunities to air their various contributions / experiences and myths.	
	5. Ask a series of questions to find out if the participants are following.	
	6. Try to simulate situations at the participants' place of work during discussions and while answering questions.	

Table 11.
Summary of session on malaria prevention.

How do we stop parasites getting into our body?

The mosquitoes that spread malaria tend to bite at night between the hours of 10 p.m. and 4 a.m. They prefer to feed on human blood. After feeding, the mosquitoes rest inside the house, usually on the walls. Common ways of preventing malaria take advantage of these characteristics of the mosquito vector.

Key elements for transmission of malaria (as discussed in module 1.3) are:

- The malaria parasite itself,
- The transmitting agent (i.e. the vector mosquito), and
- The reservoir of the disease (i.e. people carrying the parasites in their blood).

The general objective of preventive efforts are:

1. Reducing vector-host contact: Since the mosquito must feed once on an infected host to acquire the malaria parasite and once on an uninfected person to transmit it, reducing host-vector-host contact is an effective way of reducing transmission.

2. Reducing the longevity and abundance of adult mosquito population: The more the mosquito population in an area the greater is the probability of transmission. So, reducing the longevity and abundance of adult mosquito population in an area reduces probability of transmission.

3. Reducing suitable breeding sites (source reduction) wherever this is feasible and sustainable.

How effective these strategies are will greatly depend upon how assiduously they are applied. The Federal Ministry of Health in Nigeria has adopted and prioritised these prevention strategies: Insecticide Treated Nets (ITNs), the Intermittent Preventive Treatment (IPT) for pregnant women, Complementary and increasing Indoor Residual Spraying (IRS), Environmental Management and larval Source Management (to reduce breeding where significant proportions of breeding sites can be identified and targeted). They are the key prevention strategies to be discussed.

Finally, there are on-going research initiatives looking to find new ways to tackle malaria. For example, many scientists are involved in the search for new drugs and vaccines (as stated earlier), which will be safe, effective, and with affordable price tags, that could change our thinking on conquering malaria. Similarly, due to drug-resistance, particularly with *Plasmodium falciparum*, new medications are constantly being tested. A combination of all efforts towards fighting malaria put together had reduced the mortality of malaria greatly over the years; the major aim now for governments and all other partner organisations such as the WHO, Roll Back Malaria (RBM), Society for Family Health (SFH), Malaria No More (MNM), etc. is to get to a point where deaths from malaria are eliminated through effective treatment and prevention strategies.

6.2 Insecticide treated nets (ITNs)

An ITN provides effective barrier between the person who is sleeping under it and the mosquito vector. It reduces the opportunity for mosquito to bite and infect. The impregnated insecticide also acts to kill and repel any susceptible vector that rests on the net. An Integrated Vector Management System (IVMS) for malaria prevention is also in place in the country and is a combined approach involving the distribution of Insecticide Treated Nets (ITNs) as the major approach this involves all form of deliveries such as free public sector donation campaigns either jointly integrated with other health activities (such as vaccination campaigns, National immunizations) or as stand-alone campaigns, to the free public sector routine distributions such as ANC and EPI services, and the subsidised and at cost sales through hospitals, clinics and at PMV outlets.

Insecticide treated bed nets can be either conventional ITNs or Long Lasting Impregnated Nets (LLINs). Conventional ITNs, as the name implies must be treated once or twice a year (usually dependent on the duration of the transmission). LLINs are nets, whose fabrics have been impregnated with insecticides by a special technique from the source, so that the insecticidal effect is maintained for as long as the net can withstand daily usage, i.e. usually 3–5 years or about 20 washes. **Figure 4** below shows an example of an impregnated bed net hung outside to protect people from vector transmission within a garden. Total access to LLIN is the ultimate aim in public health and public sector distributions focuses on children under 5 years of age and pregnant women.

6.3 Intermittent preventive treatment (IPT) during pregnancy / special care patients

Currently, the most preferred intervention to prevent malaria in pregnancy is the use Intermittent Preventive Treatment (IPT) apart from ITNs. And this is based on the use of anti-malaria drugs that are usually given in treatment doses at some defined intervals after quickening (16 gestational weeks). This serves to reduce malaria parasitaemia which usually leads to poor pregnancy outcomes. IPT with other products like haematinics and anthelmintics are preferably provided as part of a comprehensive antenatal package. Every pregnant woman should also have access to insecticide treated nets (ITNs) in addition to the IPT, which should be used throughout the pregnancy as an additional method of malaria prevention.

Drug of Choice for Intermittent Preventive Treatment (IPT) Sulphadoxine - Pyrimethamine (SP) is a combination drug (Sulphadoxine 500 mg + Pyrimethamine 25 mg) and shall be reserved only for Intermittent Preventive Treatment (IPT).

6.4 Indoor residual spraying (IRS)

Indoor residual spraying with an insecticide is sprayed on the wall every four or six months to kill mosquitoes that rest on the wall to digest its blood meal. Before and after feeding on a person, the mosquito rests on the wall where it picks up some of the insecticide which eventually kills it. IRS is a very effective way of preventing malaria.

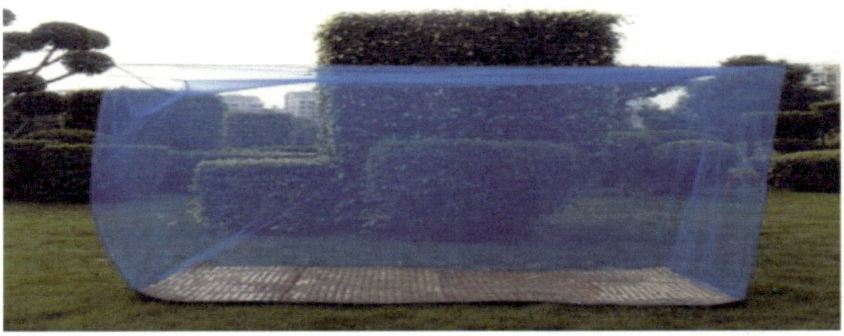

Figure 4.
An impregnated bed net (LLIN) being hanged in a garden.

Although this method is complementary to ITN distributions, it will form an important and increasing part of the preventive strategy. Scenarios that are potential focus for IRS include:

- Areas where IRS has advantages to ITNs or has a synergistic effect (e.g. in and around densely populated cities).
- Areas having a short and usually a malaria transmission season which is limited and where the addition of the sprays can make local elimination possible (e.g. the Sahel savannah in the North-East of this country).
- Areas where using treated nets shows to be difficult to implement (e.g. consistent low use rates found with some communities).
- Institutions with marked populations such as boarding schools, army and police barracks etc. the use of ITN seems more challenging in such places.

6.5 Other vector control interventions (environmental & Larval source management)

These include Environmental Management (EM) and Larval control strategies by using larvicides, predators or growth inhibitors.

6.5.1 Environmental management

Management of the environment to reduce breeding sites of the Anopheles vector usually revolves round source reduction, and this is by targeting mosquito breeding sites with the objective of reducing the availability of suitable breeding sites. This will focus on man-made breeding sites in urban and peri-urban settings, construction sites, agriculture projects etc. It should be **note THAT** Anopheles does not breed in garbage or polluted gutters. So removal of garbage / filth is good for public health in general, and reduces the number of nuisance mosquitoes. But however, it has little impact on malaria control directly. The life span of an Anopheles mosquito is between 2 and 3 weeks, if breeding is curtailed, the population of mosquitoes will drastically drop due to this short life span.

To prevent breeding of mosquitoes, every householder must ensure that there is no water collection around their houses.

6.5.2 Larvivorous fish (biological control)

Different predator fish species have been widely used to protect public health, since early 1903. One of the most widely used and successful control agent against mosquito larvae is the mosquito fish *Gambusia affinis* also called top water minnow. Another fish which has received the most attention as a mosquito control agent is *Poecilia reticulata*, the common guppy [7].

6.5.3 Chemical larviciding

Chemicals are used in breeding sites that cannot be drained, filled or where other larval control methods are impossible to implement or too expensive. This method is good only for vectors which tend to breed in semi-permanent or permanent water bodies that can be identified, and where the population of the human to be protected is sufficiently high to justify such treatment. Thus, larvicides are restricted to urban areas, barracks, labour or refugee camps and development project sites.

The residual effect of larviciding conducted varies considerably depending on the type of the breeding places and quality of the water, but is relatively short for most larvicides. Such larvicide treatment must be repeated at fairly short cycles which may vary from two to ten weeks. Temephos and Fenthion are some of the most commonly used larvicides [10].

6.5.4 Use of screens in homes

House protection with screening of windows, eaves and doors is an effective method of reducing human-vector contact, if properly implemented and maintained. Screens are popular, cheap and accessible to most members of the community.

6.5.5 Mosquito coils, repellents, protective clothing, and others

The use of protective cloths and repellents are indicated for people who are mostly outdoors during peak vector biting periods. Repellents have a very short duration of effect in most cases and are costly. Aerosols and mosquito coils are mostly popular in urban areas. Protective cloths usually covers most of the body, i.e. long sleeve shirts and jackets, protective stockings with covering trousers can provide a certain level of personal protection from mosquito.

6.6 Demonstration session

- Demonstration on the appropriate spread of the ITN to suite both indoor or outdoor use
- Demonstration on the proper method of treatment of the ITN using Deltamethrin.

6.7 Brainstorming session

- What advice would you as a PMV give a patient about prevention of malaria?

Answer:

- Use of insecticide treated materials should be encouraged.
- Mosquito screening devices in house designs and protective dressing.
- Use of insecticides and mosquito repellents.
- Environmental management especially destroying mosquito breeding sites.
- Which role can you play in the prevention and management of malaria in the community?

Answer:

Discussions should be along these lines:

- Case management aspect
- Vector control, Behaviour Change Communication
- Health education and Community participation

7. Discussion

A systematic review was conducted in 2017 on the effectiveness of different malaria intervention programmes among Patent Medicine Vendors (PMVs) by the authors of this book chapter [11]. The researchers tried to identify and review the different studies addressing poor KAP on all relevant topics that had characterised services rendered by the PMVs. The review showed that all studies analysed were effective in improving KAP despite adopting different intervention approaches for their different interventions with relatively wide range of topics all relating to malaria.

An intervention conducted in 2014 to strengthen PMV Associations for an improved malaria management [12], was also conducted in Nigeria just like the present study, but was specifically concerned with the use of RDTs for effective confirmatory test before commencement of treatment, this intervention training was embarked upon to check indiscriminate use of antimalarials without a confirmatory test. The use of RDTs was however treated in Section 3 of this training in addition to other aspects of malaria. Other studies conducted in Nigeria had a wide range of intervention focus such as PMVs knowledge and perception regarding the ACT treatment [13], improving knowledge on Pharmacovigilance [14], Influence of training on community malaria treatment and practices [15], training of rural PMVs towards improving childhood malaria treatment / referral practices [16], and primary care training for medicine vendors in rural communities of Nigeria [17].

Many other intervention trainings regarding malaria were conducted in several different malaria prone countries such as Pakistan, Kenya and Tanzania [18–24], and each had a focus on improving the services of medicine vendors, but they all had different approaches, aspects of malaria being treated and modes of delivery of intervention.

In the course of developing this training manual, inputs were considered from many malaria intervention trainings and studies, almost all the studies considered tried to improve on the knowledge and practice of respondent [13–25], while only three studies improved and assessed attitudes of respondents [12, 15, 20]. This training module however tried to improve on all aspects of knowledge, attitudes and practices of the respondents using its problem-solving approach to facilitate understanding and thereby motivating trainees by using a combination of the techniques / strategies used by all these studies and hence consolidating on their successes.

The gains of a combination of strategies cannot be overemphasised, and this had led to great successes in the fight against malaria in many parts of the malaria endemic world leading to a WHO report claiming 1.5 billion malaria cases and 7.6 million deaths have been averted since the year 2000 [26]. The African countries which shouldered more than 90% of the overall disease burden in recent years had reduced its malaria death toll by 44%, from an estimated 680,000 to 384,000 annually [26]. However, for progress to be sustained, efforts have to be intensified, particularly in those countries with the highest burden of the disease despite the environmental, economic, political and other challenges discussed.

8. Conclusion

This paper puts forward a concise training module for everyday handlers of malaria cases in sub-Saharan Africa. The training module comprising the basics in the management of malaria such as basic information, its signs, symptoms/

diagnosis, its treatment, referral and prevention as was conceptually meant for the training of Patent Medicine Vendors but its relevance extends to all other categories of health providers tasked with managing malaria. The topics and contents treated had been carefully put together to cover the relevant aspects necessary to impact a required improvement in knowledge, attitudes and practices (KAP) of the trainees and other practicing healthcare providers alike. The emphasis placed on medicine vendors is rooted to the fact that they had long been identified as the most patronised and most commonly available group of healthcare providers within the sub-Saharan African region on malaria issues, hence any intervention on their KAP will hugely influence malaria epidemiology within the sub-region.

The peculiar mode of delivery of training used across the sections of the training module included presentation of lectures, demonstration exercises, differential diagnosis to distinguish malaria from other diseases with similar presentations, quizzes / brainstorming exercises such as question and answer sessions, empathy exercises, group discussions, handling of case studies, participation in role plays, and reflections on each module with the facilitators was conceptualised due to the realisation that the medicine vendors are deficient in their knowledge, attitudes and practices with respect to malaria handling, that the various methods employed have been proved to be effective in various stand-alone trainings and that collectively employing all the various methods used will strategically improve on the KAP generally.

Acknowledgements

The authors wish to acknowledge and show gratitude for the contributions and support received from the University Putra Malaysia and the Bauchi state University, Nigeria as we set out and successfully completed this work.

Conflict of interest

No conflict of interest declared.

Author details

Yahaya Mohammed Katagum[1]*, Hayati Binti Kadir Shahar[2], Faisal Bin Ibrahim[2], Anisah Baharom[2] and Rafee Baharudin[2]

1 Department of Clinical Pharmacy, Bauchi State University, Gadau, Nigeria

2 Department of Community Health, University Putra Malaysia (UPM), Selangor, Malaysia

*Address all correspondence to: mkyahaya@basug.edu.ng; mkyahaya07@gmail.com

References

[1] World Health Organization (2019). World Malaria Report 2019. Geneva: World Health Organization. Available online from: https://www.mmv.org/newsroom/publications/world-malaria-report-2019?gclid=CjwKCAiA5IL-BRAzEiwA0lcWYsMFrfPYpExF8PXa1lpUc7agUMNavyu_eAoYlZX-Wfft1W7lsCDdqRoCX3cQAvD_BwE

[2] Fatungase, K. O., Amoran, O. E., & Alausa, K. O. (2012). The effect of health education intervention on the home management of malaria among the caregivers of children aged under 5 years in Ogun state, Nigeria. European journal of medical research, 17(1), 11.

[3] Onwujekwe, O., Uzochukwu, B., Eze, S., Obikeze, E., Okoli, C., & Ochonma, O. (2008). Improving equity in malaria treatment: Relationship of socio-economic status with health seeking as well as with perceptions of ease of using the services of different providers for the treatment of malaria in Nigeria. Malaria Journal, 7(1)

[4] Berendes S, Adeyemi O, Oladele EA, Oresanya OB, Okoh F, Valadez JJ. (2012). Are patent medicine vendor's effective agents in malaria control? Using lot quality assurance sampling to assess quality of practice in Jigawa, Nigeria. PLoS One. 2012 Sep 12;7(9): e44775.7(9), e44775.

[5] World Health Organization. (2013). Facts Sheet on World Malaria Report; 2013. World Health Organisation, Geneva. Available online: http://www.who.int/malaria/publications/world_malaria_report_2013/en/

[6] FMH, (2008): National Malaria Control Programme. Strategic Plan 2009-2013, Federal Ministry of Health. Abuja, Nigeria

[7] WHO, (2013): Training Module on Malaria Control: Case Management – Guide for Tutors. 2012. World Health Organisation, Geneva. www.who.int

[8] FMH, (2005): National Antimalarial Treatment Policy 2005. National Malaria and Vector Control Division, Federal Ministry of Health. Abuja-Nigeria.

[9] FMH, (2012): Federal Ministry of Health. 2012. National Malaria Control Programme. Training Manuals on Case Management of Malaria at the Primary Health Care Center. Service Delivery: Module 2. Abuja, Nigeria.

[10] NVBDCP, (2012): Directorate of National Vector Borne Diseases Control Programme, Directorate General of Health Services, Ministry of Health and Family Welfare, India. http://nvbdcp.gov.in/Doc/MPW-training-module.pdf

[11] Yahaya, M.K., Hayati, K. S., and Faisal, I. (2017). Effectiveness of Malaria Intervention Programmes among Patent Medicine Vendors: A Systematic Review. Malaysian Journal of Medicine and Health Sciences (ISSN 1675-8544)

[12] Future Health Systems: Strengthening patent medicine vendors' associations in Nigeria for improved malaria management (SPANIMM, 2014). Accordia Global Health Foundation and west African infectious diseases institute. Phase 1 Final Report. June 2014.

[13] Chukwuocha UM, Nwakwuo GC, Mmerole I. Artemisinin-based combination therapy: Knowledge and perceptions of patent medicine dealers in Owerri Metropolis, Imo state, Nigeria and implications for compliance with current malaria treatment protocol. Journal of Community health. 2013 Aug 1; 38(4):759-765. DOI 10.1007/s10900-013-9676-y

[14] Awodele O, Adeniran A, Awodele DF. Pharmacovigilance amongst patent medicine vendors (PMVs) in Ekiti state, Nigeria. International Journal of Risk & Safety in Medicine. 2012 Jan 1; 24(2):65-72. DOI: 10.3233/JRS-2012-0562

[15] Livinus C, Ibrahim MO, Isezuo S, Bello SO. The impact of training on malaria treatment practices: A study of patent medicine vendors in Birnin-Kebbi. Sahel Medical Journal. 2009; 12 (2).

[16] Okeke TA, Uzochukwu BS. Improving childhood malaria treatment and referral practices by training patent medicine vendors in rural south-East Nigeria. Malaria Journal. 2009 Nov 20;8 (1):260. Doi: 10.1186/1475-2875-8-260

[17] Oshiname FO, Brieger WR. Primary care training for patent medicine vendors in rural Nigeria. Social science & medicine. 1992 Dec 1; 35(12): 1477-1484.

[18] Hussain A, Ibrahim MI, Malik M. Impact of educational intervention on knowledge of dispensers working at community pharmacies in Pakistan. Pharmacy practice. 2013 Jul; 11(3):144.

[19] Abuya T, Fegan G, Rowa Y, Karisa B, Ochola S, Mutemi W, et al. Impact of ministry of health interventions on private medicine retailer knowledge and practices on anti-malarial treatment in Kenya. The American journal of tropical medicine and hygiene. 2009 Jun 1; 80(6):905-913.

[20] Goodman CA, Mutemi WM, Baya EK, Willetts A, Marsh V. The cost-effectiveness of improving malaria home management: Shopkeeper training in rural Kenya. Health policy and planning. 2006 May 8; 21(4):275-288. doi:10.1093/heapol/czl011

[21] Marsh VM, Mutemi WM, Willetts A, Bayah K, Were S, Ross A, et al. Improving malaria home treatment by training drug retailers in rural Kenya. Tropical Medicine & International Health. 2004 Apr 1; 9(4): 451-460.

[22] Abuya TO, Fegan G, Amin AA, Akhwale WS, Noor AM, Snow RW, et al. Evaluating different dimensions of programme effectiveness for private medicine retailer malaria control interventions in Kenya. PLoS One. 2010 Jan 28; 5(1):e8937. doi:10.1371/journal.pone.0008937

[23] Tavrow P, Shabahang J, Makama S. Vendor-to-vendor education to improve malaria treatment by private drug outlets in Bungoma District, Kenya. Malaria Journal. 2003 May 7; 2(1):10.

[24] Nsimba SE. Assessing the impact of educational intervention for improving management of malaria and other childhood illnesses in Kibaha District-Tanzania. East Afr J Public Health. 2007 Apr 1; 4(1):5-11.

[25] Oshiname FO, Brieger WR. Primary care training for patent medicine vendors in rural Nigeria. Social science & medicine. 1992 Dec 1; 35(12): 1477-1484.

[26] World Health Organization (2020). World Malaria Report 2020. Geneva: World Health Organization. Available online from: https://reliefweb.int/report/world/world-malaria-report-2020

Section 4

Prevention, Vector Control and Vaccines

Chapter 14

Herding and Stampeding: The Albatross of Mosquito/Malaria Control

Francis S.O. Ugwu

Abstract

Malaria is lingering globally with 3.3 billion people at risk of infection and 1.2 billion others classified as high risk. The economic burden caused by the disease and vectors is humongous globally. The epicenter is Sub-Sahara Africa which accounts for 92% of the annual death burden of 435,000 of which 61% are children of less than five years. Result of elimination activities are manifest in all other WHO regions except in Sub-Sahara Africa where efforts to control the disease/vector bear unsatisfactory testimony. This worst case scenario in the region is the handiwork of weak governments and institutions that appear to lead control strategies by showiness via information media; but in reality, they are part of the albatross that stampede the processes. Remedying the situation would require multi-tactics including arm-twisting relevant authorities in Africa by the international community and knowledge-based actions by private individuals and communities to stem the tide.

Keywords: malaria control, mosquito control, Sub-Sahara Africa

1. Introduction

Malaria occurs in all six WHO regions where about 3.3 billion people are at risk of catching the infection or development of the disease and 1.2 billion others are considered as high risk persons [1]. WHO's 2018 report shows that 219 million cases of malaria occurred worldwide consequently causing 435,000 deaths with the weight concentrated in the WHO African Region which accounted for 92% of all malaria cases and children under 5 years accounting for 61% of all deaths [2]. Nigeria as the most populous country in the region also takes his fare share of the burden – most cases were suffered by Nigerians and about 25% of global deaths were also Nigerians [3]. The prevarications of climate may worsen the foregoing data. Sharma *et al*. [4] earlier observed that the impact of malaria could be stable but may not be abetted in years of intense precipitation and flooding. Moreover, there is heterogeneity in malaria prevalence [5] so may ameliorate or exacerbate the debility or fatality associated with it. Malaria could waver in strength at the local, regional and national level, becoming more resilient by acquisition of resistance which can enhance both vectors and parasites to take deep roots and diversify into various ecotypes [5]. The point being made here is that parasites and vectors could make use of opportunities offered by climate to make their effects more or less threatening to man.

Malaria is caused by protozoan parasites which are transmitted to humans when *Anopheles* mosquito feeds on man. *P. falciparum*, *P. vivax, P. ovale, P. malariae and P. knowelsi* are five *Plasmodium* species known to infect man. Each of the specie has peculiar distribution globally, for instance, *P falciparum* dominates in Sub Sahara Africa. Clinical manifestations vary among those five species. However, *Plasmodium falciparum* cause most of the global health problems. Most merozoites are produced by this specie so causes more severe fever, anaemia, mortality [6] and accounting for 99.7% cases in WHO African Region [2]. Apart from pain and suffering during illness and subsequent death that may follow malaria, the burden on the socio-economy especially in Sub Sahara Africa is colossal [2, 7, 8].

After the discovery of malaria parasite life cycle by Ross in 1897, man had been unyielding in her efforts to eradicate them. Unfortunately, the result is a pyrrhic victory without mosquito/malaria shifting significantly from its Sub Sahara Africa hub even though there are reports of almost malaria eradication in some countries [9, 10]. For every bus, there must be a driver and every herd of cattle there must be a herder; so in every manner of success that is recorded in diseases control, there must be a driver. In well organized societies, this responsibility lies squarely on governments. Others, such as non-governmental organizations and social groups, are also important components of a successful driving crew who mobilize secondary interested parties to lubricate the process. Wherever there are such synergist drivers, any diseases control programme will be successful in significantly reducing incidence of such disease. The kernel is that there must be effective governments to herd mosquito/malaria control programmes if malaria must be eliminated in Sub Sahara Africa.

What is the current situation in Nigeria? Here the government who is supposed to nurture all anti mosquito/malaria programmes turns out to be the albatross. This happens because some persons within the government hijack governments or government programmes and upturn every strategy targeted at malaria elimination. This they do by sabotaging the conceived vision and mission by the underhand activities they engage in to divert fund meant for such projects into their bottomless pockets. They misapply the processes/programmes that work elsewhere whether it is health care, politics, commerce, industry, economy, etc. The outcomes of their clandestine activities include but not limited to a divided nation almost perpetually prosecuting internecine wars with many fronts. Would the health care sector be different? It will not because you cannot sow the wind and not reap the whirl wind.

In this paper, we attempt to present evidence that, not minding all the crisis in Nigeria, governments do provide facilities and services that appear to move mosquito/malaria control in a positive direction strategically to minimize the troubles mosquitoes/malaria impose on us. However, what is gained by constructive government maneuvers is undermined by unfolding activities of the same government that ultimately would only exacerbate the damages inflicted on Nigerians by both vectors and parasites. This scenario informs the title of this paper about the treachery in certain quarters in conformity with the adage in our place that the person herding animals may be the same person who is stampeding them.

Further, we maintain that this jeopardy is redeemable if government could change tactics. We propose to canvass, in dancing to the dictates of a global village, that anomaly anywhere in the world could be perceived as anomaly everywhere else in the world that must be tackled. This treatise intends to provoke the International Community to look inwards so as to alter her compulsive lukewarmness in internal affairs of nations such as ours where leaders plunge citizens into unending squalor, diseases and poverty. The individual citizen would also be prompted to challenge mosquito/malaria by applying simple innovations which researchers in sub Sahara Africa had made to ameliorate the pangs of mosquito malaria.

2. Government herding mosquito/malaria control and showiness

In this section we use the term 'government' generically to mean any or all levels of governments. In Nigeria there are three levels: federal, state and local governments. There is only one Federal Government which seats in Abuja, the capital city of Nigeria. The second tier consists of 36 state governments with their respective capitals spread across the country. Abuja is also the seat of the Federal Capital Territory that operates as a quasi state with its own paraphernalia of government structures. Lastly, the local governments, which number up to 774 across the federation with their respective headquarter and structure of government. We briefly consider here how government had been in the forefront in the fight against mosquitoes and malaria (**Figure 1**), albeit with showiness.

As far back as 1899, the importance of having a passionate government mounting the driver seat of mosquito/malaria control was demonstrated in Lagos. The government was led by a chief executive in the person of William MacGregor who was appointed by the Colonial Office (London) as Governor of Lagos. According to Oluwasegun [11], he was on transfer from Queensland, Australia, and he had considered Lagos a graveyard like his peers from Europe who knew that environmental

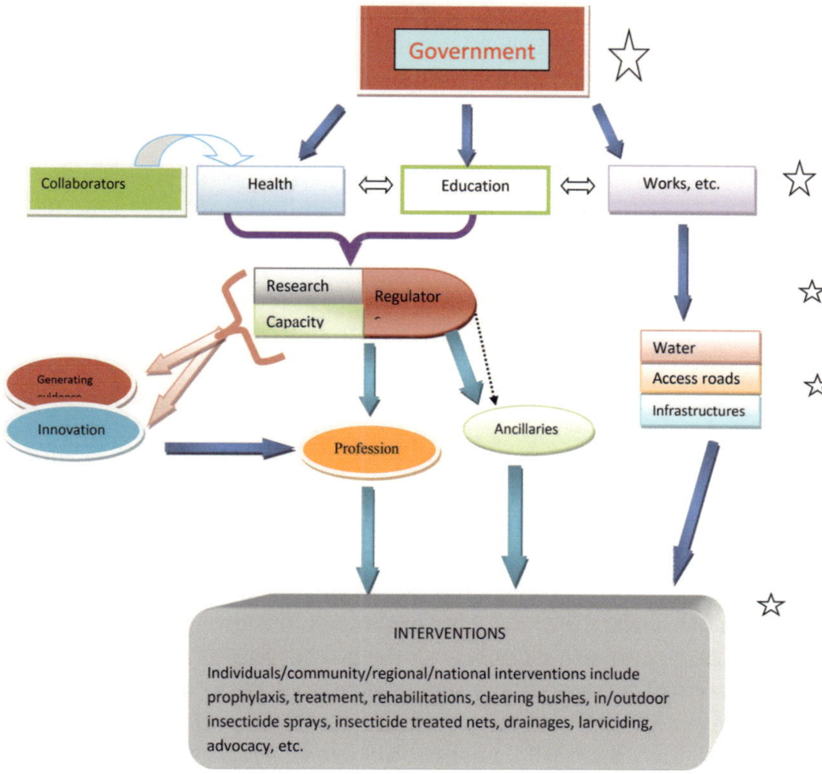

Figure 1.
Organizational framework for malaria/mosquito control based interventions. Government control is via the ministries such as Ministry of Health, Ministry of Education, etc. that are all interconnected and interwoven. Collaborators include donors, international agencies such as UNICEF/UNDP/World Bank, WHO, TDR, etc. The Nigerian state of anomie under President Buhari has highlighted security (which is normally not considered as a factor of consequence), represented by the star, is now the sine qua non or primus inter pares before any form of activity, whether as infrastructure, goods or service delivery can be embarked upon as it must superintends all government anti-malaria programs. Security became more pervasive following the emergence of criminals and fanatical religious terrorist group like Boko Haram. Ancillary refers to all other professions and their products that governments allow. The arrows pointing to it indicate both weak and strong controls: strong control via such agency as NAFDAC, weak control of native doctors, bone setters, patent medicine practitioners etc.

factors compelled it to be one of the most infamous mosquito-breeding locations on the West African Coast. As he arrived Lagos, he was confronted with a horrible statistics: malaria mortality was 71.12/1000 European population in 1898 and rose up to 87.64/1000 two years later. Consequently he decided to eliminate mosquitoes from Lagos so as to get rid of malaria. He had been advised to approach the matter by segregating the population on racial grounds, a proposal he refused to acknowledge because it would not benefit the colonialist on the long run economically and would trigger opposition from the highly educated elites in Lagos then. He perceived that there was no racial segregation and that allowing natives to live with their more enlightened Europeans would offer them education which was vital to checkmate mosquitoes/malaria. Lastly he considered it unwise to start any form of racism rather his idea was: destroy mosquito breeding, make certain modern sanitation, educate the natives on the risk of mosquitoes and the management of malaria. He began sustaining a malaria-free Lagos via land reclamation. In fact, he reclaimed the Elegbeta and Idumagbo creeks and built the MacGregor Canal.

Today, the approach to mosquito/malaria control is not different from the measures Governor William MacGregor introduced more than a century ago. He emphasized education which is still what present day researchers [12, 13] also arrived at after applying their mathematical model which states that change in human conduct (following acquisition of knowledge) will significantly reduce the burden of disease like malaria in places where the level of education is soaring; not like areas with deprived education where the disease persist. They recommended that massive and continuous health education should be combined with other forms of interventions for all persons staying within the area assaulted with malaria. The government had been unrelenting in building public schools. She also allows private schools to blossom such that today, we have lost count of the number of primary, secondary and tertiary institutions across the nation. In all these schools students are taught how to deal with mosquito/malaria. One veritable way education has helped in reducing the menace of mosquito/malaria is housing. Research has established that reduction in malaria burden and improvement in health status is attributed to health education and improved houses [14, 15]. Throughout Nigeria and particularly in Southern Nigeria, houses are so modernized that mosquitoes' entry into houses, to some extent, are excluded. In my locality thatched and mud houses had disappeared and every house built in the last 10 years has an intact ceiling in place. This implies that fewer mosquitoes get access to humans within because the usual eaves route for *Anopheles* is effectively blocked [16–19].

The government is also involved in building health centres where the sick are treated and nursed back to life. They are organized into primary, secondary and tertiary health care centres/hospitals with the last serving as schools where health care professionals are grounded. Primary care centres are located nearly in every large community today to offer the most basic health care services directed at prevention of infective diseases. These centres are also involved in distribution of drugs such as evermectin, immunization and bednets as well as treatment of uncomplicated malaria and counseling pregnant women. Secondary health centres consist of 'general hospital' where patients are given much more detailed attention. Some laboratory investigations are obtainable here as well as minor surgical services. Pregnant women gain better attention and knowledge of mosquitoes/malaria is deepened here. Tertiary hospitals offer all the foregoing services which could not be handled at the primary and secondary centres. The best of all health care professionals are concentrated here and the government designates some of them 'centre of excellence' where state of the art services and equipment are available. Governments spend a lot of money. One example of the extent of fiscal spending will suffice. The Federal Ministry of Health 2016 Appropriation Act in Naira showed that personnel cost 217,472,115,158; overhead was 3,940,432,929; capital expenditure was 28,650,342,987; while total allocation summed up to 250,062,891,075. In 2017, the various governments (federal, state and local) contributed 8% of 1.7 trillion Naira expended on malaria [20]. Governments pays for all these to support health in addition to payment through other ministries such as scholarship for students elsewhere who may end up joining the fight against malaria control such as doctors, engineers, epidemiologist, etc. who train abroad. However, government sometimes authorizes charging of minimal fees to augment running cost of health care generally [21].

Beyond building of schools, hospitals and health centres, government from time to time allow programmes designed as morale booster to mosquito and malaria control to be. One of the most popular ways this was accomplished was through the Roll Back Malaria partnership designed to achieve universal protection to all persons at risk by using appropriate interventions for prevention and treatment [22, 23]. In **Table 1**, we show some of the projects that had been popularized by direct and indirect involvement of government. She also puts in place organogram which allocate responsibilities among stake holders [24]. Government also pays for malaria management and public health jingles or allows commercial interests some space to canvass for customers throughout the country. Nowadays, both manufacturers of plant based medicines and those from numerous pharmaceutical companies (foreign and local) are allowed by governments to market their wares without hindrance. Local patent medicine stores are also allowed to proliferate and are therefore accessible to Nigerians within trekable distances.

There are also other government activities which focus on healthcare generally. Such programmes ultimately benefic malaria sufferers or indirectly assist malaria/mosquito control. The National Agency for Food Drug Administration and Control (NAFDAC) is one of such agency of the Federal Ministry of Health (**Figure 1**). The agency did a lot work to create awareness on the issue of fake, substandard, expired and adulterated drugs [25]. The agency does more work beyond the foregoing. She also monitors feedback from consumers the effects or adverse drug reactions of the drugs she permitted to be in circulation [26]. **Table 2** shows other indirect ways the governments enhance malaria/mosquito control. Most importantly, the agency had upgraded the people's knowledge that ordinary peasants must look for the "NAFDAC number" before they could pay for any medicine from the drug store or "Chemist" as they are popularly known here. All the measures above prove that government in principle is desirous of affordable, accessible and sustainable malaria/mosquito control.

We have seen that government erect physical buildings for health care services including malaria treatment. It has been observed that every successive government builds more and more houses. No incoming administration wants to build on the foundation left by his predecessor [21, 30]. The reason is for showmanship – so that the peasants would point at structures built by x's government. Such buildings soon after commissioning become just prescription houses where even asprin could not be dispensed as at when due. Such building soon get underutilized, abandoned or become overgrown with grass. Closer enquiries show that those in governments use the opportunities for awarding building contracts as avenue for looting public funds and extorting cutback from contractors.

Government control most local radio stations and citizens are inundated with the usual copious jingles of her activities ad nauseam. During the Roll Back Malaria episode, government jingles saturated the air waves that nearly everyone became away that free mosquito nets were being distributed. So when interested persons flock to the so called centre of distribution, only a hand full of bednets would be

S/no	Government Control programmes	Period	Activities executed	Observations	References
1	National Malaria control Programme (NMCP) Strategic plan 2009–2013	2009–2013	About 17 million ITNs were distributed during 2005–2007,	Only enough for 23% population	[20]
2	Procurement of artesunsate combination therapy (ACT)	2006 2007	4.5 million courses distributed. 9 million courses distributed	Far below total requirement	[20]
3	Roll Back Malaria (RBM) Initiative	2000–2005	Case management, promotion of intermittent preventive treatment (IPT), and promotion of the use of ITNs/vector management	Resistance to Chloroquine, and subsequently Sulphadoxine-Pyrimethamine (SP)	[20]
4	Topical Disease Research (TDR)	in 2006	Home management and community directed models for malaria treatment		[20]
5	Agencies like UNICEF and the Federal Ministry of Health		Propagating the distribution of these effective and long lasting ITNs to primary health centers		[20]
6	Closing up community land ponds and borrow pits				[20]
7	Spraying oil over stagnant water bodies				[20]
8	National Malaria Elimination Programme (NMEP		NMEP) is responsible for policy making and articulating broader strategies and coordination at the country level	Implementation done by state governments	[22]

Table 1.
Some malaria control programmes.

given to the selected few after prolonged delays and excuses. The reality was that the "*oga* at the top" had compromised the programme by diverting allocated mosquito nets to their accomplices who would now sell them unhindered in local market at exorbitant prices thereby making the nets unavailable to target population [31]. This may account for why some respondents in several studies angrily antagonize poor nurses at their duty post in such distribution centres without comprehending

S/no.	Activities of government	References
1	The enactment of the National Health Act, 2014. for the regulation, development and management of a National Health System, and to put in place a standard for rendering health services in Nigeria.	[27, 28]
2	The National Health Financing Policy and National Health Policy are designed to ensure universal access to health by stating mode of raising fund for the different levels of governments and to ensure fund allocation to the health sector increased up to 15% of total budget and support to primary health care (PHC).	[27, 29]
3	Creation of NAFDAC to regulate the production, distribution, sale, use of drugs and ancillary products as well as monitoring of adverse reactions.	[21, 25, 26]
4	The National Health insurance scheme (NHIS) promotes openness and more access to health to privileged minority who secure employment in the organized sector.	[21, 27, 29, 30]
5	Former president Obasanjo introduced the health sector reform to make health care accessible, equitable and congenial.	[21]

Table 2.
Indirect ways government improves malaria control.

the underhand deals that made nets not to reach those they were made for [31, 32]. If government was serious, they have all the tools at their disposal that can be put in place to ensure that pilfering of bednets cannot happen anywhere in Nigeria.

Sometimes in the past, adverts relating to health care in Nigeria were aired in American or European based media. This makes one wonder what the government or relevant institution was up to. How could such presstitution benefit Nigerians who do not have access to electricity or television sets? Even if they had, why were such adverts not placed in local media to save cost? The showmanship accompanying simple public health programme as launching a public health campaign in remote communities attracting a governor with scores of exotic jeeps and retinue of state officials, security men and politicians are simply avenue for pilfering scarce government funds because everyone who attended such fanfare would be "mobilized," euphemism for buying/bribing participants, and core civil servants who participated would be paid handsome allowances. Fraudulent commissioning programmes by government have come to be an innovative mass deception method which deepens the corruption in the system. There was an incident when a borehole was "commissioned" in a community in Udenu Local Government Area where the water seen gushing out was actually from a hidden tank somewhere! Another such "commission" was made in 2001 by no less a person than the President of the Federal Republic of Nigeria of a bore hole located in Ozalla Ezimo, a nearby community close to Obollo Afor town, that was already operational before his regime. Obasanjo, the then president came with more than 5 hundred security men and more than a thousand politicians and hangers on. Their coming arrested most economic activities in Nsukka Senatorial Zone during the period. The money spent on such frivolous visit could have been spent to prosecute the war against mosquitoes and the diseases they hawk.

3. Government as albatross stampeding mosquito/malaria control

Malaria/mosquito control can stand as the best project for health that any government in Nigeria and the rest of Sub Sahara Africa should prosecute for national/global health [33]. Governor William MacGegor embraced that concept profoundly and embarked on mosquito control with all his might. Unfortunately, his approach was abandoned soon after he took ill a few years from the time he built the canal [11]. In the past 20 years, the regime of Olushegun Obasanjo (1999–2007) was pro education and pro malaria control. His immediate successor, Musa Yaradua (2007–2010) was not healthy enough to manifest his inclination. The subsequent government of Goodluck Jonathan (2010–2015) appeared to boost education more but less so for malaria control than that of Obasanjo. The regime of Buhari (2015 – date) is a disaster for both education and mosquito/malaria control. Pregnant women and under five years children are predisposed to malaria and they suffer high mortality rate also [2, 3]. However, only 1% increase in budgetary allocation to the health sector could engender reduction of 10% of infant mortality and generally improve health outcome [34]. His government consistently scored below the mark in attaining universal health coverage provision to allocate 15% of budget to the health sector. Even when compared to other less endowed countries in west Africa such as Ghana, Gambia, Gabon and Niger, she is at the bottom [35]. Facilities at primary, secondary and tertiary hospitals are derelict; about 700 medical facilities are said to be destroyed in conflict zone. This may explain why medical tourism, even to neighbouring West African countries, is vast developing [28].

One would have expected an upsurge in malaria as a result of this gaping neglect of mosquito/malaria control during his presidency but it seems that act of God – weather conditions, willingness to survive with the residual knowledge of malaria control (use of herbs, clearing bushes, etc) may have come to the rescue of Nigerians. This is reflected in the slowing down of malaria according to WHO's record [3]. This implies that citizens are willing to contain malaria if only there is effective government support/leadership. Every government ought to be targeting malaria elimination; and according to Campbell and Steketee [33], such government must make supervision, diagnostic capacity, monitoring, and evaluation systems that is accessible and of high quality to provide timely information as cardinal requirements. So long as governments refuse to implement accepted practices of mosquito/malaria control or ignore morale boosting programmes like Roll Back Malaria, so long we would have malaria with us.

The poor performance of vector control in Nigeria is squarely attributable to whosoever is on the driver's seat. This brings the ball on the table of our leaders. It does appear that when you consider how they go about acquisition and execution of power, you would shudder. Regarding animal herder (among sheep), the Catholic Bishop of Nsukka, Fr Bishop Onah Godfrey, in a popular metaphor, said that a sheep at the rear was asked where it was being led to and it replied that the leader (herder) knows where. In the case of Nigerians, no one can vouch for our political leaders in government who used *mago-mago* (morally reprehensible means) to attain power. This author had considered their behavior like fixing their own salaries, which range between 25–30 million Naira a month, but refusing to pay 18,000 Naira minimum wage, as the pacemaker of the imbroglio raging in the country today. It is also the root of all labour unrest in the country since 1999. As at the end of November 2020, federal universities still remained closed since March 2020 to students because of mode of payment of academic staff salaries and underfunding university education. The health sector is always embroiled in strikes over payment of salaries or allowances. There would be no industrial action if there is no significant difference in the pay packet of the President and a cleaner with all other professions/workers adjusted in between accordingly. Nigerian leaders designed Nigeria for corruption so the endless catastrophe citizens suffer is the outcome of the design. In this context, mosquito and malaria control cannot be detached from all other sectors crying for attention.

DOI: http://dx.doi.org/10.5772/intechopen.96917

The present Nigerian government-citizen relationship is not different from that between the *Sarcoptes scabiei* and the dog. No matter how loud or long one shouted at the dog parasite, it will continue to suck life out of its dog host. Clearly, our leaders in government are not different from the dog parasite. In trying to rationalize why our leaders behave that way, this author was stunned by the fact that the same malaria parasites may be the remote cause why our leaders outdo parasites in exacting maximal pressure on hapless Nigerian citizens while they themselves are well ensconced in Abuja and state capitals or junketing across the globe with their families. We know that malaria parasite is a multi system parasite and it also inhabits the brain and do cause cerebral malaria. It could also camouflage itself from immune surveillance. In simple terms, it seems to enjoy some high degree of immunity that it could remain arrested in man for a long period – the same way Nigerian politicians are immuned from being accountable. It is not preposterous to suggest that it could trade genes with the host to hijack some of the host's physiological processes. Hijacking has been reported in a number of host–parasite relationships and it

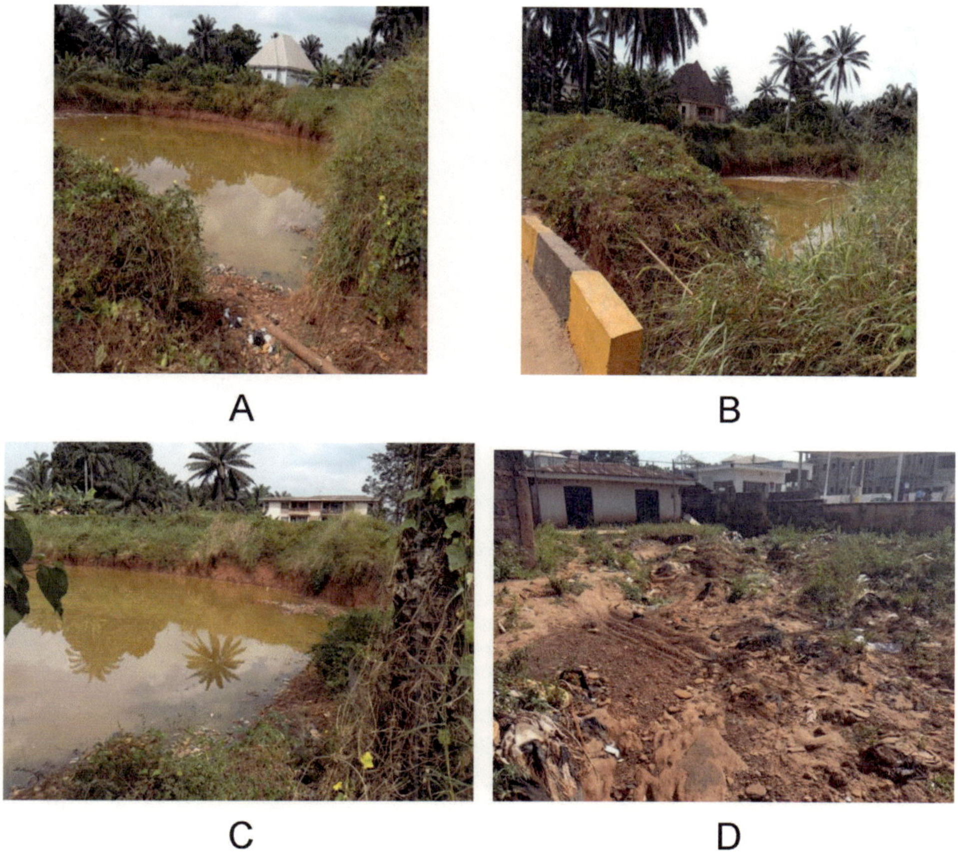

Figure 2.
Unintended consequences of flood control. (A–C) shows a pond in a residential area with houses around it. Closer look will show plastic containers as well as vegetation which provide perfect mosquito breeding milieu. The back ground story was that more than 25 years ago, the borrow pit was dug to drain Ugwuoye part of Enugu Road, Nsukka by the Local Government. Years later, the borrow pit could no longer drain the area because the government could not supervise builders who blocked the natural water ways. When that part of Enugu Road became impassable, the Enugu State Government came to the rescue by building a tunnel to drain the water which flooded the road and the rest of Ugwuoye. The deluge from the tunnel eventually sacked all the people living in the houses shown in (D). Whenever it rained, the University Road, which receives water from the place shown eroded in (D) become impassable such that cars, motor cycles and their riders were carried away. About 5 persons were said to have lost their lives to the flood since the tunnel was completed.

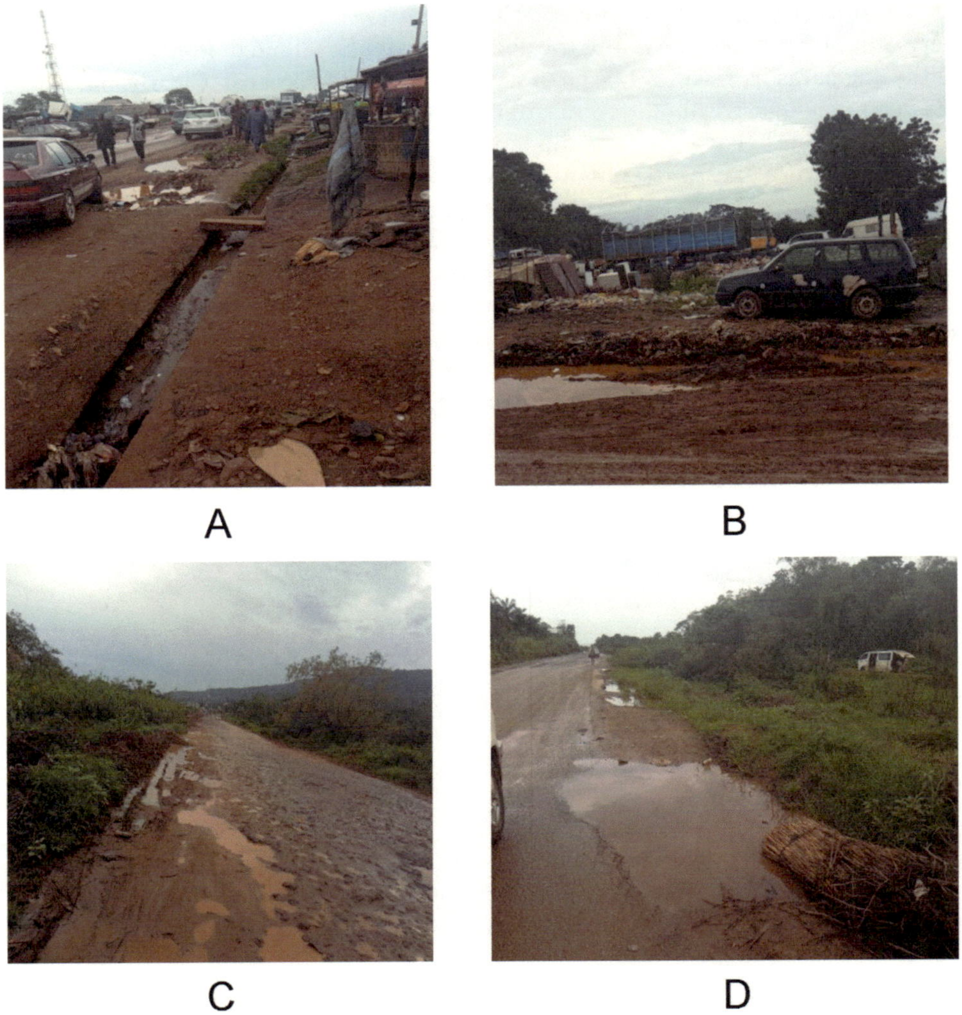

Figure 3.
A section of Enugu – Port-Harcourt Express Road, Lokpanta, Imo State. This section of the road reveal typical South Eastern Nigerian road that is supposed to be maintained by the Federal Government headed by President Mohammed Buhari. The failure of government to be functional created the observed collection of water, blocked drain, mud, solid wastes, grass, stuck vehicles, used tyres and squalid environment all of which provide perfect environment for mosquito breeding and optimized malaria transmission (A–D).

may not be different in man. Thus our leaders' have been modified to behave like parasites. And in our case, the bad policies of our leaders in governments ultimately assist parasites like *P. falciparum* to thrive.

The generation of solid waste is another albatross of malaria control. Tons of solid waste from plastics significantly impact on preponderance of mosquitoes in our country. These plastics are indiscriminately dumped in the streets, roads and into drains [36] and as shown in **Figures 2** and **3**. Solid wastes provide thousand of micro water bodies ideal for the breeding for *Anopheles*, *Aedes* and other pathogenic species of mosquitoes. When these materials are dumped on drainage they block drains and larger water bodies are formed where more mosquitoes and other pathogens would profusely breed. It is reported that when weed accompany plastics and solid wastes that malaria and its vector increase significantly [36]. What does it take to deal with solid wastes as thin sheet polyethylene? Legislation: ban them! Kenya did it [37, 38]. Large population in urban and cities throughout Nigeria is related to development of slum areas that quickly generate heaps of garbage ideal for mosquito breeding, though Nwani and Ozegbe [39] indicate that per capita/kg/annum generation is low at 204 when compared to South Africa at 730 and Ghana at 33. Such large populations not matched by increased health spending spell doom for Nigerians [34]. Given the present circumstances of funding health system, attaining competence, equity, quality and sustainable health care, financial risk security for all citizens cannot be accomplished [30].

Governments encourage trading of blames among health workers and between health workers and patients. The perennial problem in the health sector where one group of health care provider is over elevated beyond the others is a divide and rule tactics that truly undermine health care services generally and mosquito/malaria control in particular. The problems in health sector seem to be the typical fruits of corruption. The resulting very poor performances are reflected in the compendium of indicators of an ailing health sector that has nothing positive to show [40]. This sector is rife with strikes [41–43], inter-professional rivalry [44], arrogance [45], etc. All these impose unnecessary man made burden on citizens. **Table 3** shows a compendium of governments' activities which ultimately stampede malaria/mosquito control.

S/No.	Action/inaction exacerbating malaria/mosquito control	References
1	Poor allocation to healthcare: far less than the 13–15% of total budget recommended is routinely disbursed to the Federal Ministry of Health*	[20, 21, 28, 34, 35]
2	Very low health expenditure per capita: In 2017 it was US $74 less than what is recommended.	[20]
3	Neglect of primary health care (PHC) † The healthcare facilities at the Primary Health Care (PHC) level are inadequate and poorly maintained.	[20, 21, 27–29]
5	Lack of water, road, electricity, etc. Poor access roads (especially in the South East Nigeria), for example, make it difficult for patients to obtain even the paltry health care available at the nearest health care centre whether it is primary, secondary or tertiary.	[28]
6	The average health facility to population ratio is low and worse in rural areas: doctor to patient ratio, for example, is much lower than the WHO minimum standard of 1:600.	[21, 27, 34]
7	Over concentration of health facilities in cities and urban areas as a result of skewed budgetary allocation/implementation.	[21, 27, 34]
8	Government policies induce poverty: Nigeria has the highest population of extreme poverty worldwide. This was not so during pre-independence and up to early 1980s.	[21, 27, 34]
9	Not using supportive/multidisciplinary/ demand-driven models such as those of TDR to do/mirror/translate research findings of local researchers to interventions. Not strengthening research capacity in critical areas.	[46, 47]
10	Environmental/public health inspector disappearance since the 1960s.¶	Personal observation.
11	Government appears to be deceiving her citizens, the International Community and international institutions such as WHO: Government abdicates related convention she is signatory to: Nigeria allocated, between 2009–2013, as little as 3.7–5.7% of national budget instead of the 13% recommended by WHO.	[27, 29]
12	Lack of continuity, consistency and commitment (3Cs) to laid down policies, programmes and projects thereby leading to poor access to health, unemployment and poverty.	[21, 30]
13	Lack of harnessing low cost health facility from native doctors, traditional healers, etc.	[21]

S/No.	Action/inaction exacerbating malaria/mosquito control	References
14	Not making dialogue an art of governance and very poor crime management: these incapacitate families/communities from fending for themselves.⁺	[21]
15	Hospitals/health centres are without safe water, electricity, functioning equipment, adequate supply of drugs, basic diagnosing machines such as scanning and X-ray machines etc.	[28, 30]
16	Ill motivated and unsupported healthworkers	[28]
17	Uneven distribution of health care personnel	[28]
18	General insecurity and attacks on healthworkers especially in conflict zones.	[28]
19	Condoning dual loyalty of health workers who work for government and use the opportunity to divert patients from public health facilities to their private businesses.	[28]

∞Government here refers to the Nigerian Federal Government. The states and local governments mirror the federal in most of the listed activities.
**The Presidential Summit on Universal Health Coverage made the Abuja declaration that mandates member states to allocate 15% of national budget to the health sector, but the reality is that lees than half (7.4%) was available in 2014. The Federal Ministry Health indicated that 40% of health budget is expended on malaria [20].*
†PHC receive less than 10% of health budget, yet from the little, 84% is spent on non-PHC amenities [27]. Sub-optimal PHC services spell doom for up-coming generation. This negligence is akin to '10/90 disequilibrium' principle where 90% of fund is spent on 10% of less vulnerable people [48].
⁺Government by condoning insurrection as occasioned by Boko Haram, criminals and Fulani herdsmen (who insist on roaming with their cattle all over the country) engage in countless killings, abductions, ransoms taking, displacing communities, destroying crop farmers and their crops, etc. creates the environment for festering of diseases and their vectors.
¶This author's mother told him that before Nigeria's independence, health inspectors used to visit every compound to access the degree of hygiene and mosquito control compliance. "They used to check every soup pot and every clay pot used as water reservoir to ensure that they were properly covered," she said. This author had never seen, nor his home visited by such inspector since after the civil war in 1970.

Table 3.
Some activities of government which ultimately stampede malaria/mosquito control∞.

4. Why international arm-twisting tactics will improve malaria control

The International Community is sometimes perceived as a guard who stands by when a toddler engages in fireworks in a compound full of people living in thatched houses during the harmattan. The toddler lights the first house, second, third and the guard continue to look on until all the houses are completely burnt down. Then, the guard would begin to attend to charred victims and survivors and corpses. Which is cheaper – to arrest the child before he lit the houses or after? The International Community must have to reshuffle her rules that hitherto had relegated her to a passive onlooker when catastrophes come knocking under the guise of "non interference in the internal affair of member nations." For too long, she had been silent when leaders of third world countries plant strife, nurture them until they mature to genocides resulting in massive drifting of refugees from one part of the world to another. This mass movement of people evading conflicts is the same as mass movement of diseases and vectors across borders.

All the nations of the world, referred to as "The International Community" must by now be amenable to some of the lessons of Covid-19: no nation is isolated from emergent diseases and no nation could predict the spreading dynamics, morbidity and mortality of such diseases. The consequent plunging of both developed and developing nations into losing high numbers of their citizens and severe economic recession inflicted on those who survived the onslaught of Covid-19 is a lesson no one should forget. What if mosquitoes/malaria parasites should mutate and re-establish themselves as the terror they were in the days of William Mac Gregor? So all nations must begin to see health related problem anywhere in the world as a global problem that must be tackled in unison so that diseases cannot be allowed to spread.

Malaria mortality had been with Sub Sahara Africa for ages. The WHO had been publishing annual reports where numbers of deaths due to malaria are clearly shown. The International Community may have been regarding those figures as mere numbers probably because they revolved mainly in Africa whose primitive leaders unabashedly undermine their own people as it pleased them. Stopping these bad leaders is also stopping the means of generating poverty, diseases and their vectors which are not fixed but highly mobile and could spread like HIV and Covid-19.

5. Knowledge-based measures by citizens and communities to control mosquito/malaria

Knowledge based actions against malaria control is very effective in controlling mosquitoes and managing all infectious and insect borne diseases. It is also vital to controlling the vectors as had been noted and applied by Governor William MacGregor since malaria life cycle became known [11]. According to a report [20], Nigerians are already picking the gauntlet as they paid 87.8% of the 1.7 trillion Naira spent on malaria in 20 17 (excluding unquantified amounts expended paying bill from native doctors or purchasing native herbs). This is a veritable proof they could fend for themselves to rid the land of the disease and could do more if the environment is right. Knowledge based control measure evolved following the works of researchers all over the world. In Nigeria, research output in this direction is not deficient. Nigerian Universities, despite all the stumbling blocks erected by governments, continue to look inwards to find solution that will work for us for he who wears the shoe knows where it pains. Local researchers had been able to generate so much for malaria/mosquito control but are hampered by the following:

1. Civil servants follow instructions passed unto them by their superiors who are actually politicians. This author had developed several devices that could be used to control mosquitoes in-house [17–19] which are innovations that ought to attract enthusiasm by those whose responsibility it was to control malaria/mosquitoes in the Ministry of Health but he was told that window screen was not part of their job description: they were paid to disseminate bednet not window net!

2. Nigerian policy makers had been so brainwashed that they do not accept anything being projected by local researchers. Going by some informal anecdotes researchers share among themselves, they greet researchers with skepticism and scorn. They look for those packaged in Europe, China or America. They prefer importing antimalarials from China or India rather than provide the environment that would enable our own people develop them from our own resources which abound. So doing enable them to loot government treasury as they please while citizens are kept below poverty line and too poor to ask for any form of accountability from our leaders.

3. This author checked the website of the National Malaria Elimination Programme (nmcp.gov.ng/integrated-vector-management/). They had beautiful vision and mission statements regarding mosquito/malaria control. Of all the measures enunciated, door screening and window screen are conspicuously absent. Yet this government agency knows that people do not sleep in bednets because of many constraining factors [49] as only 9.7% of households own them [32], and that people misuse them [50]. Only 3.9% of pregnant women

sleep in bednets [32]. They ought to have known that house screens covers all house hold members and protect for other neglected tropical diseases [51] and devoid of all the problems associated with bednets. House screening is enforceable by the state [17]. However, if they allowed home based control devices to thrive, it could block their channel of affluence because they would not be importing nets, drugs, insecticides, etc. massively to checkmate mosquito/malaria. If the National Malaria Elimination Programme really mean to improve the people's knowledge of malaria/vector control, they would have been using their web site to inform people of current publications from local researchers that provide simple accessible, affordable and sustainable solutions that anyone could copy and apply for himself such as the ones provided for house screening [17–19].

4. The refusal by those in authority to accept new information unveiled by researchers on control measures such as insecticides could sometimes be bewildering. They apparently have negative bias against new ideas when confronted with uncertainty [52]. They had hitherto been captivated by old things they know about insecticide that any other unfolding developments are ignored. For instance, if they were initially taught that dichlorodiphenyltrichloroethane (DDT) was very good in controlling insect vector, they would be fixated with that idea and discountenance any other contrary findings that question the status quo. Informing such persons that perceived benefits of insecticides as option to tackle mosquitoes is only short lived would only provoke them to anger or alerting them on increasing reduction of *mosquito* susceptibility to insecticides such as organophosphates, organochlorine and carbamates [2, 53–55] could make them bark at you menacingly. Seriously, mosquitoes quickly acquire resistance to the foregoing insecticide that just after a few years, they would no longer be effective deterrent. Other unpalatable consequences insecticides create are environmental contamination, ecological imbalance, harm to human and animals, environment pollution, non-target organisms being affected [56, 57]. The narrative does not stop just there. As time goes on strains of mosquitoes which would even depend on the insecticide to spread to regions they were not found before would arise [58]. Therefore the best approach to deal with mosquitoes in Sub Sahara Africa is to pressure them to change their habit such that, owing to consistent denial of blood meals to them, they would change habit. Long term denial to access human blood would certainly push them to find an alternative, that is, we could habituate them to be independent of human blood meals.

6. Conclusions and recommendations

This paper, through the number of instances provided, had shown that the beginning and end of malaria/mosquito control lies in the hands of governments and persons in government in Nigeria (and everywhere mosquito/malaria are found and Nigerian-like leaders exist). They, through acts of omission and commission work in both directions, the net result being the abetment of malaria transmission, mosquito endurance and escalation of poverty and economic losses in Sub Sahara Africa, the hub of the duo, *Anopheles* species and *Plasmodium falciparum*. Looking at the Tables (1, 2 & 3), it can be inferred that what had been done to cage malaria/mosquitoes is little compared to what is yet to be done. However, we now know that some interventions can be done at various levels including the individual, community, government, collaborators and the International Community.

Now that Covid-19 has changed the game, the time has come when the International Community should focus her lenses on Sub-Sahara Africa where emerging leaders from the region must be given mosquito/malaria reduction targets which they must attain to remain in power. That is to say that who remains in power must be that leader who places global public health first among all other needs. The community must do something serious about impunity of seating governments such as the Buhari's government in Nigeria where killings is the order of the day for years and culprits are not brought to book despite the aphorism credited to the former military leader (General Abach) that the government herself must be complicit in any insurrection that exceeds 48 hours. The International Community should make an enactment that would compel seating presidents face trial in the Hague when laid down expectations are not met anywhere in the world.

The usual practice where governments in developing countries beg for more grants, loans, assistance, donations, etc. ad nauseam, which the International Community obliges them, should be re-examined. In the case of Nigeria, the earlier all the foregoing are denied her, the better. This is because all those kind gestures are misused and only end up beefing up the pockets of greedy men in governments. Those helps do not make way for sustainable long term mosquito/malaria control [24]. Our penchants for begging do bore down donor and fatigue them [33]. Sometimes it is morally wrong to give. This applies to Nigeria because she has all the resources she needs to control malaria and pathogenic mosquitoes, be it intellectual, manpower, fiscal, natural or learned capacity. There are thus required changes that must be made to turn things over to improve health financing if Nigeria must come under the universal health coverage. Such changes must include legal and regulatory frameworks, efficient use of resources through carefully planned purchasing provisions and stringent supervision [30].

Doctors claim they own the patients [45] and they must control all health institution and determine who gets what in the health sector; whereas the other health workers claim it is a team work. Government could have decided this issue long ago: either the health sector is turned to a single profession through redesigning their education and training or the health sector is organized strictly as in the game of football where the captain can be anyone in the team who has something to show as a leader. To root out mosquito/malaria, all health care professionals must work optimally and there must be no industrial action for whatever reason. There should also be no half measures in managing conflict in the health sector. According to the 2014 National Health Law, 14 days was to be allowed to resolve labour related issues resulting in strikes [28]. However, it must be borne in mid that a minute is too long to strike in the sector because, as small as the interval may seem, many lives could be lost within that interval in a country with large population such as Nigeria. So government must enable such environment by creating it using all the tools at her disposal. She could foster congenial relationships among all health workers by training them to imbue them with appropriate communication skills to be motivators rather than inhibitors [32]. There is the need for government to begin seriously to fashion two professions – lawyers and doctors to work entirely for the public by disallowing them any form of private practice. This will engender justice, peace and health, the ingredients required for sustainability development.

We indicated earlier that Buhari's government, initially voted in to fight corruption, is a disaster for education and malaria control. Under his watch, corruption grew wings and began to "fight back" ferociously such that the government has become the undisputed global gold medalist for accumulating corruption since 2015. The children of corruption under Buhari's watch in the health sector include but not limited to unmaintained utilities, infrastructures, equipment; fake, adulterated, substandard, expensive drugs; supply of "made in China" equipment and consumables; stealing government time/money by subterfuge or outright stealing/ diversion of materials and drugs; contract inflation; selective justice; cash-based instead of qualification and proficiency-based recruitment etc. [21, 28].

It is acknowledged that bills from medical tourism amounted to 359.2 billion Naira in 2018 expended mostly by public office holders and their families, clear 18.75 billion Naira higher than the health budget [28]. It is clear from the foregoing that the health budget is deliberately kept low to pave way for politicians and their collaborators. Beyond the foregoing is the shocking finding by research that every health funding apparatus in Nigeria are performing far below what is expected and that funds are not equitably allocated nor used to significantly reduce wastage, meaning that only inferior/substandard facilities/services could be what await most Nigerians thereby exposing them to unbridled high cost of health expenditures [30]. The implication is that very little is generated and that little is misused, mismanaged, stolen or wasted thus aggravating the already very bad access to health care facilities and services.

It is possible to solve Nigeria's corruption problem. One of the ways of solving problems could sometimes be to approach them from an absurd perspective. This is what this author refers to as "Sir Peter Egbo's solution." Peter, a reputable choirmaster, known throughout Igboland, would advice that one who does not know what to sing should simply wait at "amen," the end of the song. However, in this author's opinion, which can be experimented upon, adoption of Sir Peter Egbo's solution is the simplest formula to end corruption. There is no need for carving x or y agency to fight corruption as experience has shown us that such option end up aggravating corruption. Through legislative means, government can take over all lands, houses and cars. All corrupt practices in Nigeria end up being used to acquire these three. If the first two are taken over completely by government, and cars are partially taken over by governments, stolen money in private pockets would only have one way to go – investment in agriculture, manufacturing and service industries which will benefit the people because it would create infinite employment, feed the people and create congenial environment for peaceful coexistence. If this happens, no one would dare to steal government money because you cannot steal what you cannot hide or use. Only then would government and her officials take responsibility for mosquito/ malaria control. Only then could the health sector follow suit, transforming our hospitals into friendly environment for health workers and their clients [32]. Only in congenial environment would people see malaria control as one deserving all hands being on deck and willingness to insist on malaria elimination programmes [33].

In this part of the world, we cannot talk of eliminating malaria without bringing in those traditional medicine practitioners. This is necessary because the average Igbo man/woman when confronted with the first sign of malaria uses the nearest plant based anti-malaria therapy he can find, particularly in the rural areas [21]. If the condition persisted, he would go for orthodox treatment in hospital. When discharged from hospital, he still goes back to the plant based treatment he started with. This means that they are somehow attached to traditional medicine. It would be a milestone if our primary, secondary and tertiary health centres are restructured to accommodate traditional medicine. The implication is that traditional health care providers would need retraining and integration so that they and the orthodox health care providers could do their work from different perspective but with one mission: elimination of malaria in our clime. There will be many benefits derivable from such integrated health care: it will build bridges and partnership among orthodox and traditional practitioners, bring traditional medicine closer to the laboratory [59]. Orthodox drugs are perceived as chemicals with higher toxic contents, so people must be treated according to their preferences, which in our case, is natural products which must be refined to deliver optimally to fast track the control of mosquitoes and elimination of malaria.

Acknowledgements

The author is grateful to all the nameless persons who made this work possible. However, mention must be made of the management of the University of Nigeria, Nsukka, who continue to perform despite all odds. I am grateful to my colleagues and the Director, SEZBC, UNN, Prof Njoku, O. for their support. I also thank specially the management of IntechOpen who kept "panel beating" me until this work was completed. Finally, I thank my wife and family for enduring so much deprivations caused by my devotion to completing this work. May God continue to illuminate and bless his people wherever they are.

Author details

Francis S.O. Ugwu[1,2]

1 South East Zonal Biotechnology Centre, University of Nigeria, Nsukka, Nigeria

2 Zoology and Environmental Biology Department, University of Nigeria, Nsukka, Nigeria

*Address all correspondence to: francis.ugwu@unn.edu.ng; faraugwu@rocketmail.com

References

[1] WHO: World malaria report (2014). WHO Press, World Health Organization, 20 Avenue Appia, 1211 Geneva 27, Switzerland. www.who.int

[2] WHO. (2018). World Malaria Report 2018. WHO Press, World Health Organization, 20 Avenue Appia, 1211 Geneva 27, Switzerland. www.who.int

[3] WHO. (2019). World Malaria Report 2018. WHO Press, World Health Organization, 20 Avenue Appia, 1211 Geneva 27, Switzerland. www.who.int

[4] Sharma, V. P. (2012). Battling malaria iceberg incorporating strategic reforms in achieving Millennium Development Goals & malaria elimination in India. The Indian journal of medical research, *136*(6), 907.

[5] Idris, Z. M., Chan, C. W., Kongere, J., Gitaka, J., Logedi, J., Omar, A., ... & Kimura, M. (2016). High and heterogeneous prevalence of asymptomatic and sub-microscopic malaria infections on islands in Lake Victoria, Kenya. Scientific reports, 6, 36958.

[6] Zimmerman, P. A., Mehlotra, R. K., Kasehagen, L. J., & Kazura, J. W. (2004). Knowledge gaps underlying the mixed Plasmodium species infection debate. Trends in Parasitology, 9(20), 440-447.

[7] Sachs, J. D., Andrew D. Mellinger D. A., & Gallup, J. L. (2001). The geography of poverty and wealth. *Scientific American*, 284 (3), 70-75 (Published by: Scientific American, a division of Nature America, Inc.) Stable URL: http://www.jstor.org/stable/26059132

[8] Murphy S. C. & Breman J. G. (2001). Gaps in the childhood malaria burden in Africa: cerebral malaria, neurological sequelae, anemia, respiratory distress, hypoglycemia, and complications of pregnancy. *Am. J. Trop. Med. Hyg.*, 64(1,2) S, 57-67.

[9] Tatem, A. J., Smith, D. L., Gething, P. W., Kabaria, C. W., Snow, R. W., & Hay, S. I. (2010). Ranking of elimination feasibility between malaria-endemic countries. The Lancet, *376*(9752), 1579-1591.

[10] Coleman M, Al-Zahrani MH, Coleman M, Hemingway J, Omar A, et al. (2014) A Country on the Verge of Malaria Elimination – The Kingdom of Saudi Arabia. PLoS ONE 9(9): e105980. doi:10.1371/journal.pone.0105980

[11] Oluwasegun, J. M. (2017). The British mosquito eradication campaign in colonial Lagos, 1902-1950. Canadian Journal of African Studies/Revue canadienne des études africaines, *51*(2), 217-236.

[12] Musa, S., & Goni, A. N. (2018). Modelling the effect of education-based intervention in the control of malaria. Science World Journal, *13*(4), 1-7.

[13] Usman I.G., Abubakar T.U., Muhammad A.H.,Usman B.T. & Nagwari A.U. (2020). Mathematical model for the transmission dynamics and control of malaria by incorporating behavioural change. *Dutse Journal of Pure and Applied Sciences* (DUJOPAS), 6 (3), 2635-3490.

[14] Atieli, H., Menya, D., Githeko, A., & Scott, T. (2009). House design modifications reduce indoor resting malaria vector densities in rice irrigation scheme area in western Kenya. Malaria Journal, *8*(1), 108.

[15] Ayi, I., Nonaka, D., Adjovu, J. K., Hanafusa, S., Jimba, M., Bosompem, K. M., ... & Kobayashi, J. (2010). School-based participatory health education for malaria control in Ghana: engaging children as health messengers. Malaria Journal, *9*(1), 98.

[16] Morakinyo, O. M., Balogun, F. M., & Fagbamigbe, A. F. (2018). Housing type and risk of malaria among under-five children in Nigeria: evidence from the malaria indicator survey. *Malaria journal*, *17*(1), 311]

[17] Ugwu, F. S. O. (2011). Novel malaria control by strategic net-hoisting with S/O channel/grip devices. MalariaWorld J, *2*, 3.

[18] Ugwu, F. S. O., & Onu, V. C. (2012). Protecting Under-Tree Nomadic Classrooms from Haematophagous Flies with Tree Anchored Net-Tents Based on S/O Channel/Grip Devices. Nigerian Journal of Parasitology, *33*(1).

[19] Ugwu, F. S. O. (2015). Mosquito control via inbuilt net hoisting windows: the inverted S/O channel /grip device option. Malaria World Journal, *6*, (14) www.malariaworld.org.

[20] Federal Ministry of Health. National health accounts 2017. *Union Technical Report April 2019*. https://www.health.gov.ng/doc/FINAL-VERSION-NHA-2017.pdf (downloaded 16.00 hr, Feb. 24, 2021).

[21] Nwankwo, I. C., Okofor, N. I. & Olisa A. (Undated). Health Sector Reform Agenda in an Insecure Nigerian State: Issues, Problems and Prospects. *The Nigerian Journal of Sociology and Anthropology,* 11, 57-74. DOI: 10.36108/NJSA/3102/11(0150)

[22] Chukwuocha, U. M. (2012). Malaria control in Nigeria. Primary Health Care, *2*(118), 2167-1079.

[23] Ugwu, E. O., Ezechukwu, P. C., Obi, S. N., Ugwu, A. O., & Okeke, T. C. (2013). Utilization of insecticide treated nets among pregnant women in Enugu, South Eastern Nigeria. Nigerian journal of clinical practice, *16*(3), 292-296.

[24] Ukoha, N. K., Ohiri, K., Chima, C. C., Ogundeji, Y. K., Rone, A., Nwangwu, C. W., ... & Reich, M. R. (2016). Influence of organizational structure and administrative processes on the performance of state-level malaria programmes in Nigeria. *Health Systems & Reform*, *2*(4), 331-356. Health Systems & Reform, 2:4, 331-356, DOI: 10.1080/23288604.2016.1234865

[25] Amadi, L., & Amadi, M. (2014). Sustainable drug consumption, regulatory dynamics and fake drug repositioning in Nigeria: A case of NAFDAC. Sci-Afric J Sci Issues Res Essays, *2*, 412-419.

[26] Awodele, O., Aliu, R., Ali, I., Oni, Y., & Adeyeye, C. M. (2018). Patterns of adverse drug reaction signals in NAFDAC pharmacovigilance activities from January to June 2015: safety of drug use in Nigeria. Pharmacology research & perspectives, *6*(5), e00427.

[27] Uzochukwu1, B. S. C., Ughasoro, N. D., Etiaba, E., Okwuosa, C., Envuladu, E. & Onwujekwe, O. E. (2015). Health care financing in Nigeria: Implications for achieving universal health coverage. Nigerian Journal of Clinical Practice , 18(4), 437-444.

[28] Akpoghome, T. U. (2018). Examining the protection of access to and delivery of healthcare by The National Health Act 2014. *Advances in Social Sciences Research Journal*, 5(6), 521-535.DoI:10.14738/assrj.56.4802.

[29] Omotosho, O. (2017). Socio-economic and policy context of the nigerian health care financing system: a literature review *International Affairs and Global Strategy,* 53, 8-16. www.iiste.org

[30] Onwujekwe, O., Ezumah, N., Mbachu1, C., Obi, F., Ichoku, H., Uzochukwu, B. & Wang H. (2017). Exploring effectiveness of different health financing mechanisms in Nigeria; what needs to change and how can it happen? BMC Services Research, 19, 661. https://doi.org/10.1186/s12913-019-4512-4

[31] Amadi, A. N. C., Amoke, C. O., & Ganiyu, K. (2017). The status of malaria parasitemia and assessment of the use of long lasting insecticide treated bed net among Umudike Community of Umuahia, Abia State, Nigeria. Animal Research International, *14*(3), 2876-2882.

[32] Onyeneho, N. G., Idemili-Aronu, N., Okoye, I., Ugwu, C., & Iremeka, F. U. (2014). Compliance with intermittent presumptive treatment and insecticide treated nets use during pregnancy in Enugu State, Nigeria. Maternal and Child Health Journal, *18*(5), 1169-1175.

[33] Campbell, C. C., & Steketee, R. W. (2011). Malaria in Africa can be eliminated. The American journal of tropical medicine and hygiene, *85*(4), 584-585.

[34] Onisanwa, I. D., Sunday, B. S. & Adaji, M. O. (2018). Healthcare financing and health status analysis in Nigeria. Amity Journal of Healthcare Management, 3(2), 31-42.

[35] Adebisi, Y. A., Umah, J. O., Olaoye., C. O., Alaran, A. J., Sina-Odunsi, A. B. & Lucero-Prisno, D. E. Assessment of Health Budgetary Allocation and Expenditure Toward Achieving Universal Health Coverage in Nigeria. (2020). *Int J Health Life Sci*, 6(2):e102552. doi: 10.5812/ijhls.102552.0

[36] Mokuolu, O. A., Coker, A. O., & Sridhar, M. K. C. (2016). Contributions of solid wastes disposal practice to malaria prevalence in Ilorin, Nigeria. Nigerian Journal of Technological Development, *13*(1), 1-5.

[37] Horvath, B., Mallinguh, E., & Fogarassy, C. (2018). Designing business solutions for plastic waste management to enhance circular transitions in Kenya. Sustainability, *10*(5), 1664.

[38] Nwafor, N., & Walker, T. R. (2020). Plastic Bags Prohibition Bill: A developing story of crass legalism aiming to reduce plastic marine pollution in Nigeria. Marine Policy, *120*, 104160

[39] Nwani, S. E., Ozegbe A.E. (Undated). Public Health Expenditure and Health Outcomes in Nigeria.https://d1wqtxts1xzle7.cloudfront.net/57259966/Public_Health_Expenditure_and_Heath_Status_in_Nigeria.pdf?1535458808=&response-content-(downloaded 16.00 hr, Feb. 24, 2021).

[40] Eme O. I., Uche, O. A. & Uche, I. B. (2014). Building a solid health care system in Nigeria: challenges and prospects. Academic Journal of Interdisciplinary Studies, 3(6), 501-510.

[41] Akinyemi, O., & Atilola, O. (2013). Nigerian resident doctors on strike: insights from and policy implications of job satisfaction among resident doctors in a Nigerian teaching hospital. The International Journal of Health Planning and Management, *28*(1), e46-e61.

[42] Oleribe, O. O., Ezieme, I. P., Oladipo, O., Akinola, E. P., Udofia, D., & Taylor-Robinson, S. D. (2016). Industrial action by healthcare workers in Nigeria in 2013-2015: an inquiry into causes, consequences and control—a cross-sectional descriptive study. Human resources for health, *14*(1), 46.

[43] Okonta, K. E., & Okonta, O. C. (2017). Industrial crises in a Tertiary Health Institution (THI) in Nigeria: The perspective of resident doctors. *International Journal of Healthcare Management*, 1-7. https://doi.org/10.1080/20479700.2017.1397323

[44] Omisore, A. G., Adesoji, R. O., & Abioye-Kuteyi, E. A. (2017). Interprofessional Rivalry in Nigeria's Health Sector: A Comparison of Doctors and Other Health Workers' Views at a Secondary Care Center. International quarterly of community health education, *38*(1), 9-16.

[45] McFubara, K. G. (2018). Who Owns the Patient. *An Examination of the Concept of Ownership in Health Care Ethics. J Hosp Health Care Admin: JHHA-110.* DOI: 10.29011/JHHA-110. 00010

[46] Ogundahunsi, O. A. T., Vahedi, M., Kamau, E. M., Aslanyan, M., Terry, R. F. Zicker, F. & Launois . (2015). Strengthening research capacity—TDR's evolving - and middle-income countries. PLoS Negl Trop Dis, 9(1): e3380. doi:10.1371/journal.pntd.0003380

[47] TDR. (2017). TDR strategy 2018-2023: building the science of solutions. Geneva: WHO 2017. Licence CC BY-NC-SA 3.0 IGO.

[48] Morel C.M. (2000). Reaching Maturity – 25 Years of the TDR. Parasitology Today; 16, 522-528.

[49] Pulford, J., Hetzel, M. W., Bryant, M., Siba, P. M., & Mueller, I. (2011). Reported reasons for not using a mosquito net when one is available: a review of the published literature. Malaria journal, *10*(1), 83.

[50] McLean, K. A., Byanaku, A., Kubikonse, A., Tshowe, V., Katensi, S., & Lehman, A. G. (2014). Fishing with bed nets on Lake Tanganyika: a randomized survey. Malaria journal, *13*(1), 1-5.

[51] Ogoma, S. B., Lweitoijera, D. W., Ngonyani, H., Furer, B., Russell, T. L., Mukabana, W. R., ... & Moore, S. J. (2010). Screening mosquito house entry points as a potential method for integrated control of endophagic filariasis, arbovirus and malaria vectors. PLoS Negl Trop Dis, *4*(8), e773.

[52] Mueller, J. S., Melwani, S., & Goncalo, J. A. (2012). The bias against creativity: Why people desire but reject creative ideas. Psychological science, *23*(1), 13-17.

[53] Cissel Moussa B. M., Keita C., Keita D., Dengela D., Coleman J., Lucas L., ... & Beach R. (2015). Characterizing the insecticide resistance of Anopheles gambiae in Mali. Malar J, 14:327. DOI 10.1186/s12936-015-0847-4

[54] Awolola, T. S., Adeogun, A., Olakiigbe, A. K., Oyeniyi, T., Olukosi, Y. A., Okoh, H., ... & Amajoh, C. N. (2018). Pyrethroids resistance intensity and resistance mechanisms in Anopheles gambiae from malaria vector surveillance sites in Nigeria. PloS one, *13*(12), e0205230.

[55] Hancock, P. A., Hendriks, C. J., Tangena, J. A., Gibson, H., Hemingway, J., Coleman, M., ... & Moyes, C. L. (2020). Mapping trends in insecticide resistance phenotypes in African malaria vectors. PLoS biology, *18*(6), e3000633.

[56] Arivoli, S., & Samuel, T. (2011). Bioefficacy of Citrullus colocynthis (L.) Schrad (Cucurbitaceae) whole plant extracts against Anopheles stephensi, Aedes aegypti and Culex quinquefasciatus (Diptera: Culicidae). International Journal of Current Research, *3*(4), 296-304.

[57] Khan, S., Uddin, M. N., Rizwan, M., Khan, W., Farooq, M., Shah, A. S., ... & Ali, S. (2020). Mechanism of Insecticide Resistance in Insects/Pests. Polish Journal of Environmental Studies, *29*(3).

[58] Wood, O. R., Hanrahan, S., Coetzee, M., Koekemoer, L. L., & Brooke, B. D. (2010). Cuticle thickening associated with pyrethroid resistance in the major malaria vector Anopheles funestus. Parasites & vectors, *3*(1), 1-7.

[59] Uchenna, A. A., Jalal–Eddeen, O. A. C. D., Saddiq, S. D., Calista, P. U. N., Abonyi, I., Amadi, A. N., ... & Abonyi, D. O. Traditional Healers in Malaria Control Programmeme in Nsukka Zone of Enugu State Nigeria.

Chapter 15

T Cell-Based Vaccines: Hope for Malaria Elimination

Nikunj Tandel and Sarat K. Dalai

Abstract

Among the numerous infectious diseases, malaria still remains the main cause of morbidity and mortality across the world. Every year more than 200 million cases are registered and death toll is of around 4,00,000. The emergence of insecticide and drug resistance has surged an alarming situation to find an effective means to tackle it. From various approaches used for reducing the damage created by malaria to the society, developing effective vaccine has gained the attention of scientific community. The large genome size (24 MB), heterogeneity of the genes, complex life cycle in two different hosts, and expression of wide range of these genes are claimed to hinder the malaria vaccine development. It requires good understanding of the host-pathogen interaction and its correlation with the sterile protection. Recently, subunit vaccine have shown certain promising responses; however, the currently in use of RTS,S vaccine has failed to generate the long-term sterile protection as well as effector memory $CD8^{+}$T cells. However, the success of sterile protection through vaccination has been proven long back by experimental approaches, where it could be achieved using irradiated sporozoites (RAS) in rodents and humans. Similarly, GAP (genetically attenuated parasite) and CPS (chloroquine chemoprophylaxis with *Plasmodium sporozoites*) have been shown to induce sterile immunity. Despite all the developments, generation of species and stage specific-$CD8^{+}$ T cell responses has been modest. In order to generate long-lasting immune response, particularly, liver-stage specific-$CD8^{+}$ T cells, it is indeed required to study the $CD8^{+}$ T cell epitope repertoire and its implications on the host immune system. In this chapter we will discuss the current status of T cell-based vaccines and the challenges associated with it.

Keywords: Malaria, subunit vaccine, $CD8^{+}$ T cells response, sterile immunity, memory T cells

1. Introduction: Malaria pathogenesis

Since the origin of *Homo sapience* through the continuous evolution process, we have become the most successful creature on the Earth by maintaining the symbiotic relation with other species to live freely. On the other hand, there are several tiny, single/multi-cellular organisms which may not be possible to see by naked eye have created the threat for us and we have witnessed the long-fight to fulfill the basic principle of *Survival of the fittest*. Underneath all these tiny organisms, a group of species falls under the category of an *infection*, an invasion process through which they enter into the host system, and follow the multiplication/replication process that results in the release of toxins inside the body [1]. From the list of myriad infectious diseases, malaria caused by *Plasmodium* species (a parasite of

IntechOpen

Apicomplexa phylum) and transmitted through the bite of *Anopheles* female mosquitoes, still persists as the leading cause of morbidity and mortality [2, 3]. As per the latest World Malaria Report 2020, there are 229 million cases registered in more than 87 countries across the globe in 2019; it was 238 million in the year of 2000. Malaria is considered a life-threatening disease as the mortality rate is still higher, and estimated 409,000 death were reported in the last year [2]. Today half of the population lives under the risk of malaria infection and it has mainly affected the South-African region which is responsible for more than 94% cases in 2019 followed by South-East Asia and Western pacific region (**Figure 1**).

Despite the reduction in the malaria mortality rate (from 25% in 2000 to 10% in 2019), the children under the age of 5 years are the most vulnerable group (due to the lack of adequate acquired immunity) as 67% of total death in 2019 was reported in this group. Likewise, pregnant women are also at the higher risk as it quells the immune system [2, 4]. Athwart the other Apicomplexa parasites having the commodious range of metazoans for the infection, *Plasmodium* species have a restricted range in terms of specificity for insect and vertebrate hosts [5]. In humans, malaria is mainly caused by four *Plasmodium* species and, *P. falciparum* is responsible for the most severity as it has been accounted for more than 70% cases across the world (more prominent in African region-99.7%) in 2018 [2, 6] whereas, *P. vivax* is responsible for malaria infection in American region (75%) followed by South East Asia [2, 7, 8]. Other species, known as *P. ovale* [9] and *P. malariae* [10] are also responsible for the malaria infection, yet the complications are less. Recently, *P. knowlesi* is found to infect humans in Malaysia [11] however, the host specificity is not limited to the humans as reports of infection are also reported in monkeys [10].

The *Plasmodium* species carries the complex life cycle consist of two hosts: *Anopheles* mosquitoes (sexual cycle) and human (asexual cycle). The cycle begins with the bite of infected female *Anopheles* mosquitoes to the human during the blood meal and transfers sporozoites [12] into the skin. They remain at the inoculation site for a short time and further travel to the liver where they invade the liver hepatocytes. Inside the liver by tight regulation and signaling mechanism, they select the hepatocytes, invade them and mature into the schizonts. This phase of

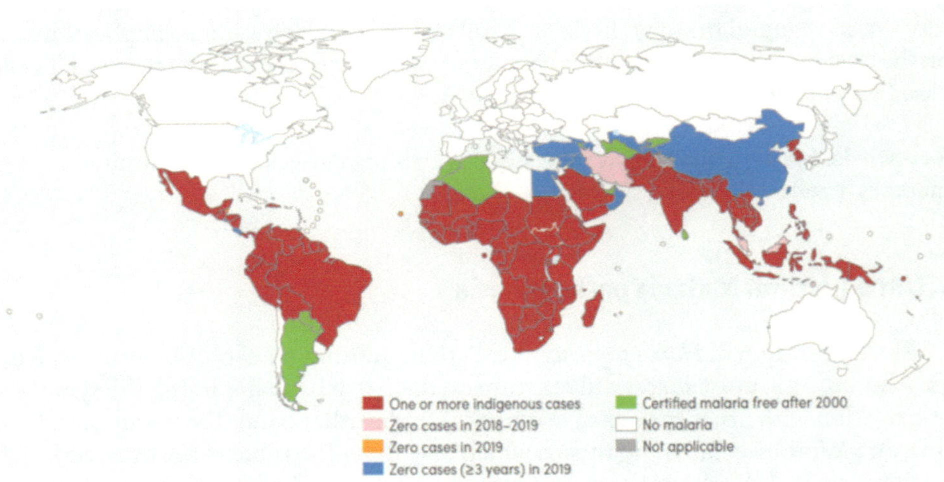

Figure 1.
Countries with indigenous cases in 2000 and their status by 2019: Countries with zero indigenous cases over at least the past 3 consecutive years are considered to have eliminated malaria. In 2019, China and El Salvador reported zero indigenous cases for the third consecutive year and have applied for WHO certification of malaria elimination; also, the Islamic Republic of Iran, Malaysia and Timor-Leste reported zero indigenous cases for the second time. Source: WHO database *(adapted with permission from [2]).*

cycle is also known as *pre-erythrocytic stage* [13]. Further, these schizonts rupture and release merozoites which come out and infect the erythrocytes (RBCs). However, *P. vivax* and *P. ovale* remain in the dormant stage in the liver for a prolonged period of time if left untreated and may relapse after several years. Once the merozoites pop-up in the blood stream, they infect the RBCs which further divide, replicate and passes through several developmental stages, ring stage-trophozoite stage-schizont formation in chronological order, and ended up in release of countless merozoites. These merozoites further infect the new RBCs and cycle continues. During this *erythrocytic stage (or blood stage)*, a number of trophozoites develop into male (micro) and female (macro) gametocytes [13]. The mature gametocytes migrate towards the dermis of skin; during the next blood meal of vector mosquitoes, they are taken-up by the mosquitoes. Formation of zygotes takes place by fertilization of micro and macro gametes in the stomach of *Anopheles* mosquito. Later, these zygotes are converted into the motile ookinetes which finally develop into the oocytes and rupture the mid-gut [13]. These oocytes evolve, unfold and materialize into sporozoites, which subsequently reach to the salivary gland of the mosquito and ready for the next cycle in human host. The phase of conversion of asexual gametocytes into mature sporozoites is also known as *sporogonic cycle* [13]. **Figure 2** depicts the basic malaria life cycle of *P. falciparum.*

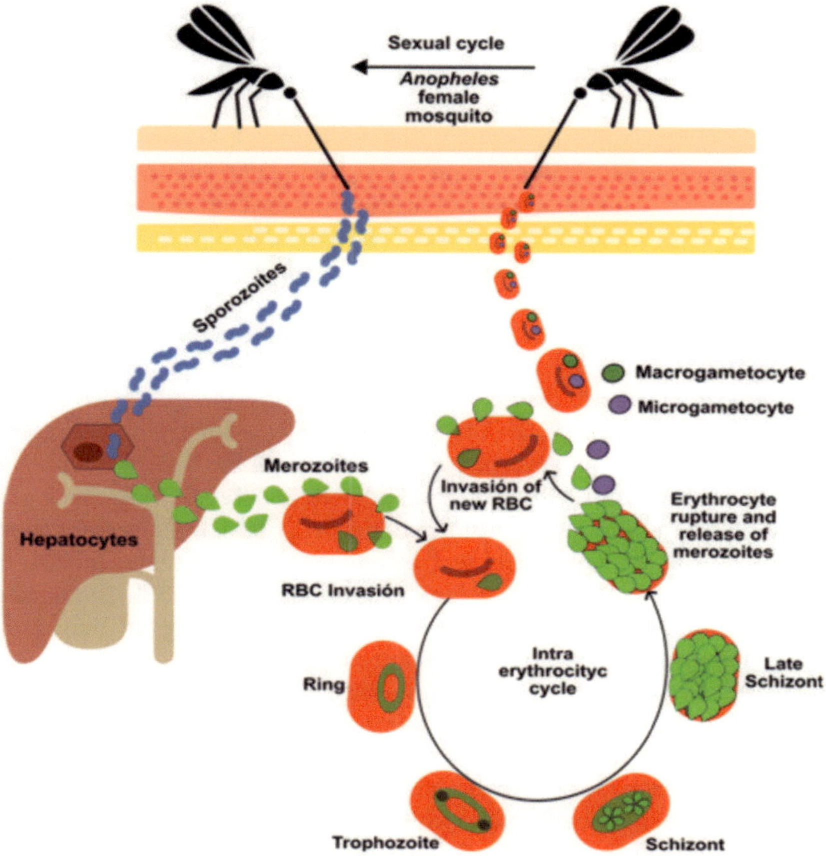

Figure 2.
The P. falciparum *life-cycle. An infected female* Anopheles *mosquito inoculates Spz as it bites a host, they then travel in the host's bloodstream and infect the hepatocytes. Merozoites are released and then invade erythrocytes, where they mature through various stages (ring, trophozoite and schizont stages) and undergo asexual multiplication (~10 or lower) every 48 h, releasing new merozoites which perpetuate the asexual cycle. Some of them enter the sexual cycle by becoming female and male gametocytes which are ingested by the mosquito when it bites an infected host, thereby starting the cycle all over again (adapted with permission from [14]).*

2. Malaria elimination and eradication: Grasping at straws

It was 1897 when Ronald Ross has identified the parasites responsible for the malaria infection and later on the development in the field of science and technology has opened up several areas to work upon and eliminate the malaria infection [15]. The basic understanding of epidemiology and entomology, host-pathogen interaction, surveillance and numerous studies have provided the information about the usage of two main prophylactic methods to curtail down the morbidity and mortality spread by malaria infection: prevention of infection and diseases by controlling the mosquitoes and usage of antimalarial therapy, respectively. As per the recommendation by WHO, insecticides-treated nets (ITNs) have been used to prevent the insect from reaching out the humans. Nonetheless, the results were discouraging as less than 2% children were protected in African region through the usage of ITNs [16]. Further, to surpass the limitation of ITNs, spraying of various insecticides (such as DDT, permethrin, deltamethrin, pyrethriods) have come into the practice, although it has only cover the tip of the iceberg [17]. To strengthen the above approaches WHO has launched the global malaria eradication program in early 1955 [18] and DDT & chloroquine have been recommended for the ITNs and prevention and treatment of infection, respectively [19]. Despite significant reduction in several developing and underdeveloped countries, the reports of *Plasmodium* resistance against the chloroquine and *Anopheles* resistance towards the DDT forced WHO to abandon the program in 1972 [20, 21]. Thereupon, several other approaches have been implemented for vector controls. However, the reports of insecticide resistance against almost all the *Anopheles* vector and resistance against 1-out-of 5 publicly used nets in more than 68 countries have created alarming situation [22]. Further, out of these 68 countries, more than 50 countries have shown the resistance against more than two or more insecticides which has added the fuel to the fire [22, 23]. To tackle the situation of resistance, noninsecticidal approach of bacterial endosymbionts [24], long-lasting insecticides nets (LLINs) and LLINs treated hammocks [25] are under development.

Likewise, the drug resistance against the frontline antimalarial drug quinine has forced the mankind to use the other drugs and combination. However, the reports of resistance against the artemisinin in Greater Mekong Subregion (GMK) in a short span of its launch [26] and unavailability of other options for artemisinin combination therapy (ACT) have invoked the bleak condition for the treatments [27]. To prevail the condition of drug resistance, scientist have opted for mass drug administration (MDA) approach in which antimalarial drugs have been recommended to the specific group of people without getting into the details of their illness. It has been further known as *targeted malaria elimination* (TME) [28, 29]. The results of this approach found to be satisfactory, however proper planning and management are the key factors for the success of MDA approach [15].

Apart from the well-known approaches, usage of antibiotics and their role to fight against the various diseases is widely accepted and therefore, azithromycin, doxycycline and clindamycin have been tested against the malaria. These antibiotics were found to be effective and also reached to the clinical phases; yet the delayed response is the major drawback due to which they cannot be utilized in mild-to-severe and severe conditions of malaria [30]. Besides, a range of antibiotics named quinoloes, tetracycline, trimethoprim, erythromycin and others are in the early stage of development as they are showing promising results which kill the parasites [31], yet it has a long way to go.

Alongside the approaches used to control the malaria infection, human body also consists of a defense mechanism which respond according to the nature of threat (humoral and cell mediated immunity). It is believed that people living in malaria endemic areas naturally develop immunity due to the continuous exposure of malaria infection. However, age, gender, geographical location, time (months to several years) and numerous other factors are considered to play a vital role in long-term protection [32–34] against malaria. Despite the characteristics of developing protection against the malaria infection naturally, the poorly understood mechanism and the long-term protection are controversial. Therefore, it is of utmost priority to gain the sterile protection against the malaria infection.

2.1 Approach of vaccine development: A ray of hope

Number of experimental approaches have been adopted to understand the *Plasmodium* species and provided us the immense knowledge about the host-pathogen interaction, and how a parasite can escape and invade the immune system for its survival. It has been well documented that during the malaria infection, the protective response vis-a-vie humoral (antibody against malaria) and cell mediated ($CD4^+$ and $CD8^+$ T cells) immunity is dampened [35]. Hence, to achieve the sterile protection against malaria infection, activation/boosting up the wings or full immune system is the fundamental target for any malaria biologist. In this direction, Nussenzwig and colleagues more than 53 years ago have used the approach of killed parasites of *P. berghei* to immunize the mice; however, they failed to generate the immune response. Therefore, approach of partial inactivation of sporozoites by X-irradiation has been used by them to achieve the protective immunity [36]. The observation of precipitation at one end of sporozoites and elevated level of the antibody (in serum) of the induced animals was correlated with the protective immunity. Further, they have observed the high level of antibody after each repetitive dose.

After successful immunization strategy of X-irradiation in non-human host, Clyde *et al.*, 1972 used the same approach for *P. falciparum* sporozoites and injected to the healthy volunteers frequently up-to 84 days, and on day 98 they were challenged with infectious sporozoites [37]. Out of three volunteers, one failed to develop the malaria infection and on day 327 anti-sporozoite antibodies were found. The result of this study has opened a new avenue for the vaccine development (usage of attenuated sporozoites) against the malaria. Later, they have extended the experiment by using two strains: *P. falciparum* and *P. vivax* and injected attenuated sporozoites [38]. The species-specific antibody formation and impact of the geographical location on the species were noticed. Also, the protection of immunized volunteers has found maximum for 3 and 6 months for the infectious sporozoites challenge of *P. falciparum* and *P. vivax*, respectively. Besides, they did not find any significant changes in the serum level of IgG and IgM [38]. In all, these data reveal the role of attenuated sporozoites in generating immune response specific to malaria, yet the long-term and species-specific immunity was remained to be unriddled. Regardless of the promising results of attenuated sporozoites approach, the tasks of rearing mosquitoes, maintaining the infection cycle and isolation of sporozoites are time-consuming, laborious and challenging. Besides, skilled-personnel for appropriate functioning and injecting the live sporozoites are the pre-requisites for the successful vaccination. On the other side, the sustainability and higher-efficacy for the long term protection is found to be limited alongside the development of naturally acquired immunity against malaria [39, 40].

As discussed earlier, it is possible that people living in malaria endemic can develop naturally acquired immunity after prolonged exposure although it could be restricted to blood-stage infection. However, induction of immunity to liver-stage (LS)infection among endemic population has not been thought to be possible because of lower infection load, heterogeneity of liver immunology of individuals and characteristics which differ from blood stage [41]. Also, among the different stages of malaria infection, blocking the transmission of human-to-mosquitoes-to-human and generation of modified mosquitoes may halt the spreading of malaria are in dire straits conditions. Similarly, to target particularly the infected RBCs containing merozoites and preventing them to infect other RBCs in the blood/symptomatic stage has been very difficult. Nonetheless, the longest exposure of infected sporozoites towards the host immune system by invading hepatocytes in the liver stage (5.5 to 7 days in humans and 48 hrs in rodents) and releasing of thousands of merozoites which further continue the blood-stage or symptomatic stage of infection makes the LS most promising stage for the target of vaccine development [14, 42], though LS-vaccine has its own limitation of tedious and challenging task of sporozoites.

Taking into the above considerations, scientific community across the globe is working on multiple targets of different stages to tackle the dire condition. At present, there are mainly three types of vaccines based on the life-cycle: the liver (pre-erythrocytic) stage (LS), asexual blood (symptomatic) stage and the third one is transmission blocking vaccines (TBV).

2.1.1 History of malaria vaccine development

The successful experimental approach of using the attenuated sporozoites (*P. berghei, P. knowlesi, P. falciparum,* and *P. vivax*) in rodents and humans [43–47] including monkeys [48] to generate the sterile and protective immune responses have unfolded the newer therapeutic options. Likewise, development of humoral-transmission blocking immunity in chicken and turkeys by immunizing killed-asexual stage parasites [49], clearance of blood-stage infection in monkeys by arming the *P. knowlesi* asexual-parasites with adjuvants [50] and significant reduction in the *P. falciparum* blood-stage infection after passive transfer of immunoglobulins from continuous exposure of malaria to naïve ones in humans [51–53] and monkeys [54] have excavated the different role of immune system. As stated above, work carried out by Clyde and colleagues corroborates the generation of protective immunity; however, requirement of large number of irradiated sporozoites was the biggest hassle. During the early 1980s, the breakthrough identification of circumsporozoite protein (CSP) as a major constituent of the sporozoite coat resulted into the sequencing and cloning of this gene followed by identification of several blood-stage antigens (Ags) led the world with the hope of early malaria vaccine [55]. Regardless of the CSP identification and other target Ags, approach of blood-stage Ags, heat-killed, lysed and formalin inactivated sporozoites and sporozoites Ags in their early clinical studies have shown the moderate immune responses and unable to reach the threshold of immunity generated by irradiated sporozoites approach [55, 56].

The advancement in the field of sequencing helped in identifying the region of CSP protein having species-specific immunodominant epitope that consists of tandem repeated sequences of amino acids, Asn-Ala-Asn-Pro-Asn-Ala-Asn-Pro-Asn-Ala-Pro $(NANP)_3$, remain conserved and found to be present in most of the people. The outcome of this work has led the pioneers to develop the approach of *synthetic peptide*. Upon synthesizing this specific epitope region $(NANP)_3$ of CSP protein, several groups have conducted the experiments in monkeys and observed the partial or complete protection [57–59]. After having promising results in monkeys, SPf66 (a synthetic peptide based vaccine from Colombia) have been tested through independent trials in Asia and Africa; however, it was found ineffective in generating protection [60]. Despite the expected results of the SPf66, it has opened an avenue to study the immune response of other prominent vaccine candidates.

Several studies have revealed the important role of CSP protein in developing immunity during the sporozoite challenge studies and become the most prominent candidate for the anti-malaria vaccine development [61]. However, the poor immunogenicity and lesser efficacy (in clinical trials) were the major concern to proceed further for CSP Ag. Therefore, Stoute *et al.*, 1997 have used a novel formulation of CSP Ag, known as RTS,S: a hybrid (fusion of CSP protein with hepatitis B surface Ag-HBs Ag) construct armed with novel adjuvants (AS02). The results were encouraging and also correlated with earlier studies [61]. This study led the foundation for the first clinical trials in Africa (in Gambia). The RTS,S/AS02 was given to the men (N = 250 & age:18–45 years) and followed up to 15 weeks. It was found to be safe and actively producing CSP specific B-and-T cell responses and also protection was not limited only to the NF54 strain of *P. falciparum* from which the vaccine has been made [62]. In subsequent studies, the involvement of $CD4^+$ and $CD8^+$ T cells, sentinels of cellular immunity against the LS infection and role of Abs specific to the sporozoites have revealed the significant role of T- and B cells against malaria infection, respectively [63].

Further, parasite-specific Ags presented by MHC I and II to the $CD8^+$ and $CD4^+$ T cells, respectively on the surface of infected hepatocytes [64–68] delineate the importance of cell mediated immunity (CMI) to target the LS infection. All the above and other experimental evidences have unveiled the prominent role of CMI in generating sterile protection. As a result, it has changed the scenario in the field of vaccine development and to generate the sterile protection via boosting up CMI through a novel approach of *plasmid DNA immunization*. In the initial stage of development, Wang *et al.*, 1998 have used the plasmid DNA bearing malaria Ag and injected into the malaria-naïve individuals. It has been shown to generate the Ag-specific, $CD8^+$ cytotoxic T lymphocytes (CTLs); however, it was found to be genetically and HLA-restricted [69]. Regardless of restricted-CTL responses, this technology has driven the field and allowed to explore different suitable options to overcome the issue of poor immunogenicity of vaccine candidate(s) against malaria infection. To boost up the T-cell specific heterologous immune response, McConeky *et al.*, 2003 have used the novel non-replicating *viral vector* (recombinant modified vaccinia virus Ankara-MVA) approach. It has shown certain level of efficacy in terms of delayed parasitemia after the challenge with sporozoites. It induced five to ten fold elevated IFN-γ producing T-cells (specific-to-Ag) compared to the plasmid DNA or recombinant MVA strategy, and the protection was independent of antibody response [70] creating the base for the preventive and therapeutic vaccine development. Thereafter, experimental results have confirmed that homologous or heterologous priming using viral vector approach could induce the CMI [71]. By using this approach, ME-TRAP, CSVAC (encodes *Pf*CSP alongside a truncated C-terminal lacking 14 amino acids of CSP GPI anchor moiety), combination of *Pf*TRAP with liver stage antigen 1 (LSA1) & LSA2 were developed and tested for their efficacy [42]. The enhanced T-cell based response is the major advantage of this approach. Nonetheless, the efficacy of different candidate(s) found to be low in malaria endemic regions. Inclusion of more target specific immunogen(s) of *Plasmodium* and or combination with RTS,S may improve the overall efficacy.

The technological advancement in the field has helped the scientific community to understand host-pathogen interaction in detail. As a result of it, numerous new and improvised approaches come into practice for the successful vaccine development. To review the status of vaccine candidates and accelerate the development of second generation malaria vaccines, several scientific meetings and forums [72, 73] were organized as well as provided the literature for the same [17, 55, 74, 75]. Therefore, here we have not discussed about all the different types of vaccines.

In early 1980s, *monoclonal Abs and recombinant-DNA* approach have also been used for several antigens followed by their cloning and efficacy testing. However, the efficacy was tested only in experimental (*in-vivo*) settings and results were not up-to the mark [76]. From the beginning, most of the vaccine development has targeted LS of malaria infection. However, people have also focused on other target of life cycle known as BS (blood stage), another approach which can kill the asexual stage of parasites. During this symptomatic stage of infection, merozoites released from the LS invade the naïve RBCs, which is followed by its multiplication and infection of the surrounding RBCs. This stage of cycle persists from 1 to 3 days depending upon the *Plasmodium* species [74].

Targeting the *blood stage* for the vaccine development is equally important as malaria symptoms occurs during this stage and it has also gained interests as results of clinical studies have confirmed the clearance of parasites in African children [51, 77] and adults in Thailand [53] after the purification and passive transfer of IgG from semi-immune African adults and *P. falciparum* infected Thai-patients, respectively. In the early 1980s, trials were conducted on monkeys by using the *P. falciparum* fully developed merozoites armed with adjuvant followed by challenge with homologous strain of *P. falciparum* [78]. Except the control monkeys, all the immunized monkeys survived and generated the strong immune response. The promising findings of the study encouraged the community to focus on development of vaccine based on blood stage resulting in more than 30 blood stage vaccine candidates that registered during 2000–2015 from the targets of the merozoites surface protein (MSP) 1 and apical membrane antigen 1(AMA-1). MSP 3 and erythrocyte binding antigen 175 (EBA-175) are some of the other BS targets which were also explored to check the efficacy. The high titer Ab was observed against most of the MSP proteins; a protein express on merozoites which further invades RBCs, and Ab-mediated cellular inhibition was noticed during the clinical trial of MSP3 in malaria endemic area [79]. In sum, the results of pre-clinical and clinical studies of BS vaccine candidates suggest that they were unable to generate the strong evidence for the protection in controlled human malaria infection (CHMI) or in natural infection.

Similarly, *in-vitro* experiments of AMA-1 have been shown to generate elevated Ab titer in two trials, but during the clinical trials of CHMI it had failed to generate the sterile protection against the homologous strain of *Plasmodium* parasites [80, 81]. Out of all the BS vaccine candidates, only GMZ2 (combination of conserved domain of MSP and glutamate-rich protein-GLURP) have shown the statistically significant efficacy in controlled trial conducted in African children [82]; however, the efficacy was around 14%. To overcome the existing issues associated with poor immunogenicity, other candidate vaccines as well as novel therapeutic options are explored and some of them are currently in pipeline. As a result of it, *P. falciparum* reticulocyte-binding protein homolog 5 (PfRH5) and AMA1-RON2 (rhoptry neck protein-2) complex are currently under experimental phases; early-stage results were found to be promising which may aid in designing the better vaccine candidate [74]. In defiance of optimistic results of BS vaccines, a narrow window period of merozoites which allow Abs to recognize and identify their epitopes during their infection cycle to RBCs (infected-to-naïve-to-infected), convoluted and complex invasion mechanism, polymorphic nature of Ags and simultaneously targeting a large number of merozoites in contrast to confined targets of LS and TBVs (transmission blocking vaccines) are the key questions which needs to be address at the earliest for the successful blood stage vaccine development.

Apart from LS and BS, researchers have also explored the third vaccine type, *transmission-blocking vaccines* (TBVs) comprising of sexual stage Ags (of gametes and/zygotes) which generate the Abs and kill the parasites during the blood-meal of mosquitoes and result in the interruption of mosquito cycle [74]. Till date, there are four major candidates, Pfs230 and Pfs48/45 of *P. falciparum* (expressed by gametocytes in human) and Pfs25 and Pfs28 (zygote surface proteins expressed in mosquitoes) are under investigation. Due to the structural nature of these Ags (cysteine-rich armed with number of 6-cys), there has been a major concern to develop the stable recombinant protein; Pfs25 is the first recombinant protein based TBVs [83] and shown the encouraging results by equal or higher Ab titer against the target of transmission [84, 85]. Apart from this, Pfs230 another TBVs is also under clinical trials as it shows the strong lysis activity against the *P. falciparum* gametes in *in-vivo* system [86]. Both the recombinant Ag based TBVs have depicted the poor immunogenicity during their immunization strategy; to boost up the immune system, approach of administration of adjuvants and or combination of both candidates together are explored and currently it is under trials [74]. Albeit the optimistic results in the early phase, safety of individuals, to cover the larger population for the herd immunity and prolonged adaptive immune response to maintain the higher Ab titer are the major challenges which need to be keep in mind for the development of next generation TBVs. Additionally, the combinational approach of LS and TBVs or BS stage and TBVs is also need to be explored to target multiple sites at a once [74]. Currently, the leading vaccine candidates for all the three different types are illustrated in below given **Figure 3**.

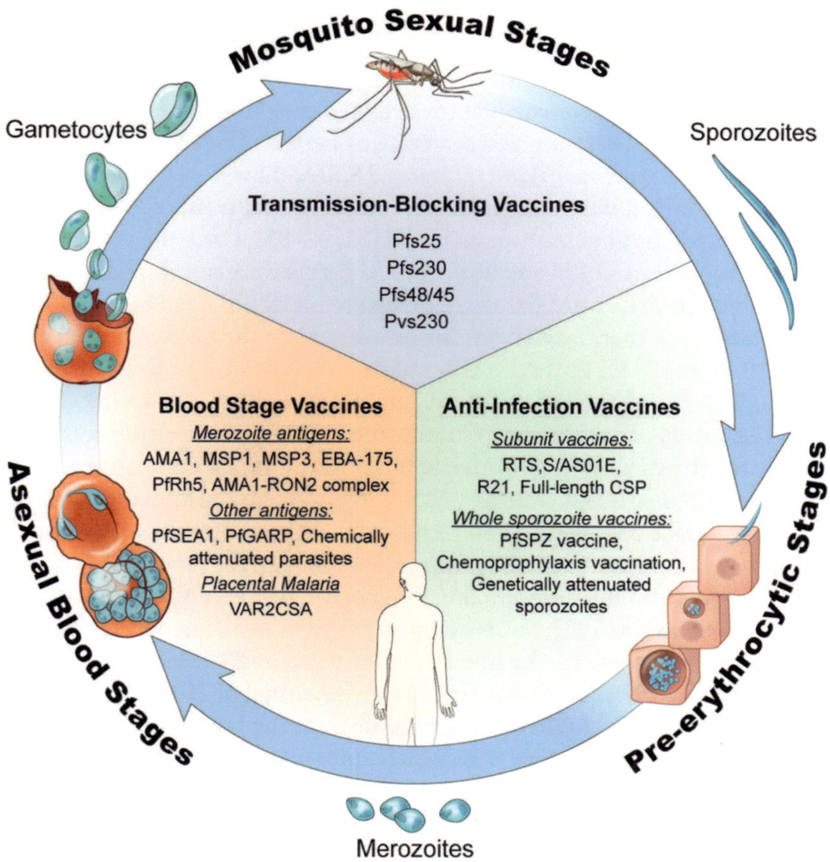

Figure 3.
Life cycle stage of Plasmodium *and vaccine candidates that target each stage (adapted with permission from [74]).*

2.1.2 RTS,S malaria vaccine: Learning lessons from gained knowledge

RTS,S (a recombinant protein based vaccine) was first developed by SmithKline Beecham Biologicals (now known as GlaxoSmithKline Vaccines) in the early 1980s, and has become the first ever licensed vaccine approved by European regulators to use against the human parasite infection in 2015 [87]. From the early experimental studies, modification has been adapted and the novel RTS,S is combined with AS01 (a liposomal formulation) or AS02 (a emulsion based formulation) adjuvant system which trigger the toll-like receptor (TLR4) mediated cytokines and appropriate co-stimulatory signaling molecules on APCs. Additionally, it also activates both wings of the immune system against the CSP and able to generate sterile protection in *Plasmodium* challenge study, led it to enter in Phase III clinical trials [14]. In a phase III study, 829 cases were treated out of 1000 malaria affected children, yet it has unable to boost up the immune system in infants [88]. In another phase III study conducted on children and infants (age group of 1–4), 56% and 65% reduction was observed in case of severe malaria, respectively [89]. The selection of CSP Ag in RTS,S vaccine is derived from the earlier reports where approach of inactivated sporozoites has generated sterile protection and provoked immune response which was mediated by CSP-specific Abs and CMI. These CSP-specific Abs withhold the penetration of sporozoites into liver hepatocytes, still they are unable to achieve the sterile protection alone and therefore, RTS,S vaccine was designed by incorporating a CSP T-cell epitopes (CMI response) alongside the B-cell epitope [90]. The prominent role of CMI in generating sterile protection against malaria infection was noticed during the phase II clinical study, in which three different adjuvant formulations (AS02, AS03 and AS04) were explored, and only formulation i.e., RTS,S/AS02 was shown to invoke the sterile immunity after the *P. falciparum* challenge [90]. Later, more focused approach was developed towards the enrichment of CMI response which further helps in designing and selection of better adjuvant system to enhance the efficacy of RTS,S vaccine [91, 92]. Thus, RTS,S/AS02 was evaluated in field trials; after prolonged study, it has been replaced with earlier adjuvant of AS01 with higher efficacy, safety and elevated immunogenicity [91, 93–95]. Once the role of T-cell started revealing in terms of protection, several assays were developed to study the phenotypic characteristics and nature & involvement of different types of T-cells in malaria infection. Further, T-cell based response against the immunization of RTS,S has been verified in CHMI & field study and further also summarized in **Table 1**.

Later on, Strategic Advisory Group of Experts on Immunization (SAGE) of WHOs and Malaria Policy Advisory Committee (MPAC) have jointly recommended a pilot study for the vaccination in Africa; it has began in Malawi, Ghana and in Kenya between the April and October, 2019 [96]. Despite the approval of RTS,S vaccination, the issue of safety in children is well-documented and therefore, combination of different novel adjuvants with change in the length of CSP-specific peptides and structural information of CSP-specific Abs may further improve the efficacy of RTS,S vaccine [97]. Subsequently, a next generation vaccine was developed (R21) and accounted for the improvised version of RTS,S as it incorporates the longer portion of *Pf*CSP C-terminal armed to N-terminal of HBs Ag. The elevated CSP-specific Ab response, higher immunogenicity at the lower doses (in *in-vivo* challenge study) and formulation with AS01 adjuvant resulted into beginning of clinical trials of phase 1/2a for its efficacy [42].

The development and efficacy of RTS,S vaccine in clinical trials and field study have confirmed the role of T-cell based sterile protection. Recent advancement in the field of genetics and structural biology has driven the area and again the older approach of *whole parasite/sporozoite* vaccine has been reintroduced to fulfill

Vaccine schedule (location)	Vaccine type	No. of samples analyzed	CMI conclusion
Malaria naïve adults			
0, 1, 6 month Belgium	RTS,S/AS02	10	CSP-specific IFN-γ ELISPOTs were induced in 8/10 subjects. RTS, S-specific IFN-γ production was induced in all subjects. LPR to CSP were induced in all subjects. CSP-specific CD8+ CTL responses were not detected
0, 1, 2 month Belgium	RTS,S/AS01 RTS,S/AS02 RTS,S	11 11 12	CS-specific CD4+ T-cell responses (i.e. cells expressing at least 2 markers among CD40L, IL-2, TNF-α, and IFN-γ) were detected in all vaccine groups with a trend for higher responses in the RTS,S/AS01 and RTS,S/AS02 groups versus the RTS,S group
CHMI studies in malaria naïve adults			
0, 2, 6 month USA	RTS,S/Alum RTS,S/AS04	10 10	One of two protected subjects had RTS,S and CSP-specific LPR and cytotoxic T-cell activity
0, 1, 7 month USA	RTS,S/AS02 RTS,S/AS03 RTS,S/AS04 RTS,S/AS02 RTS,S/AS03 RTS,S/AS04 RTS,S/AS02 RTS,S/AS03 RTS,S/AS04	07 07 08 01 05 01 07 07 06	Highest rate of protection with RTS,S/AS02 although CMI results inconclusive Inconclusive due to small sample size IFN-γ ELISPOTs associated with level of protection, ~2 weeks after Dose 3 and on DOC. Protection most frequent for RTS,S/AS02 recipients
0, 1, 2 month USA	RTS,S/AS01 RTS,S/AS02 RTS,S/AS01 RTS,S/AS02	36 44 36 44	Association between CSP-specific CD4+ T cells and protection, 2 weeks after Dose 3 and on DOC. Association between short duration IFN-γ ELISPOTs and protection. Higher frequency of CSP-specific CD4+ T cells with RTS,S/AS01 vs. RTS,S/AS02$_A$ Association between CSP-specific IL-2+ CD4+ T-cell central-memory and effector-memory populations and protection
0, 1, 2 month USA	RTS,S/AS01 (group RRR) Ad35.CS.01 (dose-1) & RTS,S/AS01 (dose-2 & 3; group ARR)	25 21	No evidence of independent association between CSP-specific CD4+ T cells or IFN-γ ELISPOTs and protection. No difference in protection between groups. CMI responses significantly greater in AAR group than in RRR group
Adults in the field			
0, 1, 6 month Gambia	RTS,S/AS02	20	CSP-specific LPR, short duration IFN-g ELISPOT levels were increased by vaccination. All 20 vaccine recipients responded to at least one of the CMI tests after Dose 3 whereas only 15/20 responded before vaccination. No CMI data on protection

Vaccine schedule (location)	Vaccine type	No. of samples analyzed	CMI conclusion
0, 1, 5 month Gambia	RTS,S/AS02 Rabies RTS,S/AS02 Rabies	16 16 ≤131 ≤119	Higher LPR in RTS,S/AS02 recipients than in rabies-vaccine recipients two weeks after Dose 3 An association between long duration IFN-γ-ELISPOT response and protection was seen across the total population of vaccine recipients and controls, and was not caused or confounded by vaccination with RTS,S/AS02. A significantly higher level of IFN- γ-ELISPOTs was also observed in RTS,S/AS02 vaccine recipients compared with rabies-vaccine recipients at 11 weeks after Dose 3.
Children in the field			
0, 1, 2 month Mozambique	RTS,S/AS02 HBsAg	≤63 ≤69	Significant induction of IL-2 secretion in CSP re-stimulation cultures in 24% of RTS,S vaccine recipients. IL-2 secretion was detected in CSP-re-stimulation cultures from 32% of individuals without a malaria episode whereas IL-2 secretion was detected in only 6% of individuals with malaria episodes ($p = 0.053$)
0, 1, 2 month Gabon	RTS,S/AS01 RTS,S/AS02	≤31 ≤32	The frequencies of IL-2^+ $CD4^+$T cells were higher than pre-immune levels in both RTS,S vaccine groups. CD40L^+ $CD4^+$ T cells were not detected. Responder rates ranged from 13–29%. No CMI data on protection
0, 1 month; 0, 1, 2 month; and 0, 1, 7 month Ghana	RTS,S/AS01 RTS,S/AS02 Rabies (0, 1, 2 month only)	≤77; ≤37; ≤73 ≤80; ≤38; ≤73 ≤45	Higher no. of IL-2^+ $CD4^+$T cells with compare to other marker positive $CD4^+$ T cells (and responder rate of 76% 1 month after dose 3 with 0, 1, 7 month schedule). CD40L^+ $CD4^+$ T cells were detected in 0, 1, 7 schedule. Highest T-cell responses were induced by a 0, 1, 7-month immunization schedule (and responder rate of 73% 1 month after dose 3 with 0, 1, 7 month schedule). RTS,S/AS01_E induced higher $CD4^+$ T-cell responses than RTS,S/AS02 for the 0, 1, 7-month schedule. No CMI data on protection
0, 1, 2 month Kenya/ Tanzania	RTS,S/AS01 Rabies RTS,S/AS01 Rabies	≤182 ≤ 197 ≤80 ≤ 98	The frequency of RTS,S-induced CSP-specific (IFNγ^-IL-2^-)TNF-α^+ $CD4^+$ T cells was associated with protection, and CSP-specific TNF-α^+ $CD4^+$ T-cell responses and anti-CSP antibody responses were synergistically associated with protection Evidence that IL-2^+-secreting CSP-stimulated memory $CD4^+$T cells can activate NK cells to secrete IFN-γ. IFN-γ ELISPOTs may include IFN-γ-secreting activated NK cells. No CMI data on protection.

Lymphoproliferative response: LPR.

Table 1.
CMI conclusions from clinical studies (adapted and modified with permission from [90]).

the criteria of generating long-lasting sterile protection with improved efficacy. Besides, radiation attenuated sporozoites (RAS) and genetically attenuated sporozoites (GAPs) and attenuated sporozoites under the drug coverage (chemoprophylaxis and sporozoite-CPS) have recently gain the interest despite the various difficulties [98].

2.2 Whole sporozoite vaccines

It has been well-documented that malaria life cycle begins with the invasion of hepatocytes (in liver) by sporozoites; if restrained its development to the LS, the immune responses to *Plasmodium* is developed. Usage of frontline-antimalarial prophylaxis to overcome the clinical manifestation or approach of attenuated parasites to arrest the life cycle at LS are the two availed options which have been explored in numerous ways (finding of specific immunogen(s) bearing B-and-T-cell based epitopes, route of administration and dosage) to empower the humoral and CMI specific response [99]. Under the beneath of sporozoite approach, there are three different ways through which protective immune responses can be achieved [42].

2.2.1 Chemo- prophylaxis and sporozoites (CPS)

Under this approach, live sporozoites are delivered alongside the available anti-malarial drugs with the aim of targeting BS infection, generation of elevated humoral response and followed by understanding the LS infection. In this direction, the first study was conducted in mice under the cover of chloroquine (CQ) and found to be protective with more number of $CD8^{+}IFN\text{-}\gamma^{+}$ T cells [100]. In the following years, the first human trial was conducted under the cover of CQ in CHMI and found to be 100% effective after homologous challenge, and more interesting, some of the volunteers remain immune for around 2 years [101]. The study of elevated immune response depicted the major role of memory T cells producing IL-2, TNF-α and IFN-γ. It has been noticed that higher dosage in homologous CHMI enhances the protection level. However, during the heterologous challenge study, protection was found to be remained limited, raising the question for its efficacy against the diversity of *Plasmodium* genus. The invention of novel antimalarial drugs have been explored, it has found and in one clinical study that usage of mefloquine (CPS-MQ) also delineate the similar results of CPS-CQ in term of its efficacy and safety [102]. Additionally, all the volunteers (naive) having the CQ under CPS category are protected from homologous CHMI challenge [103]. Other than this, next generation anti-malaria drugs are under experimental phase.

2.2.2 Radiation attenuated sporozoites (RAS)

As mentioned earlier, mice immunized with x-ray irradiated sporozoites (*P. berghei*) were unable to develop LS infection and during the challenge study they were found to be protective in nature by homologs or *P. vinckei* challenge study. The higher doses of gamma rays have the direct impact on the LS infection. Additionally, the route of inoculation also plays a critical role in success of RAS immunization. As *in-vivo* study depicted that intravenous (IV) route is more suitable with compare to subcutaneous (SQ) or intradermal (ID) route which needs 7–10 timers higher *P. yoelii* RAS for the protective immunity [14, 104]. Moreover, a study conducted in macaques showcased the superiority of IV route in inducing and generating liver-resident *P. falciparum* specific T-cells [105]. In the clinical trials with *Pf*Spz, all the

11 volunteers (immunized with irradiated mosquito's sporozoites) were protected after the first round of homologous infection challenge whereas only 2 out 10 were able to generate the sterile immune response against the heterologous challenge [106]. It portrays the vital role of RAS approach in protection against the malaria infection, yet the issue of heterogeneity needs to be addressed. In another clinical trial of CHMI, around 64% of volunteers were protected against the homologous *P. falciparum* (3D7) challenge after 19 weeks. Further, volunteers showing no parasitemia were challenged after the final immunization (33 weeks later) with the heterologous strain (7G8) and approximately 83% have shown no parasitemia [107]. The results of *Pf*SPZ (RAS) immunization confirm the limited long-lasting immune responses, although no significant increase was observed in $CD4^+$ and $CD8^+$ T cell after second or third immunization.

2.2.3 Genetically attenuated sporozoites (GAS)

To overcome the existing hurdles of RAS, novel approach of genetic manipulation was explored in *Plasmodium* species which could prevent the transition from LS to BS infection without altering major changes. In this direction, differential gene expression study was carried out to identify the target gene(s) responsible for LS to BS transition and two genes, UIS3 and UIS4 (encodes for the protein in parasitophorousvacuole membrane), were selected for the genetic manipulation [108]. In mice having *P. berghei* infection, LS development was found to be delayed in a single knock-out gene study and gained the sterile protection upon challenge which was dependent upon $CD8^+$ T cells [42]. Subsequently, it has been extended to double-knock out study and was found to induce stronger immune response by generating IFN-γ producing memory and effector $CD8^+$ T cells that persist for a period of 6 months [109].

After the success of initial GAS study, several other genes (*p36, p36(p52) and b9*) were identified which were found to remain conserved in all the *Plasmodium* species. The different gene knock-out study in animal model demonstrated a similar immune response, yet development of parasites was also observed in some of them [42]. Subsequently, a novel gene named SAP1 (sporozoite asparagine-rich protein 1) of *P. yoelii* was discovered and found to be important for the LS development. In gene knock-out study it has conferred the delay in LS development and long-lasting protection upon challenge with wild-type sporozoites [110]. Few other genes were also explored; In a comparative study with RAS which generally arrest the early LS infection, more efficient and prominent effector and memory T-cell pool was observed, due to the GAS approach that progress towards the late LS infection and may be more diverse range of Ags were present. This lead to the first clinical trial, and *P. falciparum* double knock-out (*p52 and p36*) gene was tested for its efficacy and safety. Despite the encouraging results, 1 out of 6 volunteers showed parasitemia [111]. Therefore, further development took place in GAS and triple knock-out genes (*p52, p36 and sap1*) of *P. falciparum* strain was used. There was no breakthrough parasitemia, and higher Ab titer with elevated cytokine pool of IFN-γ, IL-2 and TNF-α were observed in all the volunteers [112]. The positive outcome led to the development of another GAS vaccine with double knock-out (B9 & SLARP), and in the early phase of 1/2a it has shown poor-to-moderate immune response as only 3 out of 25 volunteers were found to achieve the sterile protection after the mosquito-bite challenge [113].

Despite the yin and yang of GAS in clinical studies, it has been considered as more accurate and doable approach with compare to RAS. Additionally, with the novel technology of CRISPR-Cas9, various attenuated sporozoites can be generated which might be more immunogenic in nature and aid in generating stronger immune response.

All the different approaches of vaccine development strongly suggest the correlation of T-cells and protection against malaria infection. And, therefore it may be a decisive player in enhancing the efficacy of vaccine. By keeping in mind the importance of T-cell, in the next section we have discussed the role of T-cell based immunity in all the stage of infection as well importance of it in developing T-cell based vaccines.

3. T-cell based immune response: A key player of vaccine development

From the very beginning, it has been well documented that T-cells play an important role in protection and generation of sterile immune response in malaria infection. Once the sporozoites enter into the host live and invade the hepatocytes, APCs process and present the *Plasmodium* peptides through MHC which result in the activation of CMI response (alongside humoral response), mainly $CD4^+$ and $CD8^+$ T cells. After the resolution of infection, all the immune sentinels undergo regulative apoptosis, except pool of memory cells. These Ag-experienced memory cells are crucial during the secondary infection of *Plasmodium* and specifically, liver-resident memory $CD8^+$ T cells serve as a first line of defense [114]. Although certain studies have confirmed that induction and expansion of memory $CD8^+$ T cells are not hampered by absence of helper $CD4^+$ T cells, the memory $CD8^+$ T cells developed under this condition are found to be short-lived [115]. Therefore, it infers that for long-lasting memory $CD8^+$ T cells which control the malaria infection, aid of helper $CD4^+$ T cells [116] and continuous exposure of Ag is required. Yet, the memory response against the malaria infection is bottleneck [115]. The TCR-MHC bearing peptide of *Plasmodium* interaction is also important in generating T-cell based response (memory pool) as polymorphic nature of residual anchor and supporting once of individual peptide may have an effect on TCR-MHC interaction [114]. With the development of sophisticated technology, the role of T-cells in malaria infection in all the different stages has been revealed. As a result, various advancements have been made in the vaccine development.

3.1 T-cell response: In early stage of sporozoites

During the blood-meal of *Anopheles* mosquitoes, infected sporozoites enter into the host, and dermis under the layer of skin is the first place where they get exposed and then transverse through the blood vessels and reach to the liver. Therefore, Ab-mediated humoral response is largely important for the early stage of infection. However, experimental animal studies have revealed that most of the injected sporozoites remain in dermis for about 6 hrs and very few of them are able to find the way through blood vessels [117]. Although the DCs (dendritic cells) mediated capturing mechanism of sporozoite Ags is poorly understood, it has been confirmed that several sporozoites crosses the network of lymphatic vessels and skin-draining lymph node where they can persist for around 24 hr after the infection [117]. Therefore, it may be possible that circulating DCs (cDCs) present in skin initiate the T-cell induction against the sporozoites. And, it has been well known that live sporozoites are capable enough of generating $CD8^+$ T cells response. Although the detailed mechanism is yet to be understood, arming the Ab-response by providing $CD8^+$ and $CD4^+$ T cells, CMI plays an important role in early detection and restraining the transition to LS infection.

3.2 T-cell response: In pre-erythrocytic stage (LS)

In continuation of early stage infection, once the sporozoites reach to the liver, LS infection cycle initiates and through a cascade of mechanisms, numbers of schizonts are formed between the periods of 5–6 days. *In-vivo* experimental study has confirmed that mouse $CD8^+$ T cells restrict the parasite development within the hepatocytes by recognizing MHC-I/peptide complexes presented by infected hepatocytes [118]. For this, perforation occurs in hepatocytes cell membrane is responsible which carry the perforin and granzymes (pro-apoptotic protease). It induces apoptosis and produces the reactive-oxygen species. Additional aid is also provided by liver macrophages and Kupffer cells that carry out the activity of Ag presentation as they face the sporozoites during their entry into the liver [119]. $CD4^+$ and $CD8^+$ T cells of CMI wing are crucial in generating sterile protection against malaria infection and it has been verified in several sporozoite-and subunit-based vaccine approaches, though in case of human it has been documented only in human peripheral blood as it is challenging and difficult to prove for LS infection because of ethical concern [114]. Howbeit, recent study carried out in non-human primates has shown 100-fold higher T-cell response (specific to protective $CD8^+$ T cells) in liver compared to peripheral blood [120]. Therefore, it is required to understand the detailed mechanism and role of $CD8^+$ T cells in protection. Li *et al.*, 2016 have developed the human immune system bearing mice and studied the role of $CD8^+$ T cells in human malaria. They have reported the direct link between the functional activities of *Pf*CSP-specific $CD8^+$ T cells and threshold achieved of protection against the malaria infection [121]. Several other *in-vivo* experiments have also shown the correlation between parasite-specific IFN-γ producing $CD8^+$ T cells and protection achieved in clinical settings [114]. It suggests that $CD4^+$ and $CD8^+$ T cells produce IFN-γ which further enhances the activity of cytotoxic $CD8^+$ T cells by elevating the Ag presentation through MHC-I. Moreover, the enhanced IFN-γ level activates other phagocytic immune sentinels, macrophages and NK cells to perform the tightly-regulated apoptosis. Throughout the protection mechanism, pool of numerous cytokines are released including IL-12 and IL-18 that are known to activate the $CD8^+$ T cells in TCR-independent manner which can kill the parasites by a mechanism of nitric oxide (NO) production [122]. The prominent role of $CD8^+$ T cells, aid of $CD4^+$ T cells in humoral and CMI response, generation and activation of cytokines and other immune cells corroborate the significance of T-cell based vaccine development.

3.3 T-cell response: In blood stage (asexual/symptomatic stage)

The release of merozoite from schizonts confirms the beginning of erythrocytic stage, where they invade the naïve RBCs, convert into trophozoites and develop thousands of merozoites which are ready to burst from the infected RBCs (iRBCs) and target the new RBCs. Due to the lack of MHC molecules, iRBCs cannot perform the Ag presentation to T cells. However, it is believed that iRBCs bind to DCs and macrophages through the receptor-ligand (of parasite) interaction and after the maturation, most of the DCs migrate to the spleen where they present the Ag via MHC-molecules to the naïve –T cells [123]. The role of DCs in the generation of BS specific Ab is studied in animal models. Experimental evidences have shown the emerging role of novel T-cell population of $\gamma\delta^+$ and $\alpha\beta^+$ in the generation of IFN-γ responses that control the BS infection of *P. falciparum* [124]. Pombo *et al.*, 2002 have studied the role of immune system by injecting low-dosage of *P. falciparum* iRBCs to the volunteers followed by challenge [125]. They have shown that iRBCs generate the $CD4^+$ and $CD8^+$ T cell specific response to the BS infection. Further characterization of T-cells confirms that majority of them are IFN-γ producing (not IL-4 or IL-10) and there was no-significant role/production of antibodies in protection [125]. It has led the foundation to understand the role of T-cell which is now equally important for BS protection.

3.4 T-cell response: Towards the blood stage sexual parasites

During the blood-stage asexual cycle, certain number of parasites come out from the RBCs cycle and develops into male and female gametocytes. Till date very little literature is available about the T-cell response against the gametocytes. The first study conducted in 1997 where purified *P. falciparum* gametocytes were injected into malaria-naïve individuals and found that activated $CD4^+$ T cells response against the gametocytes in human PBMC is similar to the response observed in asexual stage [126], except the induction of γδ T-cells. In similar line, another study was carried out in which blood of acute (not severe) infection of *P. vivax* were fed to the *Anopheles* mosquitoes and observed the pro-and-anti-inflammatory cytokines [127]. The results of this study reveal that parasite in the blood samples with the elevated anti-inflammatory IL-10 (not IFN-γ or TNF-α) were unable to develop the infection in mosquitoes. To understand the mechanism of transmission-blocking, T-cells (from immunized spleen cells of vaccinated mice) were passively transferred to Balb/c mice via IV route followed by an infection; on day 3 post-infection, ability to transmit in mosquitoes was studied [128]. It showed the reduction in 95% of transmission, and the viability of gametocytes was found significantly lower in exflagellation compared to the controls. Although the mechanism behind triggering CMI response is unclear, authors predict that it could be cytokines or secretory products released by macrophages. This study unmasks the role of T-cells in early stage of BS infection wherein Ag-specific humoral response (Ab-based) comes latter into the picture and maybe help in the development of multi-target based vaccine.

The discovery of novel T-cell populations and their role in generating sterile protection alongside the conventional T-cells at each stage of malaria infection, aid the malaria biologist especially vaccinologists to design highly efficacious vaccine based on T-cells. Therefore, we have discussed about the different T-cells and their role in antigen diversity.

3.5 T-cell and their subtypes: Role in protective immunity against malaria

The induction of *Plasmodium* specific $CD4^+$ T cells in protection against the malaria infection naturally or in different vaccination approach is well-documented [129]. As we know, the activated $CD4^+$ T cells differentiate into several subtypes which largely depend upon on the cytokine environment. The differentiation of $CD4^+$ T cells into ***Th1*** is IFN-γ and IL-12 dependent, and the role of T-bet in Th1 differentiation is also explored. The T-bet$^+$Th1 IFN-γ producing cells express the MCSF (macrophage colony stimulating factor) that aid in controlling BS infection via macrophages. In addition to this, they also release IL-2 which can directly activate the NK cells which results into the direct killing of parasite infected cells. Having the multiple characteristics of Th1 cells, IFN-γ secreting Th1 cells directly/indirectly activate the potent $CD8^+$ T cytotoxic cells via NO or higher expression of MHC-I on infected hepatocytes. In CHMI study, it has been found that the cytotoxic $CD4^+$ T cells express CD107a, IFN-γ, CD38 and granzymes B, yet the mechanism of their activation is yet to be to be understood [129].

Th2, another set of $CD4^+$ T cells that express transcription factor, GATA3 are characterized by production of IL-4 and IL-5. Although the role of Th2 in malaria infection is poorly understood, IL-4 secreting Th2 cells have a major role in B-cell class switching [130] and macrophages activity [131] in malaria infection. In different conditions of malaria infection, a population of ***T follicular helper (Tfh) cells*** is identified by the expression of chemokine receptor CXCR5, BCL-6 a transcriptional factor and programmed cell death protein 1 (PD1)-a inhibitory receptor. The *Plasmodium* specific Tfh cells mainly express the ICOS and IL-21 which helps in maturation of germinal center (GC) and aid in production of plasma and memory B cells [129]. RNA-sequencing data have confirmed that Tfh cells development is IL-6 dependent and regulated by IRF3 during the BS infection [132]. The transition of Tfh cells to any other phenotypic subsets of $CD4^+$ T cells is one of the interesting phenomena which is required to be explored as it may drive the infection on either side. There are few studies depicted the presence of ***Th17*** cells in *Plasmodium* infection that express the IL-17A. As no specific role of Th17 is found in malaria infection, IL-21 producing cells may help in GC activity and activation of $CD8^+$ T cells, further it has shown that IL-22 producing Th17 cells regulate the inflammatory mechanism in lungs and liver of malaria infected rodent system [133]. Another $CD4^+$ T cell, ***IL-27 producing $CD4^+$ T cells***, is having a dual character of pro-and-anti-inflammatory, and some of the reports have proposed their protective role in BS infection of malaria. Further it has been demonstrated that $CD4^+$ T cells can also produce the IL-17 which do not express IL-10 and IFN-γ ($CD4^+$ IFN-γ^-IL-10^-T cells) [134]. Similarly, ***IL-10 producing $CD4^+$ T cells*** and ***regulatory T cells (Treg)*** are two another sets of $CD4^+$ T cells which demarcated by their cell surface proliferative markers, their role is found to be in favor of enhancing the malaria pathogenesis, although it is yet to be defined their precise action in different stages of infection.

As $CD4^+$ T cells are important in generating strong immune response by activating humoral and CMI response, the role of ***$CD8^+$ T cells*** in malaria pathogenesis, various subunit and whole sporozoites approaches and providing protection against the infection (more defined for LS infection) makes them the most desirable target for vaccine development. Among the different types of $CD8^+$ T cells, role of liver-resident $CD8^+$ T cells is indispensible alongside the effector and memory $CD8^+$ T cells during the re-infection. Earlier studies depict the role of CD $11c^+$ DCs in priming the $CD8^+$ T cells during the LS infection [116]. Later, newly identified population of monocytes ($CD11b^+CSF1R^+CD207^+F4/80^+CD11c^+$) also found to be important in priming of $CD8^+$ T cells, which strongly support the licensing activity of $CD8^+$ T cells in the LS infection [129]. The mechanism of $CD8^+$ T cell function in interrupting LS infection is found that Fas/FasL and granzymes are the two basic armed required for the effector function of $CD8^+$ T cells which mainly produce TNF-α, IFN-γ and perforin [129].

Recently, a novel population of ***γδ T cells***, is identified which comprises of less than 5% in adult human and its role in anti-malaria immunity is yet to be revealed. The earlier studies have confirmed the proliferation of them during the *P. falciparum* or *P. vivax* infection that correlate with protection [135]. Characterization of γδ T cells shows that during the phase of mild-to-acute infection, $V\gamma9^+V\delta2^+\gamma\delta$ T cells population increase which may further curtail down during the repetitive exposure of infection [129]. The reports of rodent model used for malaria infection revealed that γδ T cells do behave like other T-cells and they are found to be present in various tissues. Additionally, they also secrete IL-21, a required cytokines for Tfh cells [136] and as a result, it can function as a bridge for innate and adaptive immunity. Their role is also found to be important in RAS immunization for effective function of $CD8^+$ T cells via production of numerous cytokines. In an experimental study of *P. chabaudi*, during the BS infection a specific type of γδ T cells ($V\gamma6.3^+\gamma\delta$ T cells) have been shown to undergo the clonal expansion and showcase the specific phenotypic profile (with different transcriptional factors) which directly play a role in protection. Thus, it may aid in better understanding the pathogenesis and designing more efficient vaccine. In all, studying the different types of T cells and their role in individual stage of malaria infection will help in vaccine development. Despite the knowledge of T-cell mediated immunity, recently polymorphic natures of *Plasmodium* Ag(s) have shown the effect on T-cell response. Therefore, it is equally important to understand the impact of antigenic nature in generating sterile protection.

3.6 T-cell response: Effect of *Plasmodium* Ag(s) diversity

It has been studied that due to the polymorphic nature of Ag(s), effector function of $CD8^+$ T cells and MHC-I peptide presentation become less prominent; as a result, during the secondary infection, it overcomes the immune system and establish LS infection [137]. Thus, with the help of sequencing technology conserved and variable epitopes of CSP and other potential target Ag(s) were found and reported [114]. Similar results were observed during RTS,S clinical trials, in which higher efficacy was observed in those children's whose parasitic infection matches the T-cell based Th2R and Th3R epitope as compared the mismatched one [138]. It has been found in another gene based vaccine study that $CD8^+$ T cells based response is restricted to HLA-I of AMA1 Ag of 3D7 strain but failed to act against the AMA1 Ag of 7G8 strain that has the difference of only single amino acid [139]. It has been strongly supported by the earlier report of CSP where single amino acid replacement have an impact on T-cell based immune response [140]. Thus, antigenic polymorphic nature and substitution of single/multiple amino acids in the epitopes may result in less interaction between T-cell peptide and MHC molecule causing the failure in generation of protective immunity.

3.7 T cells and vaccine development

The first licensed malaria vaccine RTS,S was designed by incorporating mainly B cell epitopes that induced humoral response. The Ab-mediated response may aid the induction of T-cells and evidence have shown the $CD4^+$ T cells response, yet it is unable to understand that after RTS,S vaccination why immunity is remain short-lived. It may possible that incorporation of appropriate $CD8^+$ T cells based epitope which further enhance the sterile immunity. Additionally, it is also been interesting to study the role of B cells in direct/indirect activation of $CD8^+$ T cells. On the other hand, different approaches under the roof of whole sporozoite vaccine (CPS, RAS and GAS) depicted the prominent role of $CD4^+$ and $CD8^+$ T cells in protective responses against malaria infection in rodents, whereas in humans (under CHMI study) it has been limited to peripheral blood only. Additionally, among different subsets of T-cells which play a crucial role in providing protection and signaling pathway is yet to be fully understood. As mentioned earlier, injection of attenuated sporozoites through RAS approach have shown the antimalarial immunity against LS infection. Therefore, multiple antigenic targets of LS may help in generating strong liver-resident memory T cells. These WSV approaches have their own limitation and to prevail it, another approach of viral vector bearing Ag delivery has been explored and have shown the promising results [141]. After successful pilot study, to elicit the stronger T-cell based response several other options such as usage of nanoparticle based delivery system [142] and adeno-associated virus have been tried.

As T-cell mediated immunity is having prominent role in generating sterile protection, RAS and subunit vaccine approach which can induce stage-specific T-cell

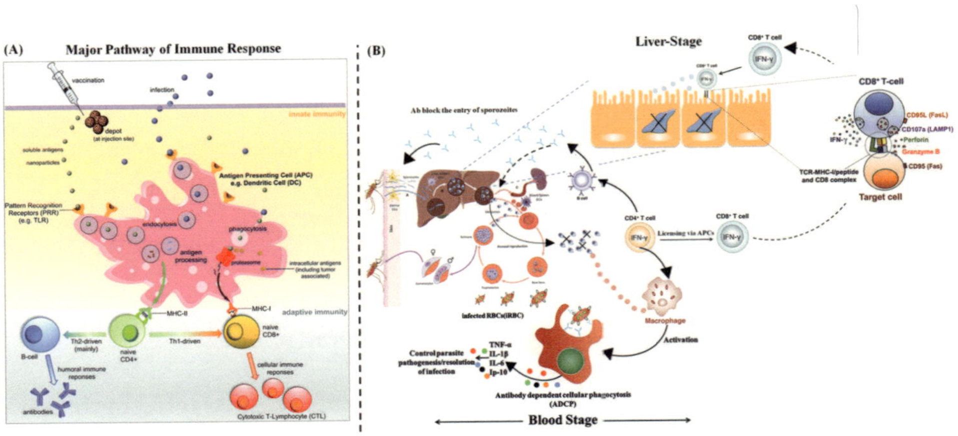

Figure 4.
(A) The major pathway of immune response and (B) at different stages of malaria infection how different immune cells can target malaria infected cells (adapted and modified from immunopaedia.org and [143–146]).

immune response and restrain the LS infection should be considered. Recently, all the experimental evidence have demonstrated that instead of using single epitope based Ag, multiple-and-stage-specific epitopes of different Ag(s) can protect and generate stage-specific sterile response, yet it has to be verified in animal settings before going for the clinical trials. Also, poor immunogenicity of stage-specific Ag(s) required screening the whole genome database and available RNA-seq. data which can predict and identify (with matched HLA-typing) B-and-T-cell based epitopes to activate the immune response in a controlled manner. To overcome the current challenges mainly in T-cell based vaccine development below-listed novel approaches may aid in better results. **Figure 4** depicted the major pathway of immune response and how they can be triggered by T-cell based vaccine.

- Reverse vaccinology
- Structural vaccinology
- Immunoinformatics
- High-throughput identification for immune protection
- Understanding the humoral and CMI response
- Selection of appropriate platform for vaccine development and delivery

4. Conclusion

Malaria still persists as a major global challenge and to fight against it several options have been explored. Despite the advancement in the field of technology, drug and insecticide resistance followed by recent threat of delayed clearance of parasite against the frontline of antimalarial(s) have created herculean situation. On the other hand, RTS,S is the only licensed vaccine against the malaria infection, which is also unable to reach the expectation in generating sterile protection. Significant role of T-cells (mainly $CD4^+$ and $CD8^+$ T-cells) is found to be a key-player against the malaria infection. To elicit the T-cell based response, novel approaches of vaccine development have been adopted and some of them are currently in pipeline of clinical trials. The older approach of WSV has recently gained the interest because of their potency to induce T-cell responses. The changes in RTS,S vaccine design via incorporating T-cell epitopes later on together with B-cells strongly support that finding of T-cell based multiple-epitope which can accelerate the immune response and aid Ab formation having immunogenicity in nature. By using the recent reverse vaccinology, structural based finding epitopes and predicted immunogen may aid in providing additional support in T-cell induction which are protective in nature.

Acknowledgements

Prof. Sarat K. Dalai would like to thank the Department of Biotechnology (DBT), New Delhi, Govt. of India for funding part of study (BT/PR34451/MED/29/1482/2019, SAN NO. 102/IFD/SAN/1633/2020-2021). Nikunj Tandel thanks the Indian Council of Medical Research (ICMR), New Delhi, Gov. of India for providing fellowship for his research (ICMR-SRF No.: 2020-7623/CMB-BMS).

Conflict of interest

The authors declare no conflict of interest.

Author details

Nikunj Tandel and Sarat K. Dalai*
Institute of Science, Nirma University, Ahmedabad, Gujarat, India

*Address all correspondence to: sarat.dalai@nirmauni.ac.in

References

[1] Watkins, K. Emerging infectious diseases: A review. Current Emergency and Hospital Medicine Reports **2018**, *6*, 86-93, doi:10.1007/s40138-018-0162-9.

[2] WHO. *World malaria report 2020: 20 yeras of global progress and challenges*; World Health Organization: 2020.

[3] Mahmoudi, S.; Keshavarz, H. Malaria vaccine development: the need for novel approaches: A review article. Iranian journal of parasitology **2018**, *13*, 1-10.

[4] Menendez, C. Malaria during pregnancy: a priority area of malaria research and control. Parasitology today **1995**, *11*, 178-183, doi:10.1016/0169-4758(95)80151-0.

[5] Martinsen, E.S.; Perkins, S.L.; Schall, J.J. A three-genome phylogeny of malaria parasites (Plasmodium and closely related genera): evolution of life-history traits and host switches. Molecular phylogenetics and evolution **2008**, *47*, 261-273.

[6] Gallup, J.L.; Sachs, J.D. The economic burden of malaria. The American journal of tropical medicine and hygiene **2001**, *64*, 85-96.

[7] Malaria, W. Key Facts. Geneva. *World Health Organization* **2020**.

[8] Guerra, C.A.; Howes, R.E.; Patil, A.P.; Gething, P.W.; Van Boeckel, T.P.; Temperley, W.H.; Kabaria, C.W.; Tatem, A.J.; Manh, B.H.; Elyazar, I.R. The international limits and population at risk of Plasmodium vivax transmission in 2009. PLoS Negl Trop Dis **2010**, *4*, e774.

[9] Win, T.T.; Jalloh, A.; Tantular, I.S.; Tsuboi, T.; Ferreira, M.U.; Kimura, M.; Kawamoto, F. Molecular analysis of Plasmodium ovale variants. Emerging infectious diseases **2004**, *10*, 1235-1240.

[10] Déchamps, S.; Maynadier, M.; Wein, S.; Gannoun-Zaki, L.; Maréchal, E.; Vial, H.J. Rodent and nonrodent malaria parasites differ in their phospholipid metabolic pathways. Journal of lipid research **2010**, *51*, 81-96.

[11] Cox-Singh, J.; Davis, T.M.; Lee, K.-S.; Shamsul, S.S.; Matusop, A.; Ratnam, S.; Rahman, H.A.; Conway, D.J.; Singh, B. Plasmodium knowlesi malaria in humans is widely distributed and potentially life threatening. Clinical infectious diseases **2008**, *46*, 165-171.

[12] Rosenberg, R.; Wirtz, R.A.; Schneider, I.; Burge, R. An estimation of the number of malaria sporozoites ejected by a feeding mosquito. Transactions of the Royal Society of Tropical Medicine and Hygiene **1990**, *84*, 209-212.

[13] Cowman, A.F.; Healer, J.; Marapana, D.; Marsh, K. Malaria: biology and disease. Cell **2016**, *167*, 610-624.

[14] Molina-Franky, J.; Cuy-Chaparro, L.; Camargo, A.; Reyes, C.; Gómez, M.; Salamanca, D.R.; Patarroyo, M.A.; Patarroyo, M.E. Plasmodium falciparum pre-erythrocytic stage vaccine development. Malaria journal **2020**, *19*, 56.

[15] Tandel, N.; Tyagi, R.K. Chapter 5 Malaria. In *Molecular Advancements in Tropical Diseases Drug Discovery*, Misra Guari, V.S., Ed. 2020; 10.1016/b978-0-12-821202-8.00005-0pp. 95-116.

[16] Monasch, R.; Reinisch, A.; Steketee, R.W.; Korenromp, E.L.; Alnwick, D.; Bergevin, Y. Child coverage with mosquito nets and malaria treatment from population-based surveys in African countries: a baseline for monitoring progress in roll back malaria. The American journal of tropical medicine and hygiene **2004**, *71*, 232-238.

[17] Skwarczynski, M.; Chandrudu, S.; Rigau-Planella, B.; Islam, M.; Cheong, Y.S.; Liu, G.; Wang, X.; Toth, I.; Hussein, W.M. Progress in the Development of Subunit Vaccines against Malaria. Vaccines **2020**, *8*, 373.

[18] Nájera, J.A.; González-Silva, M.; Alonso, P.L. Some lessons for the future from the Global Malaria Eradication Programme (1955-1969). PLoS Med **2011**, *8*, e1000412.

[19] van den Berg, H. Global status of DDT and its alternatives for use in vector control to prevent disease. Environmental health perspectives **2009**, *117*, 1656-1663.

[20] Mabaso, M.L.; Sharp, B.; Lengeler, C. Historical review of malarial control in southern African with emphasis on the use of indoor residual house-spraying. Tropical Medicine & International Health **2004**, *9*, 846-856.

[21] Tren, R.; Bate, R. *When politics kills: malaria and the DDT story*; Liberty Institute: 2000; Vol. 7.

[22] Dhiman, S. Are malaria elimination efforts on right track? An analysis of gains achieved and challenges ahead. Infectious diseases of poverty **2019**, *8*, 1-19.

[23] WHO. *Malaria: fact sheet*; World Health Organization. Regional Office for the Eastern Mediterranean: 2019.

[24] Hemingway, J.; Shretta, R.; Wells, T.N.; Bell, D.; Djimdé, A.A.; Achee, N.; Qi, G. Tools and strategies for malaria control and elimination: what do we need to achieve a grand convergence in malaria? PLoS biology **2016**, *14*, e1002380.

[25] Elimination, m.R.C.P.o.T.f.M. malERA: An updated research agenda for diagnostics, drugs, vaccines, and vector control in malaria elimination and eradication. PLoS medicine **2017**, *14*, e1002455.

[26] Kaehler, N.; Adhikari, B.; Cheah, P.Y.; Day, N.P.; Paris, D.H.; Tanner, M.; Pell, C. The promise, problems and pitfalls of mass drug administration for malaria elimination: a qualitative study with scientists and policymakers. International health **2019**, *11*, 166-176.

[27] Wang, J.; Xu, C.; Wong, Y.K.; Li, Y.; Liao, F.; Jiang, T.; Tu, Y. Artemisinin, the magic drug discovered from traditional Chinese medicine. Engineering **2019**, *5*, 32-39.

[28] Organization, W.H. *Guidelines for the treatment of malaria*; World Health Organization: 2015.

[29] Hetzel, M.W.; Genton, B. Mass drug administration for malaria elimination: do we understand the settings well enough? BMC medicine **2018**, *16*, 1-3.

[30] Dahl, E.L.; Rosenthal, P.J. Multiple antibiotics exert delayed effects against the Plasmodium falciparum apicoplast. Antimicrobial agents and chemotherapy **2007**, *51*, 3485-3490.

[31] Gaillard, T.; Madamet, M.; Tsombeng, F.F.; Dormoi, J.; Pradines, B. Antibiotics in malaria therapy: which antibiotics except tetracyclines and macrolides may be used against malaria? Malaria journal **2016**, *15*, 1-10.

[32] Greenwood, B.; Targett, G. The mysteries of immunity to malaria. Lancet **2011**, *377*, 1729-1730.

[33] Ramharter, M.; Winkler, H.; Kremsner, P.G.; Adegnika, A.A.; Willheim, M.; Winkler, S. Age-dependency of Plasmodium falciparum-specific and non-specific T cell cytokine responses in individuals from a malaria-endemic area. European cytokine network **2005**, *16*, 135-143.

[34] Doolan, D.; Dobano, C.; Baird, J. Acquired immunity to malaria. 610 Clin Microbiol Rev 22: 13-36. Table of Contents **2009**, *611*.

[35] Long, C.A.; Zavala, F. Immune responses in malaria. Cold Spring Harbor perspectives in medicine **2017**, *7*, a025577.

[36] Nussenzweig, R.S.; Vanderberg, J.; Most, H.; Orton, C. Protective Immunity produced by the Injection of X-irradiated Sporozoites of Plasmodium berghei. Nature **1967**, *216*, 160-162, doi:10.1038/216160a0.

[37] Clyde, D.F.; Most, H.; McCarthy, V.C.; Vanderberg, J.P. Immunization of man against sporozite-induced falciparum malaria. The American journal of the medical sciences **1973**, *266*, 169-177, doi:10.1097/00000441-197309000-00002.

[38] Clyde, D.F. Immunization of man against falciparum and vivax malaria by use of attenuated sporozoites. Am J Trop Med Hyg **1975**, *24*, 397-401, doi:10.4269/ajtmh.1975.24.397.

[39] Langhorne, J.; Ndungu, F.M.; Sponaas, A.-M.; Marsh, K. Immunity to malaria: more questions than answers. Nature immunology **2008**, *9*, 725-732.

[40] Tran, T.M.; Li, S.; Doumbo, S.; Doumtabe, D.; Huang, C.-Y.; Dia, S.; Bathily, A.; Sangala, J.; Kone, Y.; Traore, A. An intensive longitudinal cohort study of Malian children and adults reveals no evidence of acquired immunity to Plasmodium falciparum infection. Clinical Infectious Diseases **2013**, *57*, 40-47.

[41] Portugal, S.; Carret, C.; Recker, M.; Armitage, A.E.; Gonçalves, L.A.; Epiphanio, S.; Sullivan, D.; Roy, C.; Newbold, C.I.; Drakesmith, H. Host-mediated regulation of superinfection in malaria. Nature medicine **2011**, *17*, 732-737.

[42] Marques-da-Silva, C.; Peissig, K.; Kurup, S.P. Pre-Erythrocytic Vaccines against Malaria. Vaccines **2020**, *8*, 400.

[43] Rieckmann, K.; Beaudoin, R.L.; Cassells, J.; Sell, K. Use of attenuated sporozoites in the immunization of human volunteers against falciparum malaria. Bulletin of the World Health Organization **1979**, *57*, 261-265.

[44] Rieckmann, K.H.; Carson, P.E.; Beaudoin, R.L.; Cassells, J.S.; Sell, K.W. Sporozoite induced immunity in man against an Ethiopian strain of Plasmodium falciparum. Transactions of the Royal Society of Tropical Medicine and Hygiene **1974**, *68*, 258-259.

[45] Herrington, D.A.; Nardin, E.H.; Losonsky, G.; Bathurst, I.C.; Barr, P.J.; Hollingdale, M.R.; Edelman, R.; Levine, M.M. Safety and immunogenicity of a recombinant sporozoite malaria vaccine against Plasmodium vivax. The American journal of tropical medicine and hygiene **1991**, *45*, 695-701.

[46] Egan, J.E.; Hoffman, S.L.; Haynes, J.D.; Sadoff, J.C.; Schneider, I.; Grau, G.E.; Hollingdale, M.R.; Ballou, W.R.; Gordon, D.M. Humoral immune responses in volunteers immunized with irradiated Plasmodium falciparum sporozoites. The American journal of tropical medicine and hygiene **1993**, *49*, 166-173.

[47] Edelman, R.; Hoffman, S.L.; Davis, J.R.; Beier, M.; Sztein, M.B.; Losonsky, G.; Herrington, D.A.; Eddy, H.A.; Hollingdale, M.R.; Gordon, D.M. Long-term persistence of sterile immunity in a volunteer immunized with X-irradiated Plasmodium falciparum sporozoites. Journal of Infectious Diseases **1993**, *168*, 1066-1070.

[48] Gwadz, R.; Cochrane, A.; Nussenzweig, V.; Nussenzweig, R. Preliminary studies on vaccination of rhesus monkeys with irradiated sporozoites of Plasmodium knowlesi and characterization of surface antigens of these parasites. Bulletin of the world Health Organization **1979**, *57*, 165-173.

[49] Huff, C.G.; Marchbank, D.F.; Shiroishi, T. Changes in infectiousness of malarial gametocytes. II. Analysis of the possible causative factors. Experimental Parasitology **1958**, *7*, 399-417.

[50] Mitchell, G.H.; Butcher, G.; Cohen, S. Merozoite vaccination against Plasmodium knowlesi malaria. Immunology **1975**, *29*, 397.

[51] Cohen, S.; McGregor, I.; Carrington, S. Gamma-globulin and acquired immunity to human malaria. Nature **1961**, *192*, 733-737.

[52] Bouharoun-Tayoun, H.; Attanath, P.; Sabchareon, A.; Chongsuphajaisiddhi, T.; Druilhe, P. Antibodies that protect humans against Plasmodium falciparum blood stages do not on their own inhibit parasite growth and invasion in vitro, but act in cooperation with monocytes. The Journal of experimental medicine **1990**, *172*, 1633-1641.

[53] Sabchareon, A.; Burnouf, T.; Ouattara, D.; Attanath, P.; Bouharoun-Tayoun, H.; Chantavanich, P.; Foucault, C.; Chongsuphajaisiddhi, T.; Druilhe, P. Parasitologic and clinical human response to immunoglobulin administration in falciparum malaria. The American journal of tropical medicine and hygiene **1991**, *45*, 297-308.

[54] Diggs, C.; CL, D.; BT, W.; RM, W. The protective effect of African human immunoglobulin G in Aotus trivirgatus infected with Asian Plasmodium falciparum. Proceedings of the Helminthological Society of Washington **1972**, *39*, 449-456.

[55] Hill, A.V. Vaccines against malaria. Philosophical Transactions of the Royal Society B: Biological Sciences **2011**, *366*, 2806-2814.

[56] Doolan, D.L.; Hoffman, S.L. Pre–erythrocytic–stage immune effector mechanisms in Plasmodium spp. infections. *Philosophical Transactions of the Royal Society of London.* Series B: Biological Sciences **1997**, *352*, 1361-1367.

[57] Zavala, F.; Tam, J.P.; Hollingdale, M.R.; Cochrane, A.H.; Quakyi, I.; Nussenzweig, R.S.; Nussenzweig, V. Rationale for development of a synthetic vaccine against Plasmodium falciparum malaria. Science **1985**, *228*, 1436-1440.

[58] Good, M.F.; Maloy, W.L.; Lunde, M.N.; Margalit, H.; Cornette, J.L.; Smith, G.L.; Moss, B.; Miller, L.H.; Berzofsky, J.A. Construction of synthetic immunogen: use of new T-helper epitope on malaria circumsporozoite protein. Science **1987**, *235*, 1059-1062.

[59] Collins, W.E.; Anders, R.F.; Pappaioanou, M.; Campbell, G.H.; Brown, G.V.; Kemp, D.J.; Coppel, R.L.; Skinner, J.C.; Andrysiak, P.M.; Favaloro, J.M. Immunization of Aotus monkeys with recombinant proteins of an erythrocyte surface antigen of Plasmodium falciparum. Nature **1986**, *323*, 259-262.

[60] Patarroyo, M.E.; Amador, R.; Clavijo, P.; Moreno, A.; Guzman, F.; Romero, P.; Tascon, R.; Franco, A.; Murillo, L.A.; Ponton, G. A synthetic vaccine protects humans against challenge with asexual blood stages of Plasmodium falciparum malaria. Nature **1988**, *332*, 158-161.

[61] Stoute, J.A.; Slaoui, M.; Heppner, D.G.; Momin, P.; Kester, K.E.; Desmons, P.; Wellde, B.T.; Garçon, N.; Krzych, U.; Marchand, M. A preliminary evaluation of a recombinant circumsporozoite protein vaccine against Plasmodium falciparum malaria. New England Journal of Medicine **1997**, *336*, 86-91.

[62] Bojang, K.A.; Milligan, P.J.; Pinder, M.; Vigneron, L.; Alloueche, A.; Kester, K.E.; Ballou, W.R.; Conway, D.J.; Reece, W.H.; Gothard, P. Efficacy of RTS, S/AS02 malaria vaccine against Plasmodium falciparum infection in

semi-immune adult men in The Gambia: a randomised trial. The Lancet **2001**, *358*, 1927-1934.

[63] Schofield, L.; Ferreira, A.; Altszuler, R.; Nussenzweig, V.; Nussenzweig, R. Interferon-gamma inhibits the intrahepatocytic development of malaria parasites in vitro. The Journal of Immunology **1987**, *139*, 2020-2025.

[64] Hoffman, S.L.; Isenbarger, D.; Long, G.W.; Sedegah, M.; Szarfman, A.; Waters, L.; Hollingdale, M.R.; Van der Meide, P.H.; Finbloom, D.S.; Ballou, W.R. Sporozoite vaccine induces genetically restricted T cell elimination of malaria from hepatocytes. Science **1989**, *244*, 1078-1081.

[65] Hoffman, S.L.; Weiss, W.; Mellouk, S.; Sedegah, M. Irradiated sporozoite vaccine induces cytotoxic T lymphocytes that recognize malaria antigens on the surface of infected hepatocytes. Immunology letters **1990**, *25*, 33-38.

[66] Hoffman, S.; Isenbarger, D.; Long, G.; Sedegah, M.; Szarfman, A.; Mellouk, S.; Ballou, W. T lymphocytes from mice immunized with irradiated sporozoites eliminate malaria from hepatocytes. Bulletin of the World Health Organization **1990**, *68*, 132.

[67] Rénia, L.; Grillot, D.; Marussig, M.; Corradin, G.; Miltgen, F.; Lambert, P.; Mazier, D.; Del Giudice, G. Effector functions of circumsporozoite peptide-primed CD4+ T cell clones against Plasmodium yoelii liver stages. The Journal of Immunology **1993**, *150*, 1471-1478.

[68] Weiss, W.; Mellouk, S.; Houghten, R.A.; Sedegah, M.; Kumar, S.; Good, M.; Berzofsky, J.; Miller, L.; Hoffman, S. Cytotoxic T cells recognize a peptide from the circumsporozoite protein on malaria-infected hepatocytes. The Journal of experimental medicine **1990**, *171*, 763-773.

[69] Wang, R.; Doolan, D.L.; Le, T.P.; Hedstrom, R.C.; Coonan, K.M.; Charoenvit, Y.; Jones, T.R.; Hobart, P.; Margalith, M.; Ng, J. Induction of antigen-specific cytotoxic T lymphocytes in humans by a malaria DNA vaccine. Science **1998**, *282*, 476-480.

[70] McConkey, S.J.; Reece, W.H.; Moorthy, V.S.; Webster, D.; Dunachie, S.; Butcher, G.; Vuola, J.M.; Blanchard, T.J.; Gothard, P.; Watkins, K. Enhanced T-cell immunogenicity of plasmid DNA vaccines boosted by recombinant modified vaccinia virus Ankara in humans. Nature medicine **2003**, *9*, 729-735.

[71] Collins, K.A.; Snaith, R.; Cottingham, M.G.; Gilbert, S.C.; Hill, A.V. Enhancing protective immunity to malaria with a highly immunogenic virus-like particle vaccine. Scientific reports **2017**, *7*, 46621.

[72] Vannice, K.S.; Brown, G.V.; Akanmori, B.D.; Moorthy, V.S. MALVAC 2012 scientific forum: accelerating development of second-generation malaria vaccines. Springer: 2012.

[73] Mo, A.X.; Augustine, A.D. NIAID meeting report: Improving malaria vaccine strategies through the application of immunological principles. Vaccine **2014**, *32*, 1132-1138.

[74] Duffy, P.E.; Gorres, J.P. Malaria vaccines since 2000: progress, priorities, products. *npj Vaccines* **2020**, *5*, 1-9.

[75] Draper, S.J.; Sack, B.K.; King, C.R.; Nielsen, C.M.; Rayner, J.C.; Higgins, M.K.; Long, C.A.; Seder, R.A. Malaria vaccines: recent advances and new horizons. Cell host & microbe **2018**, *24*, 43-56.

[76] D'antonio, L.; Keshavarz-Valian, H.; Alger, N. Malaria vaccine antigen (s): detergent solubilization, partial isolation, and recovery of immunoprotective activity. Infection and immunity **1984**, *43*, 442-444.

[77] Edozien, J.; Gilles, H.; Udeozo, I. Adult and cord-blood gamma-globulin and immunity to malaria in Nigerians. Lancet **1962**, 951-955.

[78] Siddiqui, W.A. An effective immunization of experimental monkeys against a human malaria parasite, *Plasmodium falciparum*. *Science* **1977**, *197*, 388-389.

[79] Sirima, S.B.; Cousens, S.; Druilhe, P. Protection against malaria by MSP3 candidate vaccine. New England Journal of Medicine **2011**, *365*, 1062-1064.

[80] Spring, M.D.; Cummings, J.F.; Ockenhouse, C.F.; Dutta, S.; Reidler, R.; Angov, E.; Bergmann-Leitner, E.; Stewart, V.A.; Bittner, S.; Juompan, L. Phase 1/2a study of the malaria vaccine candidate apical membrane antigen-1 (AMA-1) administered in adjuvant system AS01B or AS02A. PloS one **2009**, *4*, e5254.

[81] Payne, R.O.; Milne, K.H.; Elias, S.C.; Edwards, N.J.; Douglas, A.D.; Brown, R.E.; Silk, S.E.; Biswas, S.; Miura, K.; Roberts, R. Demonstration of the blood-stage *Plasmodium falciparum* controlled human malaria infection model to assess efficacy of the *P. falciparum* apical membrane antigen 1 vaccine, FMP2. 1/AS01. The Journal of infectious diseases **2016**, *213*, 1743-1751.

[82] Sirima, S.B.; Mordmüller, B.; Milligan, P.; Ngoa, U.A.; Kironde, F.; Atuguba, F.; Tiono, A.B.; Issifou, S.; Kaddumukasa, M.; Bangre, O. A phase 2b randomized, controlled trial of the efficacy of the GMZ2 malaria vaccine in African children. Vaccine **2016**, *34*, 4536-4542.

[83] Barr, P.J.; Green, K.M.; Gibson, H.L.; Bathurst, I.C.; Quakyi, I.A.; Kaslow, D.C. Recombinant Pfs25 protein of Plasmodium falciparum elicits malaria transmission-blocking immunity in experimental animals. The Journal of experimental medicine **1991**, *174*, 1203-1208.

[84] Menon, V.; Kapulu, M.C.; Taylor, I.; Jewell, K.; Li, Y.; Hill, F.; Long, C.A.; Miura, K.; Biswas, S. Assessment of antibodies induced by multivalent transmission-blocking malaria vaccines. Frontiers in immunology **2018**, *8*, 1998.

[85] Kapulu, M.; Da, D.; Miura, K.; Li, Y.; Blagborough, A.; Churcher, T.; Nikolaeva, D.; Williams, A.R.; Goodman, A.; Sangare, I. Comparative assessment of transmission-blocking vaccine candidates against Plasmodium falciparum. Scientific reports **2015**, *5*, 11193.

[86] Read, D.; Lensen, A.; Begarnie, S.; Haley, S.; Raza, A.; Carter, R. Transmission-blocking antibodies against multiple, non-variant target epitopes of the Plasmodium falciparum gamete surface antigen Pfs230 are all complement-fixing. Parasite immunology **1994**, *16*, 511-519.

[87] Walsh, F. Malaria vaccine gets green light. BBC News Online **2015**.

[88] RTS, S.C.T.P. Efficacy and safety of the RTS, S/AS01 malaria vaccine during 18 months after vaccination: a phase 3 randomized, controlled trial in children and young infants at 11 African sites. PLoS medicine **2014**, *11*, e1001685.

[89] Bejon, P.; Lusingu, J.; Olotu, A.; Leach, A.; Lievens, M.; Vekemans, J.; Mshamu, S.; Lang, T.; Gould, J.; Dubois, M.-C. Efficacy of RTS, S/AS01E vaccine against malaria in children 5 to 17 months of age. New England Journal of Medicine **2008**, *359*, 2521-2532.

[90] Moris, P.; Jongert, E.; van der Most, R.G. Characterization of T-cell immune responses in clinical trials of the candidate RTS, S malaria vaccine. Human vaccines & immunotherapeutics **2018**, *14*, 17-27.

[91] Kester, K.E.; Cummings, J.F.; Ofori-Anyinam, O.; Ockenhouse, C.F.; Krzych, U.; Moris, P.; Schwenk, R.; Nielsen, R.A.; Debebe, Z.; Pinelis, E. Randomized,

double-blind, phase 2a trial of falciparum malaria vaccines RTS, S/AS01B and RTS, S/AS02A in malaria-naive adults: safety, efficacy, and immunologic associates of protection. Journal of Infectious Diseases **2009**, *200*, 337-346.

[92] Ockenhouse, C.F.; Regules, J.; Tosh, D.; Cowden, J.; Kathcart, A.; Cummings, J.; Paolino, K.; Moon, J.; Komisar, J.; Kamau, E. Ad35. CS. 01-RTS, S/AS01 heterologous prime boost vaccine efficacy against sporozoite challenge in healthy malaria-naive adults. PloS one **2015**, *10*, e0131571.

[93] Garcon, N.; Van Mechelen, M. Recent clinical experience with vaccines using MPL-and QS-21-containing adjuvant systems. Expert review of vaccines **2011**, *10*, 471-486.

[94] Polhemus, M.E.; Remich, S.A.; Ogutu, B.R.; Waitumbi, J.N.; Otieno, L.; Apollo, S.; Cummings, J.F.; Kester, K.E.; Ockenhouse, C.F.; Stewart, A. Evaluation of RTS, S/AS02A and RTS, S/AS01B in adults in a high malaria transmission area. PloS one **2009**, *4*, e6465.

[95] Ansong, D.; Asante, K.P.; Vekemans, J.; Owusu, S.K.; Owusu, R.; Brobby, N.A.; Dosoo, D.; Osei-Akoto, A.; Osei-Kwakye, K.; Asafo-Adjei, E. T cell responses to the RTS, S/AS01 E and RTS, S/AS02 D malaria candidate vaccines administered according to different schedules to Ghanaian children. PLoS One **2011**, *6*, e18891.

[96] Srikiatkhachorn, A. What translatable knowledge from dengue vaccine design can we pass onto future anti-parasitic vaccine development? Taylor & Francis: 2020.

[97] Langowski, M.D.; Khan, F.A.; Bitzer, A.A.; Genito, C.J.; Schrader, A.J.; Martin, M.L.; Soto, K.; Zou, X.; Hadiwidjojo, S.; Beck, Z. Optimization of a Plasmodium falciparum circumsporozoite protein repeat vaccine using the tobacco mosaic virus platform. Proceedings of the National Academy of Sciences **2020**, *117*, 3114-3122.

[98] Goh, Y.S.; McGuire, D.; Rénia, L. Vaccination with sporozoites: models and correlates of protection. Frontiers in immunology **2019**, *10*, 1227.

[99] Coelho, C.H.; Doritchamou, J.Y.A.; Zaidi, I.; Duffy, P.E. Advances in malaria vaccine development: report from the 2017 malaria vaccine symposium. NPJ vaccines **2017**, *2*, 34-34, doi:10.1038/s41541-017-0035-3.

[100] Belnoue, E.; Costa, F.T.; Frankenberg, T.; Vigário, A.M.; Voza, T.; Leroy, N.; Rodrigues, M.M.; Landau, I.; Snounou, G.; Rénia, L. Protective T cell immunity against malaria liver stage after vaccination with live sporozoites under chloroquine treatment. The Journal of Immunology **2004**, *172*, 2487-2495.

[101] Roestenberg, M.; Teirlinck, A.C.; McCall, M.B.; Teelen, K.; Makamdop, K.N.; Wiersma, J.; Arens, T.; Beckers, P.; Van Gemert, G.; van de Vegte-Bolmer, M. Long-term protection against malaria after experimental sporozoite inoculation: an open-label follow-up study. The Lancet **2011**, *377*, 1770-1776.

[102] Bijker, E.M.; Schats, R.; Obiero, J.M.; Behet, M.C.; van Gemert, G.-J.; van de Vegte-Bolmer, M.; Graumans, W.; van Lieshout, L.; Bastiaens, G.J.; Teelen, K. Sporozoite immunization of human volunteers under mefloquine prophylaxis is safe, immunogenic and protective: a double-blind randomized controlled clinical trial. PLoS One **2014**, *9*, e112910.

[103] Mordmüller, B.; Surat, G.; Lagler, H.; Chakravarty, S.; Ishizuka, A.S.; Lalremruata, A.; Gmeiner, M.; Campo, J.J.; Esen, M.; Ruben, A.J. Sterile protection against human malaria by chemoattenuated PfSPZ vaccine. Nature **2017**, *542*, 445-449.

[104] Patel, H.; Althubaiti, N.; Parmar, R.; Yadav, N.; Joshi, U.; Tyagi, R.K.; Krzych,

U.; Dalai, S.K. Parasite load stemming from immunization route determines the duration of liver-stage immunity. Parasite immunology **2019**, *41*, e12622.

[105] Epstein, J.; Tewari, K.; Lyke, K.; Sim, B.; Billingsley, P.; Laurens, M.; Gunasekera, A.; Chakravarty, S.; James, E.; Sedegah, M. Live attenuated malaria vaccine designed to protect through hepatic CD8+ T cell immunity. Science **2011**, *334*, 475-480.

[106] Hoffman, S.L.; Goh, L.M.; Luke, T.C.; Schneider, I.; Le, T.P.; Doolan, D.L.; Sacci, J.; De la Vega, P.; Dowler, M.; Paul, C. Protection of humans against malaria by immunization with radiation-attenuated Plasmodium falciparum sporozoites. The Journal of infectious diseases **2002**, *185*, 1155-1164.

[107] Lyke, K.E.; Ishizuka, A.S.; Berry, A.A.; Chakravarty, S.; DeZure, A.; Enama, M.E.; James, E.R.; Billingsley, P.F.; Gunasekera, A.; Manoj, A. Attenuated PfSPZ Vaccine induces strain-transcending T cells and durable protection against heterologous controlled human malaria infection. Proceedings of the National Academy of Sciences **2017**, *114*, 2711-2716.

[108] Kaiser, K.; Matuschewski, K.; Camargo, N.; Ross, J.; Kappe, S.H. Differential transcriptome profiling identifies Plasmodium genes encoding pre-erythrocytic stage-specific proteins. Molecular microbiology **2004**, *51*, 1221-1232.

[109] Jobe, O.; Donofrio, G.; Sun, G.; Liepinsh, D.; Schwenk, R.; Krzych, U. Immunization with radiation-attenuated Plasmodium berghei sporozoites induces liver cCD8α+ DC that activate CD8+ T cells against liver-stage malaria. PloS one **2009**, *4*, e5075.

[110] Aly, A.S.; Mikolajczak, S.A.; Rivera, H.S.; Camargo, N.; Jacobs-Lorena, V.; Labaied, M.; Coppens, I.; Kappe, S.H. Targeted deletion of SAP1 abolishes the expression of infectivity factors necessary for successful malaria parasite liver infection. Molecular microbiology **2008**, *69*, 152-163.

[111] Spring, M.; Murphy, J.; Nielsen, R.; Dowler, M.; Bennett, J.W.; Zarling, S.; Williams, J.; de la Vega, P.; Ware, L.; Komisar, J. First-in-human evaluation of genetically attenuated Plasmodium falciparum sporozoites administered by bite of Anopheles mosquitoes to adult volunteers. Vaccine **2013**, *31*, 4975-4983.

[112] Kublin, J.G.; Mikolajczak, S.A.; Sack, B.K.; Fishbaugher, M.E.; Seilie, A.; Shelton, L.; VonGoedert, T.; Firat, M.; Magee, S.; Fritzen, E. Complete attenuation of genetically engineered Plasmodium falciparum sporozoites in human subjects. Science translational medicine **2017**, *9*.

[113] Roestenberg, M.; Walk, J.; van der Boor, S.C.; Langenberg, M.C.; Hoogerwerf, M.-A.; Janse, J.J.; Manurung, M.; Yap, X.Z.; García, A.F.; Koopman, J.P.R. A double-blind, placebo-controlled phase 1/2a trial of the genetically attenuated malaria vaccine PfSPZ-GA1. Science Translational Medicine **2020**, *12*.

[114] Nlinwe, O.N.; Kusi, K.A.; Adu, B.; Sedegah, M. T-cell responses against Malaria: Effect of parasite antigen diversity and relevance for vaccine development. Vaccine **2018**, *36*, 2237-2242.

[115] Cockburn, I.A.; Chen, Y.-C.; Overstreet, M.G.; Lees, J.R.; Van Rooijen, N.; Farber, D.L.; Zavala, F. Prolonged antigen presentation is required for optimal CD8+ T cell responses against malaria liver stage parasites. PLoS Pathog **2010**, *6*, e1000877.

[116] Parmar, R.; Patel, H.; Yadav, N.; Parikh, R.; Patel, K.; Mohankrishnan, A.; Bhurani, V.; Joshi, U.; Dalai, S.K. Infectious sporozoites of Plasmodium berghei effectively activate liver CD8α+ dendritic cells. Frontiers in immunology **2018**, *9*, 192.

[117] Yamauchi, L.M.; Coppi, A.; Snounou, G.; Sinnis, P. Plasmodium sporozoites trickle out of the injection site. Cellular microbiology **2007**, *9*, 1215-1222.

[118] Bongfen, S.E.; Torgler, R.; Romero, J.F.; Renia, L.; Corradin, G. Plasmodium berghei-infected primary hepatocytes process and present the circumsporozoite protein to specific CD8+ T cells in vitro. The Journal of Immunology **2007**, *178*, 7054-7063.

[119] Tavares, J.; Formaglio, P.; Thiberge, S.; Mordelet, E.; Van Rooijen, N.; Medvinsky, A.; Ménard, R.; Amino, R. Role of host cell traversal by the malaria sporozoite during liver infection. Journal of experimental medicine **2013**, *210*, 905-915.

[120] Ishizuka, A.S.; Lyke, K.E.; DeZure, A.; Berry, A.A.; Richie, T.L.; Mendoza, F.H.; Enama, M.E.; Gordon, I.J.; Chang, L.-J.; Sarwar, U.N. Protection against malaria at 1 year and immune correlates following PfSPZ vaccination. Nature medicine **2016**, *22*, 614-623.

[121] Li, X.; Huang, J.; Zhang, M.; Funakoshi, R.; Sheetij, D.; Spaccapelo, R.; Crisanti, A.; Nussenzweig, V.; Nussenzweig, R.S.; Tsuji, M. Human CD8+ T cells mediate protective immunity induced by a human malaria vaccine in human immune system mice. Vaccine **2016**, *34*, 4501-4506.

[122] Freeman, B.E.; Hammarlund, E.; Raué, H.-P.; Slifka, M.K. Regulation of innate CD8+ T-cell activation mediated by cytokines. Proceedings of the National Academy of Sciences **2012**, *109*, 9971-9976.

[123] da Silva, H.B.; Fonseca, R.; dos Anjos Cassado, A.; de Salles, E.M.; de Menezes, M.N.; Langhorne, J.; Perez, K.R.; Cuccovia, I.M.; Ryffel, B.; Barreto, V.M. In vivo approaches reveal a key role for DCs in CD4+ T cell activation and parasite clearance during the acute phase of experimental blood-stage malaria. PLoS Pathog **2015**, *11*, e1004598.

[124] Waterfall, M.; Black, A.; Riley, E. γδ+ T cells preferentially respond to live rather than killed malaria parasites. Infection and immunity **1998**, *66*, 2393-2398.

[125] Pombo, D.J.; Lawrence, G.; Hirunpetcharat, C.; Rzepczyk, C.; Bryden, M.; Cloonan, N.; Anderson, K.; Mahakunkijcharoen, Y.; Martin, L.B.; Wilson, D. Immunity to malaria after administration of ultra-low doses of red cells infected with Plasmodium falciparum. The Lancet **2002**, *360*, 610-617.

[126] GOODIER, M.R.; TARGETT, G.A. Polyclonal T-cell responses to Plasmodium falciparum gametocytes in malaria nonexposed donors. Parasite immunology **1997**, *19*, 419-425.

[127] Abeles, S.R.; Chuquiyauri, R.; Tong, C.; Vinetz, J.M. Human host-derived cytokines associated with Plasmodium vivax transmission from acute malaria patients to Anopheles darlingi mosquitoes in the Peruvian Amazon. The American journal of tropical medicine and hygiene **2013**, *88*, 1130-1137.

[128] Harte, P.; Rogers, N.; Targett, G. Role of T cells in preventing transmission of rodent malaria. Immunology **1985**, *56*, 1.

[129] Kurup, S.P.; Butler, N.S.; Harty, J.T. T cell-mediated immunity to malaria. Nature Reviews Immunology **2019**, *19*, 457-471.

[130] von der Weid, T.; Kopf, M.; Köhler, G.; Langhorne, J. The immune response to Plasmodium chabaudi malaria in interleukin-4-deficient mice. European journal of immunology **1994**, *24*, 2285-2293.

[131] Kumaratilake, L.; Ferrante, A. IL-4 inhibits macrophage-mediated killing of Plasmodium falciparum in vitro. A possible parasite-immune evasion mechanism. The Journal of Immunology **1992**, *149*, 194-199.

[132] James, K.R.; Soon, M.S.; Sebina, I.; Fernandez-Ruiz, D.; Davey, G.; Liligeto, U.N.; Nair, A.S.; Fogg, L.G.; Edwards, C.L.; Best, S.E. IFN regulatory factor 3 balances Th1 and T follicular helper immunity during nonlethal blood-stage Plasmodium infection. The Journal of Immunology **2018**, *200*, 1443-1456.

[133] Mastelic, B.; Freitas do Rosario, A.P.; Veldhoen, M.; Renauld, J.-C.; Jarra, W.; Sponaas, A.-M.; Roetynck, S.; Stockinger, B.; Langhorne, J. IL-22 protects against liver pathology and lethality of an experimental blood-stage malaria infection. Frontiers in immunology **2012**, *3*, 85.

[134] Kimura, D.; Miyakoda, M.; Kimura, K.; Honma, K.; Hara, H.; Yoshida, H.; Yui, K. Interleukin-27-producing CD4+ T cells regulate protective immunity during malaria parasite infection. Immunity **2016**, *44*, 672-682.

[135] D'Ombrain, M.C.; Robinson, L.J.; Stanisic, D.I.; Taraika, J.; Bernard, N.; Michon, P.; Mueller, I.; Schofield, L. Association of early interferon-γ production with immunity to clinical malaria: a longitudinal study among Papua New Guinean children. Clinical Infectious Diseases **2008**, *47*, 1380-1387.

[136] Inoue, S.I.; Niikura, M.; Asahi, H.; Kawakami, Y.; Kobayashi, F. γδ T cells modulate humoral immunity against Plasmodium berghei infection. Immunology **2018**, *155*, 519-532.

[137] Gilbert, S.C.; Plebanski, M.; Harris, S.J.; Allsopp, C.E.; Thomas, R.; Layton, G.T.; Hill, A.V. A protein particle vaccine containing multiple malaria epitopes. Nature biotechnology **1997**, *15*, 1280-1284.

[138] Neafsey, D.E.; Juraska, M.; Bedford, T.; Benkeser, D.; Valim, C.; Griggs, A.; Lievens, M.; Abdulla, S.; Adjei, S.; Agbenyega, T. Genetic diversity and protective efficacy of the RTS, S/AS01 malaria vaccine. New England Journal of Medicine **2015**, *373*, 2025-2037.

[139] Sedegah, M.; Peters, B.; Hollingdale, M.R.; Ganeshan, H.D.; Huang, J.; Farooq, F.; Belmonte, M.N.; Belmonte, A.D.; Limbach, K.J.; Diggs, C. Vaccine strain-specificity of protective HLA-restricted class 1 *P. falciparum* epitopes. PLoS One **2016**, *11*, e0163026.

[140] Guttinger, M.; Caspers, P.; Takacs, B.; Trzeciak, A.; Gillessen, D.; Pink, J.; Sinigaglia, F. Human T cells recognize polymorphic and non-polymorphic regions of the Plasmodium falciparum circumsporozoite protein. The EMBO journal **1988**, *7*, 2555-2558.

[141] Ewer, K.J.; Sierra-Davidson, K.; Salman, A.M.; Illingworth, J.J.; Draper, S.J.; Biswas, S.; Hill, A.V. Progress with viral vectored malaria vaccines: A multi-stage approach involving "unnatural immunity". Vaccine **2015**, *33*, 7444-7451.

[142] Li, Y.; Leneghan, D.B.; Miura, K.; Nikolaeva, D.; Brian, I.J.; Dicks, M.D.; Fyfe, A.J.; Zakutansky, S.E.; De Cassan, S.; Long, C.A. Enhancing immunogenicity and transmission-blocking activity of malaria vaccines by fusing Pfs25 to IMX313 multimerization technology. Scientific reports **2016**, *6*, 18848.

[143] Skwarczynski, M.; Toth, I. Peptide-based synthetic vaccines. Chemical science **2016**, *7*, 842-854.

[144] Perdomo-Celis, F.; Taborda, N.A.; Rugeles, M.T. CD8+ T-cell response to HIV infection in the era of antiretroviral therapy. Frontiers in immunology **2019**, *10*, 1896.

[145] Osii, R.S.; Otto, T.D.; Garside, P.; Ndungu, F.M.; Brewer, J.M. The Impact of Malaria Parasites on Dendritic Cell–T Cell Interaction. Frontiers in Immunology **2020**, *11*, 1597.

[146] King, T.; Lamb, T. Interferon-γ: the Jekyll and Hyde of malaria. PLoS Pathog **2015**, *11*, e1005118.